AIDS:
Responses, Interventions
and Care

Social Aspects of AIDS

Series Editor: Peter Aggleton
Goldsmiths' College, University of London.

AIDS is not simply a concern for scientists, doctors and medical researchers, it has important social dimensions too. These include cultural, individual and media responses to HIV/AIDS, stigmatization and discrimination, perceptions of risk, and issues to do with counselling, care and health promotion.

This new series of books brings together work from many disciplines including psychology, sociology, cultural and media studies, anthropology, education and history. Many of the titles offer insight into contemporary research priorities and identify some of the opportunities open to those involved in care and health promotion. The series will be of interest to the general reader, those involved in education and social research, as well as scientific and medical researchers who want to examine the social aspects of AIDS.

AIDS:
Responses, Interventions and Care

Edited by
Peter Aggleton, Graham Hart
and Peter Davies

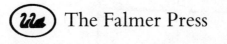 The Falmer Press

(A member of the Taylor & Francis Group)
London · New York · Philadelphia

UK   The Falmer Press, 4 John Street, London, WC1N 2ET
USA   The Falmer Press, Taylor & Francis Inc., 1900 Frost Road, Suite 101,
      Bristol, PA 19007

First published 1991

British Library Cataloguing in Publication Data
AIDS : responses, interventions and care. – (Social aspects of AIDS).
1. Man. AIDS. Social aspects
I. Aggleton, Peter *1952*– II. Hart, Graham 1957– III.
Davies, P. M. IV. Series
362.1042

ISBN 1–85000–817–X
ISBN 1–85000–872–8 pbk

Jacket design by Caroline Archer
Set in 10/13 pt Bembo by
Graphicraft Typesetters Ltd, Hong Kong

*Printed in Great Britain by
Burgess Science Press, Basingstoke*

Contents

Contents

Preface

The fourth conference on Social Aspects of AIDS took place at South Bank Polytechnic in London in March 1990, attracting a wide range of social researchers, health and social services workers and members of statutory and voluntary organizations working in the field of HIV/AIDS. The themes of the conference emphasized popular and professional responses to the epidemic, national and local interventions, and issues of care.

This book, like its predecessors (P. Aggleton and H. Homans, eds, *Social Aspects of AIDS*, Falmer Press, 1988; P. Aggleton, G. Hart and P. Davies, eds, *AIDS: Social Representations, Social Practices*, Falmer Press, 1989; and P. Aggleton, P. Davies and G. Hart, eds, *AIDS: Individual, Cultural and Policy Dimensions*, Falmer Press, 1990), contains many of the papers given at the conference. They identify the present research priorities of sociologists, psychologists, educationists and cultural theorists. They also demonstrate the diversity of work that is currently underway, as well as the quality of individual research initiatives. Rarely has so much energy been expended so productively in the pursuit of a common set of goals.

It has been our privilege as editors to work closely with contributors in preparing for the conference and in putting this book together afterwards. We would like to thank all who attended for their courage, their commitment and their critical contributions. Ours thanks go to Paul Broderick, Andrew Hunt, Heather Jones, Vijay Kumari and Michael Stephens for organizing the pre-conference publicity and arrangements on the day, and we are especially indebted to Gary Wych whose responsibility it was to undertake much of the conference administration. We are once again grateful to the Economic and Social Research Council (ESRC) for their financial support. Finally, we must thank Helen Thomas who, with endless patience and the challenge of a new wordprocessor, prepared the manuscript for publication.

Peter Aggleton, Peter Davies and Graham Hart

Chapter 1

AIDS: The Second Decade: 'Risk', Research and Modernity

Simon Watney

Perceptions of AIDS as an urgent epidemic ... are waning. (Lawrence O. Gostin)

The problems of the world come down to this: All that we can imagine is more than we want to know. (Allen Barnett)

A recent issue of *Outweek*, the leading US weekly for lesbians and gay men, contained a cartoon by Andrea Natalie, depicting a woman reading a newspaper, alongside a man with the flat-top haircut. The woman is saying:

Oh, my goodness! In this country every 18 seconds a man assaults a woman. Men rape 4000 women every DAY! 50 per cent of men batter their wives or lovers. One out of three girls is raped by a man in her family before she is eighteen. Last year men murdered — OH NO! I'd better volunteer some time at the battered women's shelter.

To which the man replies: 'Good heavens Suzy! You should be spending your volunteer hours taking care of gay men with AIDS! Don't you know there is an epidemic?!'[1]

Although there is a certain risk of seeming overly pedantic, it remains important to be able to unpick the themes that inform such cartoon jokes and anecdotes, since they speak directly and spontaneously of popular perceptions of HIV/AIDS as the first decade of the epidemic draws inexorably to a close. The sense of this cartoon, which was selected more or less at random, is based upon a strong sense of distinction between the subject of sexual violence and the subject of AIDS. It draws upon an assumed sense of irony, by which we identify the man ignoring the grim reality of rape as an issue for women. It also forcefully raises the differential status of 'knowledge' as it exists for women and for men. He is revealed as a typical chauvinist, unable to acknowledge the reality of female experience, expecting Suzy automatically to deny her position as a woman in relation to other women, and to knuckle down to the traditional nurturing role allotted to women in patriarchal societies. Yet I would suggest that it is the cartoon itself that is shockingly sexist, drawing on attitudes and assumptions that reveal both a frightening ignorance of HIV/AIDS, and an unacceptable oversimplification of the complex ways in which gender and sexuality articulate with one another and throughout the epidemic.

The latest American AIDS statistics speak baldly of a national catastrophe. Two hundred and twelve new cases of AIDS are diagnosed every day in the USA, where someone dies from AIDS every ten minutes. By the end of 1990 more than 100,000 people had already died from AIDS in the US alone. In 1991 more young Americans will die from AIDS than perished in the entire Vietnam war. Indeed, AIDS is now the leading cause of death for *all* American men aged between 25 and 44, and *all* American women aged between 15 and 33. In February 1990 the Centers for Disease Control reported a cumulative total of 11,189 women with AIDS in the United States, 52 per cent of whom were originally infected through needle-sharing, and a further 19 per cent through unprotected sex with male injecting drug users. Indeed, 28 per cent of *all* people with AIDS in America have been infected through needle-sharing, and it is currently estimated that 70 per cent of injecting drug users in some areas are already infected. Women with AIDS now make up 9 per cent of the national US total, and heterosexual transmission which accounted for only 1.2 per cent of cases in 1982, is now responsible for 4.9 per cent of the total case-load.

Yet it is clear that such statistics continue to make little impact in relation to the culturally established 'common sense' about AIDS that prevails on both sides of the Atlantic. It has never been more obvious that such 'information', on its own, has little relation to public opinion or public attitudes. From this perspective we may return to the cartoon with which this chapter began. It is initially significant that 'Suzy' is named, whilst her male companion remains an anonymous stereotype of gay masculinity. It is true that AIDS continues to have a terrible, disproportionate impact among the gay communities of the United States, but all too often this obscures the fact that for several years the majority of new cases of HIV infection have been among heterosexuals. Furthermore, gay men are casually portrayed as selfish and insensitive, 'only' concerned with the fate of other gay men. Certainly, at the end of the first decade of AIDS it is almost fashionable to depict gay men in this way, and to overlook the central fact that throughout the entire course of the epidemic it has been gay men who have struggled to alert other social groups to the potential risks of HIV infection. The professional de-gaying of non-government AIDS service organizations is more than matched by the tend-ency to minimalize the question of HIV transmission among gay men, and the terrible impact of AIDS throughout the gay communities of the West. It is, therefore, especially depressing, and alarming, that a 'feminist' cartoon, appearing in a lesbian and gay publication in New York City, reveals such ignorance and prejudice. It should not, however, surprise us, for at another level this only serves to draw attention to the continuing uneven effects of marginalization among the communities most affected by HIV/AIDS. It also draws attention to the long-term effects of conflicting information and misreporting that have so unfortunately prevailed throughout the 1980s. If people are confused and ignorant, this is hardly their fault, since few have had access to reliable sources of commentary. Nonetheless, this cannot account for the widely held belief that AIDS service organizations are run largely by and for 'white, middle-class gay men', to the deliberate exclusion of other groups. Such attitudes reveal little more than a traditional prejudice against gay men *as such*, now dressed up in the doubly distasteful rhetoric of supposedly 'progressive' analysis. Furthermore, it matters little whether such prejudice comes from the left or the right, for it is a form of prejudice that continues to put large numbers of people at increased potential risk of HIV infection by persuading them that they themselves could never be directly affected.

Yet the international statistics continue to show a worsening situation. In August 1990 the World Health Organization reported 'marked increases' of new cases of HIV throughout Asia and Latin America, together with an expanding crisis in sub-Saharan Africa that could lead to a 'dramatic upward revision' of previous estimates.[2] For example, the World Health Organization had forecast between one and 1.5 million cases of HIV in Asia by the year 2000, but an estimated 500,000 have already been reported. Three million women and children are now expected to die from AIDS around the world in the course of the 1990s. All of this returns us to the vexed question of heterosexual transmission, and the future course of the epidemic.

By June 1990 there had been 3433 cases of AIDS reported in the UK, a figure which the government's Chief Medical Officer acknowledges as a serious under-estimate of the real total (Hall, 1990). There have been 12,370 reported cases of HIV infection in the UK among men, and 1482 among women, with a further 238 ungendered cases recorded by anonymized mass screening. It is always to HIV statistics that we should look to understand the growth of the epidemic, since AIDS figures relate to transmission events that took place, on average, some ten years ago. That this is still rarely appreciated in Britain was demonstrated early in 1990, when a slight fall in the rate of AIDS-related deaths was reported in every non-gay newspaper as if this were a story about HIV transmission. The news was received with widespread relief, as if it undermined previous 'exaggerated' estimates. It was indeed good news, for it suggested that treatment and support services for people living with AIDS are slowly improving, as reflected in improved average life expectancy after an AIDS diagnosis. But this point was completely missed by journalists who seem to have very little genuine interest in the long-term prospects of people living with HIV or AIDS. What the story demonstrated was simply that ten years into the epidemic, and six years after the discovery of the Human Immunodeficiency Virus, the significance of the distinction between HIV and AIDS is *still* not recognized outside the discursive field of HIV/AIDS health promotion and direct service provision.

Putting this another way, one might well ask why it is almost impossible to imagine a cartoon depicting a man reading a newspaper alongside a woman in which the man is saying:

> Oh, my goodness! In this country there are more than 300 men in prison for sexual 'offences' that don't exist for heterosexuals. Heterosexuals killed 15 gay men in Britain last year. Homosexuality is the leading cause of suicide amongst gay teenagers. There still hasn't been a single Safer Sex advert for gay men in a national newspaper. Last week Richard Ingrams was still calling in *The Observer* for quarantine for people with HIV! *The Star* calls gay men with AIDS 'human wreckage'. How many gay men have HIV — OH NO! I'd better volunteer to work with the Terrence Higgins Trust.

To which the woman would reply:

> Good heavens Mike! You should be spending your time helping out at the black lesbians' creche at the Women's Centre! Don't you know this is a racist, sexist, patriarchal society?

Such an imaginary cartoon is only extremely unlikely because it would run the grave risk of drawing too much attention to the level of prejudice against gay men which is so sadly rife in contemporary Britain, whether among feminists or anti-feminists, racists or anti-racists, Thatcherites or anti-Thatcherites. The point is that we should not be setting up different areas of discrimination as if they were intrinsically in competition with one another. Rather, we should by trying to articulate the ways in which different types of prejudice and discrimination proliferate in relation to different institutions and different social identities, all with their distinct histories, senses of boundaries and goals (Hall, 1990).

As a gay man who has been actively involved in HIV/AIDS work in Europe and North America since the mid-1980s, it seems clear to me that in an important sense epidemiology is everything when it comes to HIV/AIDS. The single, central issue that has determined policy responses to the epidemic on both sides of the Atlantic has been the fact that our experience in Europe, such as it has been, has been overwhelmingly that of asymptomatic HIV infection. In the United States and Canada, however, experience all along has been largely that of acute care, escalating mortality statistics, and the ensuing cultural responses of mourning, anger and, increasingly, direct activism (Watney, 1990). AIDS *as such* in Europe remains largely a cultural phenomenon, even for most gay men, mediated above all by the national press and television — for the most part imagined rather than directly known from personal, lived experience. In spite of this major difference, it is clear that throughout the world responses to the epidemic have been concentrated on three broad, primary terrains: first, that of health education, or preventive medicine; second, that of treatment, care and service provision; and third, that of cultural responses, where the 'meanings' of AIDS are determined for most people.

All three terrains have been subject to massive political interference from the very beginning of the epidemic, and all three have been sites of intense contestation and polarization. Furthermore, all three share a common dependence on such research as is available to them, and hence on research policy and funding agencies. Indeed, it is no exaggeration to say that the single most important factor that will determine the course of the second decade of AIDS will be the quality and quantity of research that will inform local, national and international responses to the epidemic. Yet research does not take place in a social vacuum, and this only underscores the fact that these three areas are rarely entirely distinct from one another. Epidemiology is of use to health educators and service providers alike, just as biomedical research serves care providers, housing workers and many others. And all are, of course, influenced by the wider cultural conditions that frame popular perceptions of personal risk and research priorities alike. This is why research has been and will continue to be the single most important dynamic factor in the future management of all aspects of the epidemic. In this chapter the emphasis is on the first of these terrains — health education.

Health Education Research

Hans Moerkerk, Secretary of the Dutch Commission on AIDS Control, has distinguished three separate sets of strategies in Europe in relation to HIV/AIDS prevention (Moerkerk, 1990). First, he identifies the approach based on notions of *behaviour modification*, involving straightforward technical interventions: the provision of condoms and condom education, the establishment of needle exchange projects and so on. Second, he identifies approaches which aim at *lifestyle modification*, and attempt to work at a more sophisticated level, acknowledging the importance of social and psychological factors, community identities and so on. Third, he identifies the aim of *group cultural modification*, which employs frankly repressive techniques to supposedly prevent HIV transmission by punitive means. These might include closing down bars or saunas, harassing prostitutes or criminalizing people with HIV. As he concludes, it has been the demonstrable ineffectiveness and even counterproductiveness of this last approach that has led countries such as the Netherlands and Australia to opt for variants and combinations of the first two approaches. With Peter Aggleton, Moerkerk has also outlined the various policies adopted in Europe in some detail, noting that repressive and politically motivated measures have been applied in countries whose social, economic and political structures very considerably (Moerkerk and Aggleton, 1990).

In these terms we may distinguish at least three approaches. First, there has been a *pragmatic response* in Norway, Denmark, Switzerland and the Netherlands. These countries may be distinguished by the speed of their national response to the epidemic, and the willingness of state agencies to negotiate with and consult community organizations and non-government AIDS service organizations, preferring to establish consensus rather than impose coercive controls. As in the case of Norway, however, this approach may simply mask an underlying refusal or inability to acknowledge the cultural legitimacy of some groups, especially gay men.

Second, they identify a *political response*, which places political considerations above all others. Such may be found in West Germany, Austria, Iceland and Ireland, as well as the spectacular examples of the United Kingdom and the United States. In these countries the work of non-government AIDS service organizations preceded state interventions, and the relations between state and non-state HIV/AIDS education have often been fraught. Indeed, much of the work carried out by non-governmental organizations (NGOs) is dedicated to the task of re-education, correcting the mistakes of 'official' campaigns (Watney, 1990b). Funding has long been difficult to obtain, and self-censorship is rife, together with conflicts between different areas of work such as buddying and support services, legal work and telephone counselling. In such circumstances health education often has a low priority since it is acknowledged to be 'risky', especially when any acknowledgment of the needs and rights of gay men or injecting drug users can so easily be interpreted by hostile politicians and others as evidence of the supposed 'promotion' of immorality and drug use. Community groups and NGOs are rarely consulted by state agencies, though lip service may sometimes be paid to the value of their work, just so long as this is not specified (Watney, 1989).

Third, Moerkerk and Aggleton identify a general *biomedical approach* in countries such as Belgium, France, Spain, Italy and Greece, where governments have had little direct involvement in HIV/AIDS education, preferring to leave this work to state medical institutions, which were never designed to deal with the issues raised by the epidemic. As Moerkerk points out, in this context gay organizations (so far as they exist in the first place) are faced by the combined opposition of the political elite and the medical elite. Policies thus tend to be confused and contradictory, as politicians and doctors struggle to address groups whose very existence they would evidently prefer to forget. This is also the case in the emergent democracies of Eastern and Central Europe, whose nationalist movements are generally distinguished by a strong and explicit homophobia. For example, Poland's first AIDS service organization was ousted from its office in the Students' Union building in Warsaw by Roman Catholic Solidarity activists within weeks of moving in early in 1990. The biomedical approach still tends to regard HIV antibody testing as if it were the major means of effective prevention, and invariably reflects the well-known social prejudices of the medical professions. Indeed, one of the saddest paradoxes of the European epidemic has concerned the failure of socialized medicine in Europe to acknowledge the complexity of the societies to which it is supposed to be responsible at the level of HIV/AIDS education as much as at the level of actual care.

However, in spite of the importance of such descriptive analysis of differing health education strategies, it is equally important to understand something of the theoretical bases on which they stand. For the different models of HIV/AIDS education reviewed above have their origins in different, and generally conflicting, models of research. We may thus contrast the type of academic epidemiology which speaks confidently of 'risk groups' and 'risk behaviour' to research which attempts to make sense of people's own felt needs, pleasures and identities. For example, one recent survey of risk factors relating to seroconversion among gay and bisexual men who had attended professional education sessions listed variables including:

> age, educational level, occupation, race, type of educational session, the time between the educational session and the conversion visit, age at which volunteers began having sexual intercourse on a regular basis, numbers of all sexual partners, numbers of partners who were anally insertive, percentage of partners with whom condoms were used during receptive intercourse, the greatest amount of alcohol consumed per day, most alcohol consumed on days when drinking, frequency of use of recreational drugs, kinds of recreational drugs used, and depression. (Silvestre *et al.*, 1989: 648)

What is so startlingly absent from this long list is any awareness of the possible role of sexual identity or social self-esteem, factors which are on the contrary foregrounded in research conducted from a fuller understanding of the complex, variable relations among information, attitudes, identity and behaviour. In this respect one may immediately contrast research undertaken by researchers who have little or no knowledge or understanding of the social worlds of lesbians and gay men and research which deliberately employs gay men in order to be effective. One may also distinguish between research conducted in academic departments for publication or conference reports and research which is specifically designed to answer questions raised by health educators working in the field. Yet in practice, very little HIV/AIDS health education research is conducted in relation to the immediate needs of health educators working in European AIDS service organizations in the voluntary sector. This means that much of their work is essentially ad hoc, and is rarely evaluated. A vicious circle is thus established so that the most effective interventions are the least researched, and therefore are not written up or officially acknowledged. They thus stand little chance of influencing 'official' campaigns, and valuable experience is not communicated nationally or internationally.

Academic research in Europe still tends to treat its subjects as more or less exotic deviants, and the fluidity and complexity of sexual and drug-using behaviour are not recognized because of the rigid dependence on categories such as prostitution, homosexuality and so on. A visitor from outer space would undoubtedly have the greatest difficulty un⁻ :rstanding almost any aspect of sexuality in modern Britain if they had only read the epidemiological literature available in the medical journals. Fortunately, there are some exceptions to the general rule. For example, Hilary Kinell's work in Birmingham provides important data on risk factors for HIV infection among women in the sex industry because it is especially sensitive to the ways in which 'information' is actually interpreted (Kinnell, 1991). Thus while only 4 per cent of her sample of women failed to identify unprotected anal sex as a risk factor for men, 33 per cent failed to identify this as a risk for women. Messages which simply talk about 'anal sex' may be 'understood', and may be reflected in quantitative surveys, but nonetheless there may be little relation between the results of surveys whose questions are ill-conceived and actual risk factors in the lives of those being questioned. Kinnell's work also demonstrates a significant correlation between anti-gay attitudes and risk behaviour, though very few surveys ever include questions about attitudes towards homosexuality on the part of heterosexuals, although this has long been recognized as an important issue by gay health educators.

Kinnell's work similarly calls into question the familiar epidemiological obsession with the issue of numbers of sexual partners, usually understood as an intrinsic independent risk factor. For example, her survey reveals that younger women aged between 17 and 22 tend to have many more clients than older women, but are much better informed and take far fewer risks. Older women, with fewer partners, are often involved in casual work in order to support children, pay the poll-tax and so on. The available sociology of prostitution clearly shows that prostitutes are generally well informed about sexually transmitted diseases, and sexual health, since this relates so directly to their ability to work. Yet as Judith B. Cohen has pointed out, researchers still frequently speak of clients being 'exposed to' prostitutes and thence HIV infection as if they were the sexual equivalent to a leaky nuclear reactor (Cohen, 1989). In this manner moralism interferes with the task of researching strategies for developing effective health promotion. As recently as April 1990 a London magistrate jailed an 18-year-old seropositive mother for loitering, commenting that: 'Any man who takes his chances with a prostitute on the street deserves what he gets.'[3] It seems apparent that the major risk factor for prostitutes continues to be prejudice and the effects of criminalization, which continue to portray male clients as 'victims' and to disregard the question of how sex industry workers can themselves be protected. In this respect much epidemiology resembles traditional forms of policing and surveillance rather than affording a means of effective health education.[4]

The epidemiological scapegoating of prostitutes is repeated throughout the field of HIV/AIDS research, in relation to the social groups who initially proved most vulnerable to HIV. By reinforcing the ideological categories of 'prostitution', 'homosexuality' and 'drug abuse', the opportunity to call into question the methods of behavioural psychology and statistical sociology has been lost. This is largely because academic methodology is *threatened* by what we learn from the study of the epidemic: that sexual and drug using behaviours are not immutably fixed and stable within clearly defined and identifiable social groups; that the categories of sexual 'science' constitute a complex biopolitics which is perhaps the most fundamental level at which social life is managed, organized and 'thought'; and that the meaning of 'sex' and sexual categories is not natural but cultural. What is most remarkable in all of this, however, is the extent to which psychosocial research has ignored the lived experience and entitlements of those it regards as members of 'risk groups', and how closely such research tends to align itself with the interests of those it perceives to be fundamentally *not* at risk from HIV. Researchers themselves are almost invariably inscribed within this latter group. Hence the paradox of the massive degree of individualism that characterizes so much 'official' HIV/AIDS education. For it is only as long as HIV can be successfully presented as a risk to be faced by isolated individuals, who are understood to be able to make *moral* choices to protect themselves, independently of all other social or personal factors, that the larger abstract categories of 'sexuality' may be protected. In other words, the unequal power relations between heterosexuality and homosexuality are protected and even reinforced by research that presents heterosexuals with HIV as if they are *exceptions*, or indeed not heterosexual, as in the obvious example of most injecting drug users. Indeed, in the epidemiology of HIV/AIDS, injecting drug use usually appears as if it were a *sexual* category, distinct from heterosexuality. Thus British HIV statistics as published still fail to establish the vital point that the majority of people with HIV in the United Kingdom are indeed heterosexuals. What is immediately erased from this perspective is the range of ways in which anyone might become vulnerable to HIV. It remains intensely significant that the simple message that HIV is *potentially* a risk to everyone, across all social and sexual boundaries, is so frequently heard as if it were being claimed that everyone is *equally* at risk. What is being protected in such examples, and what kinds of defences are in play, remains far from clear. Suffice it to say that the precise mechanisms whereby such reversals and double standards are inscribed throughout the field of psychosocial research remain in urgent need of detailed elaboration and theoretical analysis. The most important question remains the ways in which the findings of research might be promptly translated into effective health education initiatives.

In Britain, as in many other countries, much of the most useful research, especially in relation to safer sex, has long tended to take place in an ad hoc fashion, undertaken by health educators themselves who are generally gay men, lesbians or feminists, working far away from the established centres of academic social science, either in Departments of Education or of Cultural Studies, or else entirely outside the formal academic world — either for reasons of choice, or because state funding is still not available to such 'risky' projects.

There is a sad irony in the fact that the explosion of research into 'homosexual behaviour' or 'the homosexual lifestyle' has so very little relevance to the immediate, pressing needs of gay men living in the real world of an epidemic. This is largely because gay men's sexuality is so often abstracted and isolated from the rest of their lives, including all questions of class and the contingent world of anti-gay prejudice. Yet far away from the grim day-to-day realities of the epidemic and of increasing homophobia, the question of the moral responsibility of the social sciences in the AIDS crisis is rarely raised, save by the objects of research who thus reveal themselves as 'non-compliant'. The dangerous myth of value-free research continues to legitimate costly and expensive research that is both scientifically and ethically dubious. This is not to question the need for quantitative research into all aspects of human sexuality. However, in the midst of an epidemic such projects can only be justified if they can demonstrate concrete implications for the development of effective health education strategies. If this is not always the case, social scientists cannot be surprised if they are attacked as academic tourists, thriving professionally as 'scientific' spectators on the misery of others — misery that it should be *their* primary responsibility to attempt to minimize. Nonetheless, as we enter the 1990s there is still precious little evidence that most academic psychosocial HIV/AIDS research concerning gay men or other 'risk groups' has their health or well-being anywhere among its aims or objectives.

Fortunately, there are good examples of research which has been specifically designed in relation to immediate concrete needs. Thus we may distinguish the work of Lavinia Crooks and her colleagues at the University of Wollongong, which is closely tied to the work of the AIDS Council of New South Wales, and the Australian Federation of AIDS Organisations (AFAO). This research project has produced much valuable work on the needs of specialized counselling for carers, and especially on the needs of carers who are themselves HIV antibody positive. I am not aware of a single research project in Britain which betrays the slightest awareness that such people even exist, let alone that they might have special needs and entitlements in relation to which social scientists might be able to make genuinely helpful contributions. Another impressive research project is located at Macquarie University, also in New South Wales. The work of Gary Dowsett and his colleagues in the Social Aspects of the Prevention of AIDS

(SAPA) project has few international parallels in its sensitivity to the changing cultural contexts in which safer sex education takes place, contexts that must be fully appreciated if such education is to be effective rather than merely cosmetic.[5] In a recent paper on 'Unsafe Anal Sexual Practice among Homosexual and Bisexual Men' they conclude that:

> We noted at the start of the paper the symbolic significance of anal intercourse both in repressive laws and in gay men's claims for sexual liberation. So far as gay social life can be understood as a 'sexual community', this is a practice which has had a significant role in creating identities and social links.... From this point of view, insisting on a total safe sex regime may be counterproductive. Over rigid rules are impractical; invite blow-outs, whose net effect may be greater risk than a more moderate regime from the start. (Connell *et al.*, 1989: 19–20)

Such work has especially significant implications for safer sex education, not least by pointing to the special needs of those on low incomes, those who have few friends or who have little access to the types of gay community institutions where safer sex is learned as a cultural, community-based aspect of gay identity and gay pride. Such research points:

> ...to the need to foster group support for change, to work through existing patterns of interpersonal relationships. This has been the approach of many gay community organizations...and it needs to be more widely known that there is social-scientific backing for this approach. We need to move beyond the individualistic approach of much official health education and academic AIDS research, towards collective, social strategies of change. The aim of such work is not so much to change individual 'attitudes' or 'health behaviours' as to move whole networks of people towards safer practice and encourage the social processes among them which can sustain the prevention. (Connell *et al.*, 1989: 21)

British and American research strongly supports more recent Australian findings that: 'Men who are isolated from others like themselves and are unattached to gay community in any form are those least likely to change' (Kippax *et al.*, 1990: 44). Moreover, such research also repeatedly demonstrates the change to safer sex outside primary long-term sexual relationships among gay men, within which unsafe sex is far from uncommon. Yet this is not remotely surprising. Nor is it in any way unique to gay men. However, when similar studies were reported at both the Fifth and Sixth International Conferences on AIDS, press reaction outside the gay press spoke uniformly of supposedly irresponsible gay men 'slipping' or 'giving up' safer sex.[6] Yet there is a vast amount of international evidence that demonstrates with frightening clarity how very few sexually active heterosexual men have even considered starting to have safer sex in the first place.

The starkest of double standards are at work here, since it has never for one moment been suggested that heterosexuals might consider giving up penetrative sexual intercourse in the way that is so routinely expected of gay men. For example, the practice of anal sex is still evidently regarded as an intrinsic risk factor in much epidemiological analysis, independently of any question of condom use, although vaginal intercourse as such is never regarded in this manner, and its culturally sanctioned acceptability is entirely taken for granted in official surveys.[7] Excellent research has been conducted in Britain at Bristol Polytechnic, and at South Bank Polytechnic in London, but beyond this there is little evidence of any systematic linkage between academic researchers and the sites in which health education initiatives are developed. Furthermore, by their very nature, British non-government AIDS service organizations are unlikely to be aware of the possibility that social scientific research might be of immediate help in their work, since there are so few professional social scientists involved in the voluntary sector. This highly regrettable situation has been made worse by the policy of the government's main funding agencies, including the Economic and Social Research Council (ESRC), only to fund quantitative research. One leading female researcher working on an ESRC funded project concerned with attitudes and beliefs among female prostitutes told me recently that although she hoped her work might 'be of some use', she had not stopped even to consider its possible implications for the purposes of health education among the very women with whom she was working. Indeed, she was quite indignant in the face of what she evidently regarded as my vulgar, reductive question.

Such studies are typically conducted by interviewing cohorts of subjects attending sexually transmitted disease clinics, who are provided with psychological and information-oriented questionnaires, on the basis of which it is asserted that changes in sexual behaviour may be detected. This type of research is literally obsessed with isolating scientific 'indicators' of sexual behaviour in relation to HIV transmission, but as I have already argued, these usually relate far more to conventions of sociological enquiry than to the actual lived experience of the people being questioned, who are casually dehumanized by being viewed behind the thick protective curtains of orthodox academic deviancy theory. Indeed, such research is often the sociological equivalent to barrier-nursing, and is generally about as appropriate. It should certainly be recognized that academic sociology is one of the strongest bastions of anti-gay prejudice, rationalized and legitimated within the narrow world of academic life by its own working methods and the beliefs on which they are based. Indeed, there can be few social groups less well equipped to appreciate the needs of health education in relation to the AIDS crisis than British social scientists, especially those coming from backgrounds in 'pure' statistics.

In this context one might well contrast British academic research into safer sex to recent Norwegian work conducted by Annick Prieur and her colleagues at the University of Oslo. What is so rare and impressive about Prieur's work is its commitment to *listening* to what her subjects were telling her, and her willingness to check what she was hearing against her own academic and personal preconceptions. Thus her survey on unsafe sex among young gay men in Oslo ends on a personal note, all too rare in such published research findings:

> When we started this research, some of us were surprised that gay men still had unsafe sex. Why can't they change their sex life? It must be more important to survive than to keep on having sex in the same way as before? It was primarily we women who were astonished. We were distanced from gay men's sex life, and we didn't know what it meant to have your entire sexlife labelled as something dangerous. It was easy for us only to conceive of negative reasons for having unsafe sex. We are used to thinking that every evil is caused by another evil. If this were true, continued practice of unsafe sex would be caused by lack of self control, by drinking, drugs, or just plain madness. This is a view that stems from a simple rational choice model. If people don't behave 'rationally' that must be because they have lost their reason. But the world is not that simple ... a wider understanding of rationality is needed: including longing and love as motives for action. (Prieur *et al.*, 1990: 12)

Such an approach can only derive from a truly open-minded willingness to try to understand the situation in which so many men who have sex with other men find themselves. Not that the circumlocution 'men who have sex with men' does much more than suggest *something* about the variable social and cultural conditions in which homosexual desire is lived in widely differing circumstances. The ceaseless quest for scientifically verifiable 'indicators' and 'objective correlates' is pointless if these only serve further to blind social scientists to the complex realities of sexual desire, identities and behaviour in grossly puritanical, moralistic and anti-gay societies. Effective HIV prevention can only take place when local factors such as the proximity of gay bars and clubs, the patterns of distribution of gay newspapers and magazines, local policing policies and so on have been adequately researched and their consequences understood and factored into health educational initiatives. Above all, it is the availability of a sense of belonging to some kind of community that will always determine the development of a resilient sense of self-esteem which is demonstrably the sine qua non of safer sex education, not just for gay men — though this is a principal lesson from the gay response to AIDS — but for everyone. We await the emergence of the sociology of longing and of love with bated breath.

Conclusions

In the meantime we could do worse than pay close attention to the extraordinary critique of the response of the social sciences to an earlier twentieth century catastrophe, contained in Zygmunt Bauman's book, *Modernity and the Holocaust*. Bauman argues that the Holocaust is either regarded as if it were a discrete incident in the history of the Jews, or else from a more Durkheimian perspective an example of the failure of modernity to contain a universal capacity for evil, which broke through the veneer of German civilization in the form of Nazism — thus conveniently letting everyone else off the hook. Writing of the complex ways in which soldiers, journalists, statisticians and other functionaries came quite easily to regard Jews as less than human, he observes that:

> Dehumanized objects cannot possibly possess a 'cause', much less a 'just' one; they can have no 'interests' to be considered, indeed no claim to subjectivity. Human objects became therefore a 'nuisance factor'. Their obstreperousness further strengthens the self-esteem and the bonds of comradeship that unite the functionaries. The latter see themselves now as companions in a difficult struggle, calling for courage, self-sacrifice and selfless dedication to the cause. It is not the objects of bureaucratic action, but its subjects who suffer and deserve compassion and moral praise.... Dehumanization of the objects and positive moral self-evaluation reinforce each other. The functionaries may faithfully serve any goal while their moral conscience remains unimpaired. (Bauman, 1989: 104)

I do not wish to appear to be making casual or impertinent analogies between the treatment of the Jews, gypsies, gay men and others, and the events that have determined the first decade of the AIDS crisis. However, it would be entirely inconsistent and unproductive to argue, with Bauman, that the Holocaust was precisely a result of the conditions that constitute modernity, and then imagine that such an analysis can have nothing to say about the history of the present. Bauman argues that the Holocaust could only have come about as a result of a combination of factors including social and psychological tensions deriving from the new, and rigid boundary-drawing tendencies under the conditions of modernization and the subjectivities these produced, the breakdown of a sense of traditional order, the hardening of nation states and nationalisms, the role of scientific rhetoric in legitimating the ambitions of political and other would-be social engineers, the emergence of modern forms of racism, and their relation to the possibility of a technology of genocide. This is not to claim for one moment either that the AIDS crisis is in any simple sense 'like' the Holocaust, or that anti-Semitism is in any simple sense 'like' the fears of difference that seemingly fuel much anti-gay prejudice. Nonetheless, it is impossible not to note the growing homologies between social policy in the field of HIV/AIDS related education and policies that determine the direction of biomedical research, epidemiology and popular cultural interpretations of the epidemic which continue to regard people with HIV/AIDS as culpable, and less than human.

Besides, we know that power is not a single, unitary force that merely flows through different sites of struggle creating different forms of oppression in the same way, and by the same means. Our analysis of the forces at work in the many institutions which 'manage' the epidemic must be at least as supple and nimble as Bauman's reading of anti-Semitism, following as it does in the mighty footsteps of Hannah Arendt.[8] Indeed, the categories of sexuality and the identities that they engender, including the steady escalation of anti-gay prejudice in countries like Britain or Poland or the Soviet Union which in important ways have *yet to achieve* modernity in the sense described by Bauman, are themselves a central and indispensable element within the wider, evolving disposition of modernization.

Anti-gay prejudice is no more *necessary* to modernity than anti-Semitism. It is, however, a characteristic and predictable feature of certain aspects of the changes in domesticity, child-raising, pedagogy in schools, medical practice, and social science, which are themselves not the products but the *means* of centralized, bureaucratic modernity, whatever different forms it may have assumed in the intersection with different national histories. Who, for example, could possibly have predicted the widespread passivity among gay men in relation to the practices of clinical medicine throughout the epidemic in Western Europe that results from the client mentality produced within cradle-to-grave welfare and national health services? Who could have imagined that, on the contrary, the epidemic would stimulate the most urgent confrontation with institutionalized medicine in the modern period in the United States? Who could have imagined the sheer scale of the failures of governments, national medical research institutes, health education agencies, journalists, religious leaders, politicians and sociologists alike, to acknowledge the enormity of the disaster that confronts gay men and injecting drug users, haemophiliacs and the poor and disadvantaged of the earth?

I sometimes hear the message that 'things could be worse', but this can only come from those who continue to place their faith in the supposedly disinterested forces of social democratic consensus and morality. As we enter the second decade of the epidemic it seems imperative that we find time to consider, in all the necessary sobriety we can muster, the long-term consequences of the categories and identities of 'sexuality' in relation to the lives at stake in the ongoing struggles against state censorship, the unavailability of private or public funding, the continuing design of unethical and thus unscientific protocols for the conduct of clinical trials, the refusal to legislate against HIV/AIDS-related discrimination (however flagrant), the sheer, relentless violence of the response to humane health education, medical research and cultural agencies.

Five years ago I began to write about AIDS on the basis of my own appalled and initially unbelieving perception that the social constituencies associated with AIDS were widely regarded, in their entirety, as disposable. For a long time I found it well nigh impossible to accept the accumulating evidence before me. In the meantime little has changed, and I see no reason to revise my earlier judgment. As we enter the second decade of AIDS, I can see no evidence whatsoever that countries such as Britain and the United States have even begun to grasp what the first decade was really like, and this alone provides no grounds for optimism concerning the ability to identify and attempt to reverse the pitiless forces of dehumanization resulting from the cultural exaggeration of sexual otherness, or the direct effects of the marginalization this entails for *everyone* involved, that seem at this time to be indispensable elements in the 'successful' working of contemporary modernity. As the epidemic worsens, we shall see whether AIDS continues to be accepted as a minor cost of modernity, or whether other moral and ethical forces in our societies will be brought in to challenge this 'morality'. Certainly new battle lines are currently being established between rival pictures of human morality, and these will doubtless be increasingly involved in direct confrontation throughout the 1990s. The great issues of abortion, embryo research, marriage, censorship and sexual morality will continue to intersect with the issues raised by the epidemic in ever more complex conjunctions. But of these AIDS is likely to prove by far the most controversial, for the simple reason that it has the power to condense almost all the other issues into itself, and is thus radically overdetermined as a site on which conflict is likely to take place. We will not know that this struggle for the right to diversity has been won until our respective societies, including our governments and doctors, and teachers, and journalists and social scientists are able to accept, quite casually, that gay men simply like sex just like everyone else. Given the great distance of that ideal, imaginary goal, we cannot afford to be complacent or delude ourselves that 'common sense' will ultimately, inevitably, prevail. Unfortunately, it would appear that the dominant common sense of the United Kingdom has little or no interest in the fate of gay men. This, during an epidemic, guarantees otherwise avoidable increases in HIV infection, and otherwise avoidable human suffering on a dreadful scale. One can only enter the 1990s with profound forebodings, for while we know that the future is not fixed, we also know that the evidence of the 1980s strongly suggests a worsening crisis ahead.

Notes

1 *Outweek*, 59, 15 August 1990, p. 5.
2 'Sharp Rise in AIDS Infection is Reported in Third World', *New York Times*, 2 August 1990, p. A. 18.
3 'Prostitute with AIDS Sent to Jail', *The Times*, 21 April 1990; see also 'You Deserve to Die If You Go with a Hooker', *The Star*, 21 April 1990.

4   The modern *locus classicus* for this debate remains Michel Foucault.
5   The Social Aspects of the Prevention of AIDS Project is located at Macquarie University, New South Wales 2109, Australia.
6   Jack O'Sullivan, 'Young Homosexuals "Giving Up Safe Sex" in Setback on AIDS', *The Independent*, 20 April 1990.
7   For one typical such article, see R. Fitzpatrick *et al.* (1989) 'High Risk Sexual Behaviour and Condom Use in a Sample of Homosexual and Bisexual Men,' *Health Trends*, 21, pp. 76–9. However, for an important and rare critique of orthodox epidemiological methods in relation to HIV/AIDS, see J.P. Vandenbroucke (1989) 'An Autopsy of Epidemiological Methods: The Case of 'Poppers' in the Early Epidemic of the Acquired Immune Deficiency Syndrome (AIDS)', *American Journal of Epidemiology*, 129, 3, pp. 455–7.
8   See, for example, Hannah Arendt (1963) *Eichman in Jerusalem: A Report on the Banality of Evil*, Harmondsworth, Penguin.

References

ARENDT, H. (1977) *Eichman in Jerusalem: A Report on the Banality of Evil*, Harmondsworth, Penguin.

BARNETT, A. (1990) *The Body and Its Dangers and Other Stories*, New York, St Martin's Press.

BAUMAN, Z. (1989) *Modernity and the Holocaust*, Cambridge, Polity Press.

COHEN, J.B. (1989) 'Overstating the Risk of AIDS: Scapegoating Prostitutes', *Focus*, University of California Regents, 4, 2, 2–3.

CONNELL, R.W., *et al.* (1989) 'Unsafe Anal Sexual Practice among Homosexual and Bisexual Men', *Social Aspects of the Prevention of AIDS, Study A*, Report 7, Sydney, Macquarie University, School of Behavioural Sciences.

FITZPATRICK, R., *et al.* (1989) 'High Risk Sexual Behaviour and Condom Use in a Sample of Homosexual and Bisexual Men', *Health Trends*, 21, 76–79.

FOUCAULT, M. (1984) *The History of Sexuality: An Introduction*, Harmondsworth, Penguin.

GOSTIN, L.O. (1990) 'Preface: Hospitals, Health Care Professionals, and Persons with AIDS', in L.O. GOSTIN (Ed.), *AIDS and the Health Care System*, New Haven and London, Yale University Press.

HALL, S. (1990) 'Cultural Identity and Diaspora', in J. RUTHERFORD (Ed.), *Identity: Community, Culture, Difference*, London, Lawrence and Wishart.

KINNELL, H. (1991) 'Prostitute's Perceptions of Risk and Factors Related to Risk-Taking', in AGGLETON, P., HART, G. and DAVIES, P. (Eds) (1991) *AIDS: Responses, Interventions and Care*, London, Falmer Press, pp. 79–94.

KIPPAX, S., *et al.* (1990) 'The Importance of Gay Community in the Prevention of HIV Transmission', mimeo, Sydney, University of Macquarie, School of Behavioural Sciences.

MOERKERK, H. (1990) 'AIDS Prevention in Europe: The Gay Response', paper given at the First European Conference on HIV and Homosexuality, Copenhagen.

MOERKERK, H. and AGGLETON, P. (1990) 'AIDS Prevention Strategies in Europe', in P. AGGLETON, G. HART and P. DAVIES (Eds), *AIDS: Individual, Cultural and Policy Dimensions*, Lewes, Falmer Press.

O'SULLIVAN, J. (1990) 'Young Homosexuals "Giving Up Safe Sex" in Setback on AIDS', *The Independent*, 20 April.

PRIEUR, A., *et al.* (1990) 'Gay Men: Reasons for Continued Practice of Unsafe Sex', paper presented at the First European Conference on HIV and Homosexuality, Copenhagen.

SILVESTRE, A.J., *et al.* (1989) 'Factors Related to Seroconversion among Homosexual and Bisexual Men after Attending a Risk-reduction Educational Session, *AIDS*, 3, 647–650.

VANDENBROUCKE, J.P. (1989) 'An Autopsy of Epidemiological Methods: The Case of "Poppers" in the Early Epidemic of the Acquired Immune Deficiency Syndrome (AIDS)', *American Journal of Epidemiology*, 129, 3, 455–457.

WATNEY, S. (1989) 'Introduction', in E. CARTER and S. WATNEY (Eds), *Taking Liberties: AIDS and Cultural Politics*, London, Serpent's Tail Press.

Watney, S. (1990a) 'Safer Sex as Community Practice', in P. AGGLETON, G. HART and P. DAVIES (Eds), *AIDS: Individual, Cultural and Policy Dimensions*, Lewes, Falmer Press.

WATNEY, S. (1990b) 'Foreword: The Persistence of Memory', in L. KRAMER, *Reports from the Holocaust: The Making of an AIDS Activist*, Harmondsworth, Penguin.

Chapter 2

Changing to Safer Sex: Personality, Logic and Habit

Mitchell Cohen

In New York, Paris, San Francisco, Amsterdam, London and several other large urban centres throughout developed countries, the percentage of gay men who become HIV positive each year has fallen to a low point of less than 2 per cent. One reason for this decline in the incidence of HIV infection has been a dramatic change in behaviour from unsafe to safer sex.[1] While an ongoing infection rate of between one and two in a hundred still borders on epidemic proportions, and while there is some evidence of a slight upturn in the number of men becoming infected by HIV, the overall picture is one of unprecedented change in gay men's sexual behaviour.

In this chapter the rise and fall of the HIV epidemic and its relationship to behaviour change will first be discussed. It will be evident that considerable behaviour change occurred in several gay communities long before many cases of AIDS were diagnosed in those communities, long before many men had died, and even before the causes and consequences of AIDS were fully known. At the same time it will become clear that some men continue to practise unprotected anal sex despite an awareness that this is a leading mode of transmission of HIV infection and the knowledge that AIDS is likely to be fatal. Having looked at this evidence, theories of sexual behaviour change will be examined within three broad frameworks: those that emphasize personality traits, those that emphasize logical information processing, and those that emphasize habits. Finally, recommendations will be made about HIV/AIDS prevention strategies based on these three frameworks. In particular, reasons will be given why community-based activities are effective; why eroticized safer sex campaigns may be more effective than more cut-and-dried informational campaigns; why partner and peer pressure are effective agents of change; why inaccurate beliefs continue to be a major factor in continued unsafe sex; and why, especially during the final stages of the HIV epidemic, the reinforcement of safer sex activity is as important as persuasive messages advocating behaviour change.

Figure 2.1 Annual Incidence of HIV Infection

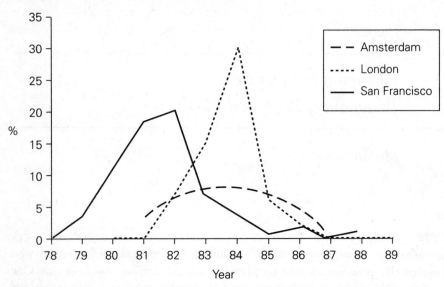

Amsterdam: Van Griensven (1989c). *N* = 1431;685 Hepatitis B vaccine trial; recruited between November 1980 and November 1982, and 746 healthy homosexual men recruited October 84 onwards from the homosexual community. *London*: Jenkins, P. (1990) and personal conversaton. *N* = 318; recruited January 1982–March 1985 from St Mary's GUM STD clinic, and volunteers recruited through gay newspaper.
San Francisco: Hessol, N., *et al.* (1989) and personal conversation. *N* = 320; Hepatitis B vaccine trial; recruited through San Franscisco City Clinic, seronegative for Hepatitis B at recruitment.

Behaviour Change and the Decline of HIV

Figure 2.1 shows the incidence of HIV infection among cohorts of gay men in San Francisco, London and Amsterdam. Projections of HIV infection from several other cities show a similar pattern of rapid increase and then decrease of HIV infection among gay men.[2] Given that most men sero-convert within six months of becoming infected, the relatively rapid rise and then decline of HIV infection indicates that something must have happened very early in the HIV epidemic to change the rate of new HIV infections.

One reason for the decline in the incidence of HIV infection is that as the epidemic has developed there have been fewer and fewer 'hosts' to attack.[3] This occurred because those men who engaged frequently in unsafe sex were the first to become infected *and* because many men removed themselves from being at risk for HIV infection by changing to safer sex (Martin, 1987; Dowsett, 1989; Coates *et al.*, 1988b; Winkelstein *et al.*, 1987a, 1987b; Van Griensven *et al.*, 1989a; Carne *et al.*, 1987; Aggleton, Coxon and Weatherburn, 1989). HIV has peaked at different levels among similar gay cohorts in the same city and in different cities. A likely explanation for this is the different timing of levels of compliance with safer sexual practices.

During the time that the incidence of HIV was decreasing, several scientific studies recorded a sharp decrease in unprotected anal sex (Table 2.1) and increased use of condoms (Table 2.2), and there is a growing body of evidence that the decreased incidence of HIV infection was most directly due to the change from unprotected anal sex to safer sex. For example, in a study in New York (Martin *et al.*, 1989) 22 per cent of the men who reported having stopped receptive anal intercourse in 1985 were HIV seropositive in 1987, whereas 48 per cent of the men who said they did *not* stop were seropositive two years later.

In addition to these changes gay men have reported less anonymous sex. Bathhouses, movies and cruising areas continue to exist, but they are less popular, and the sex that takes place there is much more likely to be safer sex (Martin, 1987; Martin *et al.*, 1989; Van Griensven *et al.*, 1987; Connell *et al.*, 1988c). Gay men also report a growing number of primary relationships that tend to last longer, and with multiple partners there is much greater likelihood of safer sex. This change is most likely due to both anxiety over AIDS and the ageing of a large segment of the gay population which, along with other 'baby boomers', seems to be searching for more stable relationships.

Why Gay Men Changed to Safer Sex

There is no single reason why gay men should change to safer sex or continue to practise unsafe sex. Two very common explanations for the change to safer sex are: (1) because the men involved learned that AIDS was caused by unprotected anal sex and was likely to be fatal; and (2) because the men involved knew someone who had ARC/AIDS or had died of AIDS. The evidence reviewed below indicates that these are, at best, only partial explanations, and there are several other factors which lead to continuing unsafe sex, adopting safer sex and continuing safer sex.

The factors found to be empirically related to changing sexual behaviours can be clustered into three frameworks. The *personality framework* describes relationships between selected psychological factors which are involved in the development of a self-concept, and which influence sexual behaviour. The *rational man framework* focuses on the cognitive processing of information and the impact of awareness, attitudes and beliefs about safer and unsafe sexual practices. The *cybernetic framework* focuses on the power that external stimuli, particularly normative influences, have in changing a sexual habit.

The literature reviewed in relation to these three frameworks comes from qualitative and quantitative studies carries out in over fifteen cities in ten countries.

Table 2.1 Changes in Risk Behaviour

Study	Location	Assessment period	Study groups	1978	1979	1980	1981	1982	1983	1984	1985	1986	1987
								Change					
McKusick et al. (AIDS Behavioral Research Project)	San Francisco	30 days								22.3% a 34.7% b		7.2%	
Winkelstein et al. (San Francisco Men's Health Study)	San Francisco	6 months	2 2 1							14.4% a 39.6% b 43%	5.8% 13.3% 37%	15.4%	8% 3%
Doll et al. (Hep B/AIDS Cohort)	San Francisco	4 months	4	10.9 a 12.9 b							0.4% 1%		
Stall et al. (Secondary Analysis of Communication Technologies)	San Francisco									30.5%	13.2%	10.2%	6.9%
Stall et al. (AIDS Behavioral Research Project)	San Francisco									38.7%	21.1%	19.1%	15.5%
Puckett et al. (Secondary Analysis of AIDS Behavioral Research Project)			4 3							18% 69%	12% 81%		
Larry Bye (Communication Technologies)	San Francisco	30 days								M = 2.6c			
Larry Bye (Communication Technologies)	Los Angeles	30 days	4									M = 1.6a	
Klein et al.	Los Angeles	6 months	Physicians: Students:							79% a 90% b 79% a 84% b		35.3% 46.5% 60.9% 67.3%	M = 0.3

Study	Location	Time period	Study group	Data
Martin	New York	annual		M = 70a, M = 85b
Siegal et al.	New York	30 days		M = 20, M = 25; 59.9% a, 87.4% c; 48.1%, 71.7%
Fox et al.	MACS — Baltimore, Chicago, Los Angeles, Pittsburgh	6 months		71% a, 80% b; 51%, 55%
Johnson and McGrath	Texas	30 days		
Joseph et al.	Chicago	6 months		40% c, 54.1% a; 10%, 48%; 25.1% a
Kelly et al.	Mississippi	12 months	4	
Jones et al.	New Mexico	12 months	4	M = 19.4a; 70% a
Carne	UK, Middlesex	12 months		27%, 41%; 8%, 16%
Van Griensven et al.	Netherlands, Amsterdam	6 months	7	73%, 44%; 61%, 29%
National Gay Magazine	Holland	12 months	8	70% c; 59%
Connell	Australia		4	83% a, 71% a
Schechter et al. (VLAS)	Canada, Vancouver	6 months	8, 5, 6	63%, 26%, 64%, 55%

Change:
(a) denotes unprotected receptive anal intercourse
(b) denotes unprotected insertive anal intercourse
(c) denotes both/either where distinction was not made

Study Groups:
1 — HIV positive only
2 — HIV negative only
3 — steady partners
4 — non-steady partners (sexual contact only once or twice)
5 — steady HIV +
6 — steady HIV –
7 — non-steady HIV +
8 — non-steady HIV –

Table 2.2   Condom Use

Study	Baseline	Last assessment	Change (percentage)
San Francisco			
McKusick *et al.*	1982	1984	
(AIDS Behavioral	14.1%	23.8%	+0.7
Research Project — 1985)			
Larry Bye (Communicaton	1984	1987	0
Technologies 1987 — CDC)	0.03[1]	0.3	
	23%	23%	
	1984	1985	
Pucket *et al.*	18%[7]	26.7%[2]	
New York			
Martin (1987)	1980–81	1985–55	
Active	1%	20%	19
Receptive	2%	19%	8.5
Other areas			
MACS	1984	1986	
(Baltimore, Chicago,	13%	29%[2]	1.2
Los Angeles, Pittsburgh)			
Schechter *et al.*	1984–85	1986–87	
(VLAS)	21%[23]	55%[235]	
	28%[4]	76%[246]	
		84%[236]	
		98[246]	
Joseph *et al.*	1984	1985	
	16.51%[4]	26.7[2]	

Notes: 1 mean frequency usage per secondary partner
2 receptive anal intercourse
3 seronegatives
4 seropositives
5 regular partners
6 casual partners
7 anal insertive without condom

It is important to recognize that most scientific studies on HIV/AIDS in gay communities relate to periods well after the peak of the HIV epidemic. Although some of the studies ask men to recall their behaviour in the early 1980s, there is little evidence about the reasons gay men changed to safer sex when HIV was spreading most rapidly.

This chapter does not include a framework which incorporates social and class factors. There is no question that class often determines the resources spent on AIDS prevention, and that different classes attribute different meanings to sexual

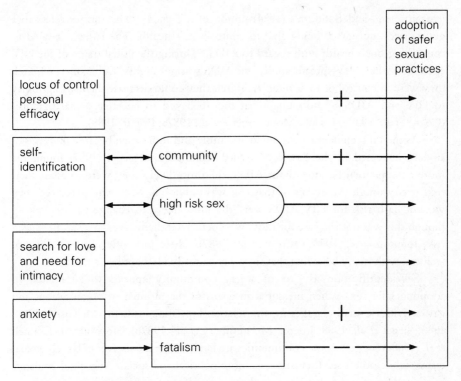

Figure 2.2   Personality Framework

behaviour and homosexuality. Unfortunately, few studies systematically analyze the impact of social and class factors on behaviour change.[4] The overwhelming majority of studies have been done among urban, white, middle-class, self-defined gay men, and there is scant evidence on sexual behaviour change in gay ethnic and rural communities. In some respects most studies are like spotlights illuminating a small part of a large stage during an act of a play. Not only is it impossible to see the beginning of the play, but even much of the existing action is hidden well outside the beam of the light.

The Personality Framework

The personality framework emphasizes the relationship between a person's self-concept and behaviour change toward safer sex. As indicated in Figure 2.2, key components of self-concept include a person's sense of internal control over his environment, self-identification with the gay community or with particular sexual practices, search for love and intimacy, and his levels of anxiety and fatalism about AIDS. The top box in Figure 2.2 represents an amalgam of Rotter's (1966) *internal locus of control* and Bandura's (1984) notion of *self-efficacy*. The former refers to a generalized concept of being able to control one's health. The latter is related to controlling one's health with regard to AIDS.[5] During the initial stages of the HIV epidemic, when HIV spread rapidly but AIDS was not highly visible, men who felt they were in control of their own health felt they could decrease their susceptibility to HIV and AIDS by adopting what they believed to be safer sexual practices (Coates *et al.*, 1988b; Joseph, Montgomery *et al.*, 1987a; Prieur, 1988).

As the HIV epidemic progressed and more and more men became ill, levels of anxiety increased in the gay community. Bauman and Siegel (1987) found the more anxious men became about AIDS, the more likely they were to assess their risk, even though the extent of that risk was unknown. Men who perceived they were at high risk for HIV/AIDS were the most likely to change to safer sex — though this was not the case for those who perceived themselves to be at the *highest* risk) Johnson *et al.*, 1988; Ostrow *et al.*, 1987). These men often had a feeling of fatalism, with many believing that they were already HIV antibody positive.

Self-identification as part of a gay community appears to be related to adopting safer sex. When measured in terms of the number of organizations and gay activities a man engages in, the relationship is inconsistent (McKusick *et al.*, 1985; Siegal *et al.*, 1988; Joseph, Montgomery *et al.*, 1987b). However, as Connell *et al.* (1988c) suggest, some communities are likely to see themselves in largely sexual terms, while others see themselves as more political and social. Anecdotal evidence in a number of cities demonstrates how a handful of early adopters of safer sex, who had a strong sense of self-efficacy and a strong identification within their gay communities, acted as agents of change by starting community-based organizations (CBOs) such as the Terrence Higgins Trust in London, the Gay Men's Health Crisis in New York, AIDES in Paris, Bobby Goldsmith in Sydney, the San Francisco AIDS Foundation and the Swiss AIDS Foundation.

By the time the incidence of HIV dropped to its lowest level, most gay men had high levels of knowledge about the modes of transmission. Yet, for men who did not have access to a gay community, such as those in many small towns, villages and rural areas, and for those men whose gay identification was pre-dominantly sexual, the need to affirm their gay identity often overwhelmed known dangers about unsafe sex (Bye, 1988b; Prieur, 1988; Pollak, 1989).

Another personality characteristic related to continuing unsafe sex is the search for intimacy and love. One man in Prieur's (1988) study places this need in perspective: 'The whole point of being fucked is that it should go inside you, otherwise you haven't really given him all of yourself.' There is also some evidence to suggest that as relationships mature there is a growing need to express intimacy and trust in a partner, and this can lead to unsafe sex, regardless of level of knowledge about HIV and AIDS. However, some men appear to balance their need for intimacy with their awareness of risk. The next framework provides some insight into why this awareness may, or may not, be effective.

The Rational Man Framework

Information processing and reasoning underlie the rational man framework, which asserts that men change to safer sex following a logical evaluation of information. An underlying assumption here is that *awareness* of information about HIV/AIDS leads to *beliefs* about the accuracy of that information, which result in positive *attitudes* toward safer sex. These lead, in turn, to safer sex. Awareness is defined as knowing about a piece of information. Belief refers to the degree of certainly that the piece of information is true. Attitudes refer to the positive or negative feelings a person has toward the information. (This three component process is similar to the concepts articulated by Fishbein and Ajzen (1975) and to the *predisposing factors* in Green *et al.*'s (1980) PRECEDE model. To illustrate these concepts, three hypotheses have been suggested for the finding that condoms are not consistently used. One hypothesis suggests that persons who are *unaware* of condoms or do not know how to use them will not use them. A second hypothesis is that those who are less likely to *believe* that condoms are effective are less likely to use condoms. A third hypothesis is that those who *like* condoms are more likely to use them than those who dislike condoms. While each appears to be a common-sense explanation, the predictive power of negative attitudes towards condom use appears to be greater than either awareness or beliefs.

As is indicated at the bottom of Figure 2.3, the overwhelming majority of studies do not find any relationship between awareness (usually referred to as 'knowledge') of unsafe sex practices and the change to safer sex (Connell *et al.*, 1988b; Joseph, Montgomery *et al.*, 1987b; Prieur, 1988; Coates *et al.*, 1988b; Fitzpatrick *et al.*, 1989; Martin, 1986; Becker and Joseph, 1988). Also most of these studies do not show a relationship between knowing friends/lovers with AIDS/ARC and a change to safer sex. This may be because most scientific studies were done quite late in the HIV epidemic. Figure 2.4 plots the cumulative number of AIDS cases against the incidence of HIV infection curves for San Francisco and London. It shows that considerable behaviour change started even before HIV was known to be the virus causing AIDS (1984), long before many cases of AIDS were diagnosed in these communities and long before men knew with certainty the causes of AIDS of its consequences. Although almost no studies investigate these initial stages of the epidemic, for a large number of these early adopters *uncertainty* about the cause and consequences of AIDS must have provided a stimulus to change.

What the studies do show, however, is that basic information about unsafe sex spread quickly through the gay communities. Four to five years after the start of the epidemic, HIV was spreading quickly and large numbers of men began showing symptoms of AIDS. At this time — when most scientific studies were just beginning — virtually every gay man studied knew the basics about unsafe and safer sex, and most knew or had known someone who had ARC/AIDS. For example, Bochow (1990) finds in his recent study of gay men in West Germany, a

Figure 2.3   *Rational Man Framework*

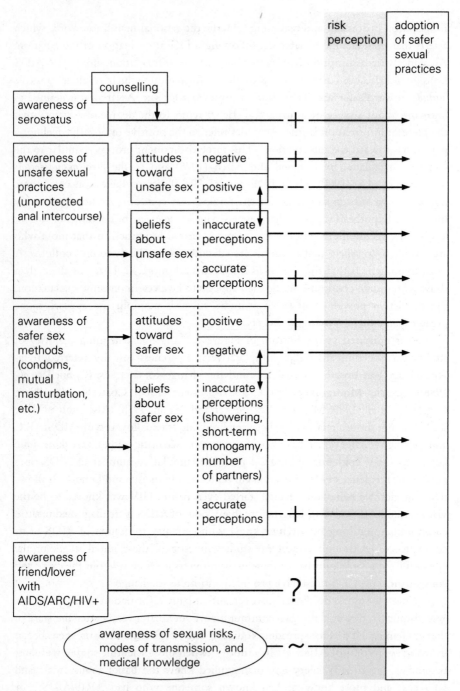

Figure 2.4   *Incidence of HIV and Prevalence of AIDS among Cohorts*

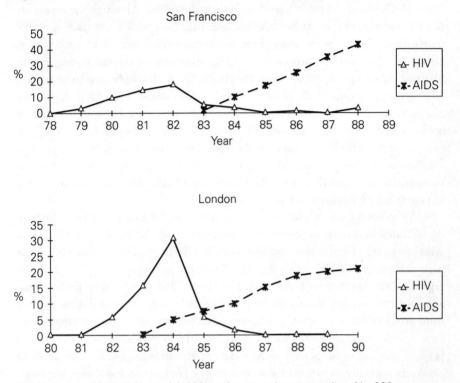

San Francisco: Hessol, N. *et al*. (1989) and personal conversation. *N* = 320; Hepatitis B vaccine trial; recruited through San Francisco City Clinic; seronegative for Hepatitis B at recruitment.
London: Jenkins; P. (1990) and personal conversation. *N* = 318; recruited January 1982–March 1985 from St Mary's GUM STD clinic, and volunteers recruited through gay newspaper.

country which is further behind in the HIV epidemic, that there is a relationship between knowing someone with AIDS/ARC and adopting safer sex.

Another reason for the lack of relationship between knowledge and behaviour change was the methods used to measure knowledge. Typically, knowledge was measured by adding up awareness of different transmission modes, symptoms and medical treatment. It was assumed that, like weights on a scale, the 'heavier' the awareness, the more likely it was that the scales would tip to safer sex. The adage, 'it's not how much you know, but what you know', may be more appropriate.

Awareness of information that leads to an increase in perceived susceptibility to AIDS appears to have an impact on changing behaviour. For example, during the period when HIV was spreading rapidly among gay men, several studies found that those who were aware of their HIV serostatus were more likely to change to safer sex than those who did not (Bye, 1988b; Winkelstein *et al.*, 1987b; Fox *et al.*, 1987; McCusker *et al.*, 1987; Van Griensven *et al.*, 1989b). Although the results are mixed, the majority of studies also indicate that men who know they are HIV seropositive change more than those who know they are HIV seronegative. However, these studies indicate that while awareness of serostatus might have hastened the change, it did not *cause* the change. In all the studies the trend toward safer sex was already well established, and a few studies indicate that, for late adopters of safer sex, knowledge of HIV serostatus gained through testing is unlikely to be related to change (Ostrow *et al.*, 1987; Martin *et al.*, 1989). To complicate the relationship, none of the studies took into account the independent effects of counselling. Consequently, it may be counselling alone, testing alone, or a combination of counselling with the knowledge of HIV serostatus that causes the change to safer sex (Fitzpatrick *et al.*, 1989).

Awareness of unsafe and safer sex practices may not in itself lead to adoption. As indicated in the second group of boxes down from the top in Figure 2.3, men who are aware of unsafe sex and like it are less likely to perceive that they are at high risk and less likely to practise safer sex than men who do not like anal sex, regardless of the perceived risk. Based on Connell *et al.*'s (1988b) findings that awareness of safer sex and an awareness of unsafe sex are separate dimensions, the third group of boxes in Figure 2.3 indicates that men who are aware of safer sex *and* have a positive attitude toward it are more likely to have an increased perception of personal risk and to adopt safer sexual practices. Returning to our hypotheses about condoms, virtually all studies show that in gay populations most men are aware that condoms provide protection against HIV. Yet they are not consistently used, because many men just do not like them (Valdiserri and Lyter, 1988; Staub, 1988; Bye, 1985; Connell *et al.*, 1988c).

In addition to positive attitudes, men have to believe that protected anal sex or non-penetrative sexual practices are the major means of HIV prevention and that other forms of prevention are not effective. Awareness of safer sex methods accompanied by incorrect beliefs about their efficacy can often result in rationalization of the continuation of unsafe sex or the adoption of ineffective methods of HIV prevention. Even the most educated and knowledgeable persons misinterpret, selectively perceive, or rationalize information in order to confirm their own biases and behaviours.[6] For example, although awareness of condoms is almost universal, studies indicate that some persons do not use them because they do not believe they are effective. On the other hand, if men believe that inefficacious methods are effective, they are more likely to engage in them. Inaccurate perceptions about safer sex methods are widespread (McKusick *et al.*, 1985; Joseph, Montgomery *et al.*, 1987b), and Bauman and Siegal (1987) found that 70 per cent of the men in their study reported engaging in behaviours which they believed reduced their risk but actually made little difference.

Some inaccurate perceptions such as showering before and after sex and the efficacy of douching appear to be based on a misunderstanding that HIV infection starts on contact with the blood.[7] Other misperceptions are based on an inaccurate understanding of transmission probability, such as reducing the number of partners without engaging in protected anal sex. In a community with an infection rate of 30–50 per cent, reducing the number of partners is unlikely to reduce greatly the risk of HIV infection.

The largest number of rationalizations appears to be based on the poor understanding of the eight to ten years it takes for HIV to manifest itself as AIDS. First, while many men report monogamous relationships as their response to reducing their risk, in many instances monogamy was reported in terms of months, not years. Given the time lag involved, unprotected anal sex practised with short-term monogamous partners who are seropositive or of unknown HIV status is a high risk activity. Second, some believe that they have developed immunity. Third, for some young gay men, there is an inaccurate perception that AIDS is an older man's disease. Finally, the lack of understanding about the lag between HIV and AIDS, combined with awareness of the falling HIV rate, is likely to be misinterpreted by some as an end to the need for safer sex. However, despite the fact that the number of seroconversions has declined, the likelihood of becoming HIV positive from unprotected anal sex remains high because there continue to be large numbers of sexually active seropositive persons.

The Cybernetic Framework

Unsafe sexual habits are hard to break. They are often resistant both to high levels of awareness of safe and unsafe sexual practices and to belief in the efficacy of safer sex methods. The cybernetic framework suggests that when unsafe sex becomes a habit, the momentum of that behaviour will continue until some force is strong enough to alter its course. The best predictor of unsafe sex is the previous practice of unsafe sex (McCusker *et al.*, 1989b; Martin, 1986; Connell *et al.*, 1988a).[8] The cybernetic framework is derived from stimulus-response (S-R) theories and the mechanistic process associated with conditioning based on strength of habit, reinforcement and punishments. Like more current S-R theories, such as Bandura's *social cognitive* theory, the cybernetic framework suggests that learning comes directly through the experience of safe or unsafe sexual practices and through modelling the behaviour of others (Rosenstock *et al.*, 1988). The most powerful stimuli are often external, coming from social groups, peers and sexual partners, rather than internal, stemming from personal awareness of information. On the one hand, a man conforming to the sexual behaviour of his partner or peers can be rewarded by their acceptance and the gratification of pleasing others, while a man who does not conform risks punishment through social rejection and isolation. Similarly, for those for whom sexual stimuli have an addictive component (Ostrow

Figure 2.5 *The Cybernetic Framework*

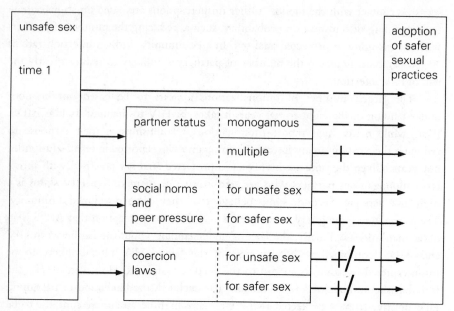

and Joseph, 1986), the reward for engaging in unsafe sex is the act of sex itself and the punishment is withholding of sex. This framework is applicable to an understanding of most behaviour modification programmes, where external forces such as peer *pressure* and public commitments are used to change strong habitual (or addictive) behaviour, and peer *support* is used to reinforce that change.

For younger gay men or men coming out, the cybernetic framework suggests that much of their sexual behaviour is learned from modelling the behaviour of other gay men. Where the model is unsafe sex, there is likely to be pressure to engage in unsafe sex; where the model is safer sex, there is a greater likelihood of safer sex.

A finding from several studies, indicated by the 'partner status' box in Figure 2.5, is that more unsafe sex occurs within a primary relationship than between men who are not in a primary relationship or between men who also have sex *outside* their primary relationship (Bye, 1987; McCusker *et al.*, 1985; Martin *et al.*, 1989; Connell *et al.*, 1988a). In some instances, as suggested by the rational man framework, this is a calculated risk, often based on inaccurate information. In other instances, however, it may reflect the fact that neither partner wanted to be 'punished' by withholding sex or causing potential conflict within the relationship.

The box in Figure 2.5 under partner status suggests the importance of peer and social pressure. In communities such as San Francisco and New York in the late 1970s and early 1980s, multiple partners and unsafe sex became, for a large number of men, the social norm. At the same time there was a growing cohesion within gay communities. As the HIV epidemic increased, Martin (1986), Valdiserri *et al.* (1989), Aggleton *et al.* (1989) and others report that having multiple partners was related to greater *change* to safer sex, and at the same time a higher overall incidence of unsafe sex. The rapid decline in the HIV incidence in some gay communities may reflect the presence of gay 'ghettos' where there was greater social interaction and political presence. In theory a more socially cohesive network may find it more difficult to accept behavioural change but, once started, the diffusion of change due to social norms and peer pressure may occur more rapidly. This hypothesis remains to be tested, and in any case it is a matter of degree, since in all communities with gay cohorts the level of HIV infections declined and there was some level of gay-run HIV prevention.

For those men more committed to continuing unsafe sexual practices, and for those men who have sex with men but who are not part of the gay community, bathhouses, movies and cruising areas are likely to provide an opportunity for unsafe sex. The cybernetic framework suggests that when unsafe sex is the norm in these settings, men will engage in unsafe sex rather than feel socially isolated or rejected. Anecdotal evidence suggests that, when these locations exist within a gay centre, they are likely in time to reflect the safer sex norms of that wider gay community. However, in similar locations in more rural settings, unsafe sex is likely to continue at a higher level.

Stimulants, such as drugs and alcohol, are another factor in this framework, acting as aphrodisiacs or reducing social barriers to sexual encounters. Most of the evidence to date indicates that getting 'high' increases the likelihood of engaging in unsafe sexual activities (Stall *et al.*, 1986; Bye, 1987; Connell *et al.*, 1987, Prieur, 1988; Van Griensven *et al.*, 1987). Yet as the social norm changes to safer sex, alcohol and drugs may have different effects. In theory, if both partners have the habit of safer sex, the most likely outcome of a sexual encounter will be safe, regardless of stimulants. However, where there is disagreement about the preferred type of sex, being 'high' can lead to unsafe sexual behaviour. On the other hand, there is some chance that stimulants may lessen anxieties about safer sex and, among groups where safer sex is the norm, it may help people to break out of a pattern of unsafe sexual behaviour.

The role of perceived or actual coercion to engage in safe or unsafe sex is also addressed by the cybernetic framework, especially in situations involving initiates with more experienced partners, or in settings, such as prisons, where there may be those who hold more dominant roles and those who are more submissive. Laws, club codes, or rules in the military or workplace are clearly based on the belief that punishment provides a strong stimulus. Needless to say, these methods of promoting safer sex are surrounded by serious ethical questions about coercion and confidentiality. In some instances, legal constraints designed to promote behaviour change may actually perpetuate unsafe sexual practices by driving those who would seek assistance underground. For example, mandatory testing, unless accompanied by strict assurances of anonymity and confidentiality, may be seen as a means of classifying and listing men which could, directly or indirectly, lead to discrimination in employment, insurance, housing and social activities. In addition, these laws may act as barriers to the development of community support groups, which have been shown to be effective agents in promoting behaviour change.

Recommendations for HIV/AIDS Prevention Programmes

The personality, rational man and cybernetic frameworks highlight different factors affecting the adoption of safer sexual practices which can be the focus of HIV/AIDS prevention programmes. In the development of such a programme, one of the first tasks is to determine the pattern and phase of the HIV epidemic for a specific group, either through precise epidemiologic information, or through less precise information about 'markers' such as the incidence of anal gonorrhoea. The target audience should then be identified by its relevant traits. For gay men, such traits can include sexual preferences, intellectual pursuits, geographic area, ethnic or age groups, recreational activities, etc.

On a practical basis, it is very difficult to determine the pattern of HIV infection in different gay subpopulations, as most of the evidence now comes from cohorts recruited through the gay community, gay press, physicians and STD clinics. This only emphasizes the need to obtain information about HIV incidence outside the 'gay ghettos' — in minority ethnic communities, among rural and small town gays, and among those men who do not affiliate with a gay community.

The personality framework suggests that, in the early stages of the epidemic, there will be a core of gay men who believe they have control over their own health and can make efficacious changes in behaviour. They are likely to be more anxious about their own health and that of their friends and community. For these people, preliminary and basic information about HIV and AIDS appears to enable a change in behaviour. The energies of these early adopters of safer sex can be harnessed by providing them with the financial, legal and moral support to begin CBOs which can build community cohesion and create new channels of communication such as safer sex seminars, social events and recreational activities. They can often mobilize at a faster pace than government organizations and are often subject to fewer restrictions regarding health education material. Community activism is clearly good for HIV/AIDS prevention.

The cybernetic framework suggests that CBOs are likely to be effective because they act as new interpersonal and social networks in the gay community, fuelling normative change and peer pressure towards safer sex, and because they can provide the peer support that reinforces continued safer sex. The volunteers they attract are likely to change to safer sex, not only because they are persuaded of the risk of unsafe sexual practices, but also because safer sex becomes their group norm.

The rational man framework suggests that, early in the epidemic, effective information is that which increases anxiety *and* provides safer sex as a way of relieving that anxiety (Job, 1988). The messages will have greater impact if they come from within the gay community, rather than from less trusted medical or political sources. This information can be circulated through existing media such as gay newspapers and magazines, and, where they exist, radio and cable TV. If the past is a guide, mainstream mass media will rarely cover AIDS during the initial stages of the HIV epidemic, and then only from a predominantly moral and medical perspective (Albert, 1988; Herzlich and Pierret, 1989). More targeted media are able more effectively to disseminate educational messages as identifiable risk factors become clear. Newly created specialized newsletters, brochures, pamphlets, posters and videos can be effective in conveying in-depth erotic or other specialized messages, and they can be effectively disseminated through channels such as social and political clubs, bars, saunas, cruising areas, gay centres, literary, business and sports groups.

Once change has started, as the rational man framework suggests, information should quickly go beyond basic messages about unsafe sex and the use of condoms. Such information spreads quickly, but appears to be unrelated to behaviour change during the middle and later stages of the HIV epidemic; *awareness* of information does not mean that men *accept* or *believe* it. Many traditional health educators believe that the most effective way to teach men about HIV/AIDS prevention is through educational lectures and the production of commercials distributed through the mass media. These educators anticipate that once men are aware of the reasons why unsafe sex leads to HIV/AIDS, the only logical choice is a change to safer sexual practices. Unfortunately, little attention is given to whether messages are believed or considered appealing by the audience. Messages should be designed to promote positive attitudes toward, as well as awareness of, safer sex methods (Ross and Rosser, 1989). Erotic formats are one method of doing this. But regardless of their quality, the literature, videos, etc. will not be effective for some men, for whom personalized programmes, such as workshops on safer sex and eroticizing safer sex, are more likely to be effective.

HIV/AIDS prevention programmes must create believable messages and address misperceptions about methods of safer sex: incorrect beliefs are often associated with rationalizing the continuation of unsafe sexual practices or the adoption of ineffective methods. It is necessary to make clear that unprotected anal sex is the major conduit for HIV. The transfer of epidemiological information directly into health prevention messages is the source of much inaccurate information. For example, the earliest brochures and pamphlets, while effective in disseminating information, reflected the prevailing uncertainty of the risk associated with deep kissing and oral sex, and advised against them. In retrospect, this made it difficult to emphasize that anal sex was, by far, the highest risk factor. Many men thus avoided change which they found overly difficult or because messages were perceived as false. Perhaps the most widely adopted, and the most misleading, advice given early in the HIV epidemic was the reduction of the number of partners. During the height of the HIV epidemic, this precaution, unaccompanied by safer sex practices, often provided minimal reduction in risk. Although much later material provided less ambiguous information about risk, these early messages still continue to fuel many inaccurate perceptions which lead to underestimation of personal risk, and the continued practice of unsafe sex.

Many inaccurate perceptions are based on a poor understanding of the time lag between being infected and developing AIDS, including the perceived efficacy of short-term monogamous relationships, or of reducing the number of partners, and the possibility of detecting HIV status by a physical inspection of potential partners. For younger gay men or those just establishing a gay sexual identity, there is a need to emphasize the risk of sex among peers. Inaccurate perceptions based on a misunderstanding of the way HIV infects, such as the efficacy of douching and showering, must also be reversed. During the tail of the epidemic there is a constant need to emphasize that, despite the fact that the number of sero-conversions has declined, the likelihood of becoming HIV positive from unprotected anal sex remains high because there continue to be large numbers of sexually active sero-positive men.

There is little research on the efficacy of different HIV/AIDS prevention messages, but communications research does provide some leads. Frightening messages are likely to raise anxiety — which may be related to behaviour change *if* information about effective safer sex methods is also provided as a way of resolving this anxiety. Without knowledge and a willingness to adopt safer sex methods, however, heightened anxiety may lead to avoidance, rationalization and in some instances a fatalistic attitude. Each of these is negatively related to the adoption of safer sex and may lead to psychological problems. In the development of safer sex messages, a particular effort must be made to use language and graphics that are understood by the target audience. The few studies which have evaluated the content and level of HIV/AIDS health promotion literature have found that the majority of messages have been written for an audience with high school education and above (Siegal *et al.*, 1986; Hochhauser, 1987). For lower socio-economic groups, different material may prove to be more effective. There is likely to be no single effective approach for all men, so it is desirable to use multiple approaches and to test the comprehension of messages within the target subgroups. In general, some subgroups are likely to respond to highly emotional messages, while others respond to more rational content. Finally, whatever the message, its proper distribution plays as important a role as its content.

Although there is considerable ongoing debate about the preventive benefit of

HIV testing, the statistical evidence is convincing that testing, *with* assurances of anonymity, *and* counselling can have a positive impact on behaviour change during the middle of the HIV epidemic. However, while testing may increase the *pace* of change by alerting a person to their risk of HIV, it is not the *cause* of that change. Mandatory testing, as well as other prevention efforts based on legal edicts, are likely to be counterproductive as they may drive men who need assistance away from health providers because they fear employment, health care, housing and social discrimination.

As the HIV epidemic enters its later stages, an awareness of information, attitudes and beliefs is less likely to provide adequate motivation for behaviour change for those men who have not yet adopted consistent safer sex. These men will be most likely to change when their partners and peers apply pressure. For others, the need for acceptance or intimacy may be expressed by unsafe sex, regardless of risk. These men are likely to be difficult to convince. Among those with low self-esteem and a weak sense of self-efficacy the demands of others may take precedence over rational reasons for safer sex. For these, programmes which increase self-esteem and self-empowerment, such as partner negotiation workshops, safer sex workshops and peer counselling, may be effective interventions. Also, certain behaviour modification programmes where enjoyable safer methods are substituted for unsafe methods are likely to be effective.

In all stages of the HIV epidemic the use of alcohol and drugs is likely to be related to engaging in unsafe sexual practices. As the norm in the subgroup changes to safer sex, these disinhibitors may lead to more, but not necessarily unsafe, sex. HIV prevention should be a part of all drug and alcohol rehabilitation programmes. Safer sex messages and condoms should also be available where liquor is sold and consumed, and bartenders and outreach workers can be trained to provide advice and condoms.

Finally, the cybernetic framework suggests the importance of reinforcement in the continuation of safer sex. Mass media and interpersonal HIV/AIDS prevention programmes must insist on the need for safer sex, while legitimating a change in social norms and reinforcing the large change that has already occurred. Groups and associations developed to spread the message must also focus on safer sex *maintenance* programmes.

While by no means exhaustive, this last section demonstrates that the analytic framework discussed in this chapter, combined with an *awareness* of the stage of the HIV epidemic and the make-up of the subgroup affected, can assist in shortening the curve of the HIV epidemic by increasing the number of men who take themselves out of the available pool for HIV infection through a modification of unsafe sexual behaviour. It cautions against expensive mass media awareness campaigns late in the epidemic, when most people are already aware that unprotected anal sex is a major cause of AIDS and that condoms are a means of prevention, but demonstrates the effectiveness of CBOs and community participation. It also suggests that the development of positive attitudes toward safer sex and the correction of inaccurate perceptions about effective safer sex methods remain a challenge for HIV/AIDS prevention programmes. Finally, it warns about the likely recurrence of HIV in certain subgroups. For young men developing a gay identity and for those who have not yet made safer sex a habit, there is considerable likelihood of unsafe sex; thus programmes reinforcing behaviour change will remain necessary if gay communities are to maintain their low levels of new infection.

Acknowledgments

The original literature review for this article was supported by WHO/GPA. The theoretical development was done while the author was at a post at INSERM Unit 21, where Dr J. Chwalow has been of particular assistance. Marguerite Guiguet and Dr A-J. Valleron at INSERM Unit 263 have provided invaluable feedback and support for this work. Bob Stern has patiently provided editorial assistance.

Notes

1 'Unsafe sex' as used in this chapter refers to unprotected anal intercourse. 'Safer sex' includes consistent use of condoms with anal sex, oral sex, non-penetrative sex and abstinence. There is some argument about whether or not HIV can be acquired through oral sex. Most studies show no relationship, and there are only a few instances of suspected HIV transmission through oral sex (Coates *et al.*, 1988a, 1988b; Van Griensven *et al.*, 1987).

2 In the US, cohorts in New York (NY Blood Center — C. Stevens; Colombia School of Public Health — John Martin), Los Angeles, Chicago, Baltimore, Washington (MACS study — Joseph) started too late to show the level of increase, but each show decline to less than 1 per cent by 1987. In France, using the back method of calculation, homosexual populations in Paris indicate a sharp decline in HIV (INSERM, unit 263), and data from Oslo show dramatic decreases in HIV infection.

3 Other reasons might have been that the virus mutated into a less contagious form or that men developed a natural immunity. Neither of these is true for HIV, although there is some evidence that co-factors contribute to susceptibility to HIV infection.

4 Michael Pollak's work in France and Michael Bochow's work in West Germany are exceptions. For them, social class is a major factor, and their sampling method allowed them to have a number of homosexual men outside the gay ghettos.

5 Bandura later suggested two components of self-efficacy. The first, *efficacy expectation*, is the belief that one is capable of engaging in safer sex; the second, *outcome expectation*, is the belief that safer sex will significantly reduce the chance of HIV infection and AIDS. This framework refers only to efficacy expectations. The rational man framework incorporates the concept of outcome expectations.

6 The process of selective perception is more fully described in McQuire (1969), and the process of rationalization in Festinger's (1957) theory of cognitive dissonance.

7   These practices may actually increase the risk due to irritation of the rectal membranes, increasing the likelihood of viral transfer if semen is introduced (Coates *et al.*, 1988a).
8   It is called a 'cybernetic' framework because it describes behaviour patterns analogous to those of robots, where the same actions are repeated until reprogramming occurs.

References

AGGLETON, P.J., COXON, A. and WEATHERBURN, P. (1989) 'AIDS Health Promotion Activities Targeted at Homosexually Active Men in London (UK): A Briefing Document Prepared for WHO/GPA', Institute of Behavioural Research into AIDS, University of Wales, UK.

ALBERT, E. (1988) 'The Response of the Press to Acquired Immune Deficiency Syndrome', in Feldman and Johnson (Eds), *Social Dimensions of AIDS: Method and Theory*, New York, Praeger.

BANDURA, A. (1984) 'Self-efficacy: Toward a Unifying Theory of Behavioural Change', *Psychological Review*, 84, 191–215.

BAUMAN L. and SIEGEL, K. (1987) 'Misperception among Gay Men of the Risk for AIDS Associated with Their Sexual Bebaviour', *Journal of Applied Social Psychology*, 17, 3, 329–350.

BECKER M. and JOSEPH, J. (1988) 'AIDS and Behavioural Change to Reduce Risk: A Review', *American Journal of Public Health*, 778, 4, 394–410.

BOCHOW, M. (1989) *AIDS und Schwule*, Berlin, AIDS-FORUM D.A.H. Brand IV.

BOCHOW, M. (1990) 'Oral Report Presented at Assessing AIDS Prevention in the Homo/Bisexual Community: A European Comparison', EEC Conference, 27–28 April.

BYE, L. (1985) 'Designing an Effective AIDS Prevention Campaign Strategy for San Francisco: Results of the Second Probability Sample of the Urban Gay Male Community', San Francisco, San Francisco AIDS Foundation.

BYE, L. (1987) 'A Report on Designing an Effective AIDS Prevention Campaign Strategy for San Francisco: Results of the Second Probability Sample of the Urban Gay Male Community', San Francisco, San Francisco AIDS Foundation.

BYE, L. (1988a) 'Moving beyond Counselling and Knowledge-enhancing Interventions: A Plea for Community Level AIDS Prevention Strategies', position paper prepared for the CDC, Atlanta, Ga., US.

BYE, L. (1988b) 'Focus-Group Research Influencing AIDS Risk Behaviour Change among Homosexual and Bisexual Men in the United States', prepared for Lynda Doll, Center for Infectious Disease Control, CDC, Atlanta, Ga., US.

CARNE, C.A., JOHNSON, A.M., WELLER, I.V.D. *et al.* (1987) 'Prevalence of Antibodies to HIV, Gonorrhea Rates and Changed Sexual Behaviour in Homosexual Men in London', *Lancet*, 1, 656–658.

COATES, R., CALZAVARA, L., *et al.* (1988a) 'Risk Factors for HIV Infection in Male Sexual Contacts of Men with AIDS or AIDS-Related Condition', *Journal of Epidemiology*, 128, 729–736.

COATES, T., STALL, R., HOFF, C., *et al.* (1988b) 'Changes in Sexual Behaviour of Gay Bisexual Men Since the Beginning of the AIDS Epidemic', unpublished manuscript prepared for the CDC, Atlanta, Ga., US.

CONNELL R.W., CRAWFORD, J., KIPPAX, S., *et al.* (1988a) 'Social Aspects of the Prevention of AIDS: Report 1: Methods and Sample', Macquarie University, Australia.

CONNELL, R.W., KIPPAX, S., CRAWFORD, J., *et al.* (1988b) 'Social Aspects of the Prevention of AIDS: Report 2: Information about AIDS: The Accuracy of Knowledge Possessed by Gay and Bisexual Men', Macquarie University, Australia.

CONNELL, R.W., CRAWFORD, J., *et al.* (1988c) 'Social Aspects of the Prevention of AIDS. Facing the Epidemic: Changes in the Sexual and Social Lives of Gay and Bisexual Men in Response to the AIDS Crisis, and Their Implications for AIDS Prevention Strategies', Macquarie University, Australia.

DOLL, L., DARROW, W., et al. (1987) 'Self-Reported Changes in Sexual Behaviours in Gay and Bisexual Men from the San Francisco City Clinic Cohort', IInd International Conference on AIDS, Washington, D.C.

DOWSETT, G.W. (1989) 'AIDS Prevention Strategies for Gay and Bisexual Men in Sydney, Australia', report prepared for WHO/GPA, Geneva.

FESTINGER, L. (1957) *A Theory of Cognitive Dissonance*, Evanston, Ill., Row Peterson.

FISHBEIN, M. and AJZEN, I. (1957) *Beliefs, Attitudes and Behaviour*, Reading, Mass., Addison-Wesley.

FITZPATRICK, R., BOULTON, M. and HART, G. (1989) 'Gay Men's Sexual Behaviour in Response to AIDS', in P. AGGLETON, G. HART and P. DAVIES (Eds), *AIDS: Social Representations Social Practices*, Lewes, Falmer Press.

FOX, R., ODAKA N., et al. (1987) 'Effect of HIV Antibody Disclosure on Subsequent Sexual Activity in Homosexual Men', *AIDS*, 1, 241–246.

GREEN, L., KREUTER, M., DEEDS, S. and PARTRIDGE, K. (1980) *Health Education Planning: A Diagnostic Approach*, Palo Alto, Calif., Mayfield.

HENNENKERNS, C., BURING, J. and MAYRENT, S. (Eds) *Epidemiology in Medicine*, Boston, Mass., Little Brown Company.

HERZLICH, C. and PIERRET, J. (1989) 'The Construction of Social Phenomenon: AIDS in the French Press', *Social Science and Medicine*, 29, 1235–1242.

HESSOL, N., LIFSON, A., O'MALLEY, P., DOLL, L., JAFFEE, H. and RUTHERFORD, G. (1989) 'Prevalence, Incidence and Progression of HIV Infection in Homosexual and Bisexual Men in Hepatitis B Vaccine Trials, 1978–1988', *American Journal of Epidemiology*, 130, 1167–1175.

HOCHHAUSER, M. (1987) 'Readability of AIDS Educational Materials', paper presented at the Ninety-fifth Annual Convention of the American Psychological Association.

JENKINS, P. (1990) 'Eight Year Prospective Study HIV Infection/Sexual Behaviour in a Cohort of Homosexual Men', paper presented at the Fourth Conference on Social Aspects of AIDS, South Bank Polytechnic, London.

JOB R.F. (1988) 'Effective and Ineffective Use of Fear in Health Promotion Campaigns', *American Journal of Public Health*, 78, 163–167.

JOHNSON, R., OSTROW, D., et al. (1988) 'Educational Strategies for Prevention of Sexually Transmitted HIV', unpublished manuscript, Ann Arbor, Mich., Institute for Social Research.

JONES, C.C., WATKIN, H., GERETY, B., et al. (1987) 'Persistence of High Risk Sexual Activity among Homosexual Men in an Area of Low Incidence of the AIDS', *Sexually Transmitted Diseases*, 14, 79–82.

JOSEPH, J., MONTGOMERY, S., et al. (1987a) 'Perceived Risk of AIDS: Assessing the Behavioral and Psychological Consequences in a Cohort of Gay Men', *Journal of Social Psychology*, 17, 216–230.

JOSEPH, J., MONTGOMERY, S., et al. (1987b) Magnitude and Determinants of Behavioral Risk Reduction: Longitudinal Analysis of a Cohort at Risk for AIDS', *Psychology and Health*, 1, 73–86.

KELLY, J.A. and ST LAWRENCE, J.S. (1987) 'Risk Factors for Seroconversion to HIV among Male Homosexuals', *Lancet*, 1, 345–349.

McCUSKER, J., ZAPKA, J., STODDARD, A., MAYER, K., AVRUNIN, J. and SALTZMAN, S. (1987) 'Determinants and Effects of HIV Antibody Test Disclosure', paper presented at Third International Conference on AIDS, Washington, D.C.

McCUSKER, J., STODDARD, A., ZAPKA, J., ZORN, M. and MAYER, K. (1989b) 'Predictors of AIDS-preventive Behaviour among Homosexually Active Men: A Longitudinal Study', *AIDS*, 3, 443–448.

McCUSKER, J., ZAPKA, J., STODDARD, A. and MAYER, K. (1989b) 'Responses to the AIDS

Epidemic among Homosexually Active Men: Factors Associated with Preventive Behaviour', *Patient Education and Counseling*, 13, 15–30.

McKusick, L., Horstman, W., *et al.* (1985) 'AIDS and Sexual Behaviour Reported by Gay Men in San Francisco', *American Journal of Public Health*, 75, 493–496.

McKusick, L., Coates, T., Wiley, J., Morin, S. and Stall, R. (1987) 'Prevention of HIV Infection among Gay and Bisexual Men: Two Longitudinal Studies', *Third International Conference on AIDS*, Washington, D.C.

McQuire, W. (1969) 'The Nature of Attitudes and Attitude Change', in G. Lindzey and E. Aronson (Eds), *Handbook of Social Psychology*, Vol. 3, Reading, Mass., Addison-Wesley.

Martin, J.L. (1986) 'AIDS Risk Reduction Recommendations and Sexual Behaviour Patterns among Gay Men: A Multifactorial Categorical Approach to Assessing Change', *Health Education Quarterly*, 134, 4, 347–358.

Martin, J.L. (1987) 'The Impact of AIDS on Gay Male Sexual Behaviour Patterns in New York', *American Journal of Public Health*, 77, 578–581.

Martin, J.L. (1988) 'Psychological Consequences of AIDS-related Bereavement among Gay Men', *Journal of Consulting and Clinical Psychology*, 56, 6.

Martin, J., Dean, L., Garcia, M. and Hall, W. (1989) 'The Impact of AIDS on a Gay Community: Changes in Sexual Behaviour, Substance Use and Mental Health', *American Journal of Community Psychology*.

Ostrow, D., Joseph, J., *et al.* (1986) 'Psychosocial Aspects of AIDS Risk', *Psychopharmacology Bulletin*, 678–683.

Ostrow, D., Joseph, J., *et al.* (1987) 'Disclosure of HIV Antibody Status: Behavioural and Mental Correlates', manuscript submitted to *AIDS Education Prevention*.

Pollak, M. (1989) 'AIDS Prevention Activities and Their Impact on Attitudes and Behaviour: The Case of French Homo and Bisexuals', report prepared for WHO/GPA, Geneva.

Puckett, S. (1985) 'Self-reported Behavioral Changes among Homosexuals and Bisexual Men — San Francisco', *Morbidity and Mortality Weekly Reports*, 34, 40.

Rosenstock, I., Strecher, V. and Becker, M. (1988) 'Social Learning Theory and the Health Belief Model', *Health Education Quarterly*, 15, 2, 175–183.

Ross, M. and Rosser, B. (1989) 'Education and AIDS Risk: A Review', *Health Education Research*, 4, 273–284.

Rotter, J. (1966) 'Generalized Expectancies for Internal vs. External Control of Reinforcements', *Psychological Monographs*, 80.

Schechter, M., Crabib, K., *et al.* (1988) 'Patterns of Sexual Behaviour and Condom Use in a Cohort of Homosexual Men', *American Journal of Public Health*, 78, 1535–1538.

Siegal, K., Grodsky, P. and Herman, A. (1986) 'AIDS Risk-reduction Guidelines: A Review and Analysis', *Journal of Community Health*, 11, 4, 233–243.

Siegal, K., Bauman, L., Christ, G. and Krown, S. (1988) 'Patterns of Change in Sexual Behaviour among Gay Men in New York City', *Archives of Sexual Behaviour*, 17, 481–496.

Stall, R. (1988) 'The Prevention of HIV Infection Associated with Drug and Alcohol Use during Sexual Activity', unpublished manuscript, San Francisco.

Stall, R. and Wiley, J. (1989) 'A Comparison of Alcohol and Drug Use Patterns of Homosexual and Heterosexual Men: The San Francisco Men's Health Study', *Drug and Alcohol Dependence*, 22, 63–73.

Stall, R., McKusick, L., Wiley, J., Coates, T. and Ostrow, D. (1986) 'Alcohol and Drug Use during Sexual Activity and Compliance with Safe Sex Guidelines for AIDS: The AIDS Behavioral Research Project', *Health Education Quarterly*, 13, 359–371.

Stall, R., Coates, T. and Colleen, H. (1988a) 'Behavioral Risk Reduction for HIV Infection among Gay and Bisexual Men', *Journal of the American Psychological Association*, 43.

STALL, R., BYE, L., CAPELL, F., CATANIA, J., COATES, T., *et al.* (1988b) 'Changes in Sexual Risk for HIV Infection among Gay Men in San Francisco from 1984–87: The Communication Technology and AIDS Behavioral Research Project Cohorts', unpublished manuscript, San Francisco.

STAUB, R. (1988) *Homosexulle und AIDS der Versuch Einter Bewasltigung*, Zurich, Swiss AIDS Foundation.

VALDISERRI, R. and LYTER, D. (1988) 'Variables Influencing Condom Use in a Cohort of Gay and Bisexual Men', *American Journal of Public Health*, 78, 801–805.

VALDISERRI, R. and LYTER, D. (1989) 'AIDS Prevention in Homosexual and Bisexual Men: Results of a Randomized Trial Evaluating Two Risk Reduction Interventions', *AIDS*, 3, 21–26.

VAN GRIENSVEN, G.J.P., TIELMAN, R., GOUDSMIT, J., *et al.* (1987) 'Risk Factors and Prevalence of HIV Antibodies in Homosexual Men in the Netherlands', *American Journal of Epidemiology*, 125, 1048–157.

VAN GRIENSVEN, G.J.P., DE VROOME, E., TIELMAN, R., GOUDSMIT, J., VAN DER NOORDAA, J. DE WOLF, F. and COUTINHO, R. (1988) 'Impact of HIV Antibody Testing on Changes in Sexual behaviour among Homosexual Men in the Netherlands', *American Journal of Public Health*, 78, 1575–1577.

VAN GRIENSVEN, G.J.P., VROMME, E., GOUDSMIT, J., *et al.* (1989a) 'Changes in Sexual Behaviour Corresponding with Strong Decline in HIV Incidence among Homosexual Men', *British Medical Journal*, 289, 218–221.

VAN GRIENSVEN, G.J.P., VROMME, R., TIELMAN, R., *et al.* (1989b) 'Effects of HIV Antibody Knowledge of High Risk Sexual Behaviour with Steady and Nonsteady Sexual Partners among Homosexual Men', *American Journal of Epidemiology*, 129, 596–603.

VAN GRIENSVEN, G.J.P., VAN DEN HOEK, J. LEENTVAAR and COUTINHO, R. (1989c) 'Surrogate Markers for HIV Incidence among Homosexual Men', *Journal of Infectious Diseases*, 159, 6, 1157–58.

WINKELSTEIN, W., GRANT, R., WILEY, J., *et al.* (1986) 'Reduction of HIV Virus Transmission in San Francisco 1982–1985', *The 2nd International Conference on AIDS*, Paris.

WINKELSTEIN, W., SAMUEL, M., *et al.* (1987a) 'The San Francisco Men's Health Study: Reduction in HIV Transmission among Homosexual/Bisexual Men, 1982–86', *American Journal of Public Health*, 77, 685–689.

WINKELSTEIN, W., LYMAN, D., *et al.* (1987b) 'Sexual Practices and Risk of Infection by the HIV', *Journal of the American Medical Association*, 257, 321–325.

Chapter 3

What Is a Sexual Encounter?

Andrew Hunt and Peter Davies

Some ten years into the HIV/AIDS epidemic, a prominent member of the AIDS 'industry' can write: 'there is evidence that amongst some groups of homosexuals there are high rates of partner change... This high rate of partner change has presumably contributed to the rapid rate of infection amongst homosexual men...' (Johnson, 1988: 151). It would seem that the message that HIV has a different probability of transmission for different sexual acts and the corollary that it is not the number of partners but the range of practices that needs to be modified has yet to percolate even to parts of the 'expert' community, let alone the lay audience for health education material. Implicit in this statement, however, is an even more depressing perception: that a sexual partner is a sexual partner is a sexual partner. The perception is depressing because hopes for a set of sex-positive responses to AIDS depend on a willingness radically to deconstruct, and subsequently reconstruct, our sexual experiences and to explore new manifestations of desire in response to the challenges that HIV presents.

The notion of a sexual encounter is central to the study of sexual behaviour in general and to the epidemiology of a sexually transmitted virus in particular. The question, 'How many sexual partners have you had?' is asked explicitly or implicitly in all studies of sexual behaviour. A moment's thought should, however, suffice to convince that the question, 'who is a partner?' begs the question, 'what counts as sex?' However, the meaning of 'sexual partner' is usually taken for granted and very few of these studies define what is meant (see Coxon, 1988; Wellings, 1989). Occasionally, euphemisms such as 'to sleep with' are substituted for the word 'sex' without destroying, it is assumed, the robustness of the category. Implicit in this assumption is the idea that sexual behaviour is a well defined and unanimously agreed cognitive category associated with an unambiguous and logically watertight language. There is a further implication, more deeply embedded in the assumption, that there is only one way of having sex, namely vaginal (or anal) penetration.

The separation between the notion of 'partner' and consideration of sexual practices pervades sex research. Kinsey *et al.* in their volume on men (1948) famously concentrated on orgasm as the marker of sexual behaviour and classify that by 'outlet', a formulation which confounds sexual activity (for example, masturbation), partner choice (homosexual, bestial) and social formation (prostitution). Even in the studies of gay men undertaken in the 1970s questions about partners and about sexual repertoire are kept distinct. For example, Bell and Weinberg (1978:85) present their findings on the reported numbers of sexual partners without a discussion of the meaning of the term; subsequently (1978:106ff) they present information about what they refer to clinically as 'sexual techniques'. While these studies, by looking at sexual behaviours, do not assume that sex implies penetration, they nevertheless presume a universal understanding of the term 'partner'.

This logical separation of the partner from the sexual activities carries forward into the studies undertaken to assess the impact of AIDS on sexual behaviour and predict the future spread of the virus. One of Project SIGMA's earliest contributions to the debates about AIDS in Britain was to comment on the problem of reconciling the relatively slow spread of HIV through homosexual contact with the large numbers of sexual partners reported in studies of gay men carried out before AIDS (Coxon, 1985:18–20).[1] For example, Bell and Weinberg (1978:312) report that over half their white male sample had more than twenty-five sexual partners in the year before interview. Such numbers would generate a rate of spread far faster than that which was recorded even in the early days of the epidemic, before the massive changes in their sexual behaviour made by gay men in the mid-1980s (see, for example, McManus and McEvoy, 1987).

The recognition that individual sexual activities are differentially implicated in the spread of HIV means that any epidemiology of the virus must start with these sexual acts as its logical primitives. Much of the confusion, including the pervasive and highly consequential notion of 'risk groups', arises from the failure to recognize this simple fact. Attempts to equate the physical processes of viral transmission with social identities or labels have had pernicious consequences commented on at length in this volume, earlier volumes in the series and elsewhere (see especially Crimp, 1989). Taking the notion that sexual acts are the prime focus of interest has a number of important consequences in the prosecution of research.

Sexual acts do not, by and large, appear randomly across time and space: they are socially defined, constrained and controlled. The first level of aggregation of sexual acts is into the encounter or session, which we define as a (non-empty) sequence of sexual acts which occurs within a space of time in the same situation. The notion of 'partner' can only be defined in terms of these entities (acts and sessions) as someone who participates in a session with another person, although a session may only involve one person, so not every session has an associated partner.

This recognition that the notion of partner is at least a second-order concept (and arguably third order) also leaves the way open to aggregate sessions by other criteria, for example, the context of the session (see Davies and Weatherburn,

Ch. 8, this volume). However, it does not exhaust the problems associated with talking about sex, since it begs the question, 'what is sex?'

Broadly, there are three classes of answer to this question. The first is to ignore it, to assume that the imprecision of the language is a trivial problem which will be swept up in the sampling process. This approach assumes that any differences in meaning will be minor and will accumulate in the error that remains when the statistical model of choice has been fitted. The second approach is to impose on the terms a set of strictly defined meanings proceeding from the deliberations of researchers or emerging from a pilot study. This has the advantage, at least in principle, of providing a common currency for discussion. The third approach is to investigate in depth the meanings which the various terms have in use by ordinary people and to use these as the basis of subsequent talk and investigation. It is an investigation of this last type which is reported in this chapter.

A number of particular problems remain. First, we are, as a culture, still extremely reticent about sex, and the available vocabularies contain little or nothing between the 'coarse and vulgar' vernacular and the obscure Latinate vocabulary of Ellis and Kraft-Ebing. Second, and much more importantly, the notion of a sexual act is itself far from uniform. Clearly, there are some acts whose occurrence will always be deemed sexual. There are others whose 'sexual' nature is entirely dependent on context: they are sexual because they occur in a sexual context. Third, the list of sexual acts, though presumably in principle finite, is at least very large, the only bounds being those dictated by a failure of the imagination or lack of suppleness.

Despite all these problems, we do — some of us at great length — manage to talk about sex. It seemed reasonable to investigate what it was we were talking about when we talked about sex. So we decided to ask the men whom we were interviewing what they thought they — and we — meant when we talked about sex.

Methods

Project SIGMA is a longitudinal study of a non-clinic-based cohort of homosexually active men. A total of 930 men were recruited, by a variety of means including response to a postal questionnaire in the gay press, recruitment in gay pubs, clubs and social and political organizations, and contacts of the above (see Davies *et al.*, 1990). These respondents came from ten main sites across England and Wales: London, Cardiff, Newcastle, Teesside, Portsmouth, Leeds, Norwich, Birmingham, Liverpool, Bristol. No respondents were recruited from clinic-based environments; thus, in terms of social and sexual activity they represent a wide cross section of the male homosexually active community.

All respondents were interviewed about their sexual behaviour and history, social attitudes and behaviour, health, knowledge of and attitudes towards AIDS/ HIV. Respondents were asked, but not required, to provide blood and/or saliva for testing for HIV. Refusal to provide blood did not exclude respondents from the study.

The median age of the cohort is 29 years and 50 per cent of the cohort are aged between 23 and 38 years; 26 per cent report having one regular sexual partner, 32 per cent have one regular partner and others (either regular or casual) and the remaining 42 per cent have no regular sexual partner. In general, the men are gay-identified and happy with this identity and are from a white, well educated background (for a more detailed discussion, see Davies *et al.*, 1990).

Each respondent was asked the following question:

> Suppose someone asked you 'How many sexual partners have you had this month?', what must have happened sexually for someone to 'count' as your sexual partner?

Most initial reactions to this question were of surprise that it needed to be asked at all; most of the respondents thought it obvious. However, everyone did offer an answer which was recorded verbatim by the interviewer. There seems to be no interviewer effect in the responses, though there is a possibility that the way the answer was given may have been affected by interaction between the interviewer and respondent.

Two judges, working independently, sorted the responses into an unspecified number of categories, which they then labelled. It was agreed that responses could be 'double counted', that is deemed to fall into more than one category. When the results of this sorting exercise were compared, there was minimal disagreement between the judges on the nature and labels of the emergent categories. The only major difference was that one judge conflated two categories distinguished by the other. The content of the categories — which responses fell into which groups — was also marked by a high (and surprising) degree of unanimity. The gross disagreement between the judges on the allocations, measured by the normalized pairbonds statistic (Arabie, 1972) is .075, indicating that 7.5 per cent of the responses would have to be reallocated from one sorting to render it identical to the other.

Findings

Broadly speaking, the responses fall into one of two groups: either physical (that is, pertaining to some form of actual physical contact) or affective (that is, descriptions which are highly contextual or which refer to emotional states) in a ratio of about three to one. There are no differences by age ($t = 0.098$, $p = 0.46$) or relationship type ($X^2 = 2.574$, df $= 2$, $p = 0.28$). The results are summarized in Table 3.1.

Table 3.1 Counts of Categories Noted by Respondents When Asked to Define a Sexual Partner

Category	Number	Percentage[1]
Genital contact	449	48.2
of which:		
penetration[2]	57	6.1
anal sex	49	5.3
Orgasm	241	25.9
Bed/naked/sleep with	208	22.3
Physical contact	69	7.4
Eroticism/arousal	25	2.7
Aim for orgasm	15	1.6
Must see more than once	14	1.5
Privacy	4	0.5

Notes: 1 Some people mentioned more than one category so percentages total more than 100.
2 Penetration includes both oral and anal sex.

Some responses fit into more than one category so that a response which reads, 'We have to go to bed and I have to ejaculate' is counted in both the categories 'go to bed with' and 'orgasm'. The counts are reported as percentages of the number of respondents and the total adds to more than 100.

Nearly half the respondents mentioned some genital contact, specified either generally (for example, as 'genital contact') or in relation to a specific act (for example, wanking or sucking). Of these, fifty-seven (6 per cent) specified that the contact had to include penetration of some sort, and of these forty-nine (5 per cent) specified anal intercourse (either as the insertor or the insertee). For the large majority of respondents, therefore, penetration need not occur for sex to happen.

While many respondents simply stated that some sort of genital contact is required for sex, others mentioned specific acts. About 10 per cent of responses defined or implied a hierarchy of acts: 'From groping, up to sucking or fucking', 'Anything beyond kissing', 'Masturbation or fucking or sucking', and 'Close petting and up the scale.' The order implicit in these responses is relatively precise and reflects a view of sex as a staged process: kissing, then groping, then wanking, then sucking, culminating in anal intercourse. However, it is far from clear at what point 'sex' is deemed to have begun.

For a few, anal intercourse is the most important marker: 'Fucking is the basic criteria', 'Someone you have sex with, real sex, fucking', and 'It has to be full sex, fucking.' These responses are examples of the view that 'real' and 'full' sex are the same thing as anal (or vaginal) intercourse and anything short of these is not to be considered 'proper' sex. In contrast, some responses were much less precisely defined: 'Kissing. Broad parameters. There must be a flavour of eroticism.' Here genital contact is not specified, but the encounter must be erotic, which begs the further question of what is considered erotic.

For some people, 'A good cuddle can be sexual with someone mutually attractive', 'Orgasm is not essential.' Nothing overtly sexual is mentioned here, but the context of the 'cuddle' is important. Orgasm is explicitly referred to as inconsequential. On the other hand, an actual orgasm for one or both partners (but usually the respondent) was mentioned by about a quarter of the respondents as being essential for an encounter to be counted as sex: 'Orgasm inside them', or 'One or both of us to reach orgasm.' For others, the intention of orgasm was all that was required: 'Physical interaction with aim of at least one orgasm', or 'An attempt at orgasm with a partner.'

Some form of physical contact not otherwise specified was mentioned by 7.4 per cent (sixty-nine) of respondents. In common with almost all of the responses, this excludes sex over the telephone (an increasingly popular safer sex alternative) and any mutual self-masturbation which takes place. However, a few of the responses spoke of a situation which is erotic or by which the respondent is aroused (twenty-five, 2.7 per cent), and in these cases no actual contact was implied: 'I must have reached orgasm in some privacy (e.g. not cottaging) — there must be body contact.' In this response an orgasm is essential, but the respondent explicitly notes that sex must happen in private, and as an example excludes sex in toilets. It illustrates, however, the importance of the setting of the encounter to many of the respondents. Other categories mentioned were sleeping with someone, being naked or unclothed with someone and going to bed with someone (208, 22.3 per cent). This may be seen simply as reflecting a popular euphemism for sexual intercourse, but it may indicate that the respondent distinguishes 'partners' from, say, 'contacts'. In other words that term may exclude casual sexual encounters.

In the following examples going to bed or sleeping with someone is essential: 'Either going to bed and indulging in some intimacy or partial or full removal of clothing somewhere else. Orgasm is not important', 'Sleeping with someone, more than just a quick thrill.' Other contexts may also be important: 'Someone I see regularly and have a mutually satisfying relationship with', 'There must be clear signs of mutual sexual interest, almost always kissing and some cock play with a view to orgasm, usually involving bondage.' In this last response it appears that bondage must usually be involved for a sexual encounter, and both parties must show some sexual interest in one another. By way of contrast the next person always demands some sado-masochistic (SM) context to the sex, and that need not include genital contact: 'Bondage and other SM activities even without genital contact.' Here sex may not even be directed towards an ultimate orgasm.

Some responses are difficult to categorize: 'That involves someone putting his hands down my trousers', and even, it must be admitted, rather bizarre, 'Must go to the cinema.'

Implications and Conclusions

It is clear from these data, therefore, that the notion of a sexual partner and the logically anterior notion of sex are far from specific in their reference and far from unanimously understood. It seems that there are, broadly speaking, two referents for the term 'sexual partner'. The first is someone with whom sex occurs in the context of love or affection — not exactly a lover, which carries further overtones of commitment, but someone with whom sex carries an emotional charge. The second notion subsumes the first in that it refers merely to someone with whom sexual behaviour takes place. What is immediately pertinent is that there is no agreement on where the boundary between the sexual and the non-sexual falls. Many men volunteered the notion of a hierarchy of sexual acts — broadly manual, oral, anal or some subset of such — but there was no agreement on the point in this hierarchy at which sex — or 'real sex' — begins.

This should remind us of two general features of language: its fuzziness and its ambiguity. Language is fuzzy in the sense that its relationship to the world of experience is not well described using Aristotelian logic. Axiomatic in such a system, which underpins most of our science and mathematics, is the notion that we can distinguish absolutely between those things which 'count' as, say a chair, and those which do not. This 'law of the excluded middle' requires that we do not allow things which are 'neither one thing nor another'. Yet even on such a mundane level, such certainty is difficult. Is a chaise longue a chair or a settee? In the case of something as diverse as human behaviour the problems, as we have seen, multiply. The concept of fuzziness, implicit in Wittgenstein's (1973) family resemblance theory of meaning and mathematically expounded by Zadeh (1975), goes some way towards superseding the law of the excluded middle. Rather than regarding the process of classification as attaching to an object an absolute probability of inclusion (1) or exclusion (0), fuzzy set theory attaches a probability which indicates the likelihood of that object belonging to that class. The higher this 'inclusion probability', the greater the likelihood.

This logic is a better description of the way that human beings operate in their everyday world than the Aristotelian model (Kaufmann, 1975, but see also Rich, 1983:173–99), partly at least because it recognizes ambiguity as a fundamental feature of language. The particular subset of language with which we are concerned, that relating to the sexual, is particularly ambiguous. On the most simple level the meanings of the term 'partner' in the sentences, 'I'd like you to meet my partner' and 'How many partners have you had?' are quite different. At a more rarefied level Douglas (1960) has argued persuasively that the ambiguity of experience generates many of the discourses of danger, purity and wholeness which swirl about notions of sexuality.

At the level at which we are concerned, that is, with the practical problems of talking about sex, it is important that it is not possible to prefer a priori one of the options discussed at the beginning of this chapter: allowing the respondent to choose his own definitions; imposing a standard definition; or working towards a common definition, through the use of focused groups, interviews, etc. For the effect of these strategies is not to eliminate ambiguities; it is to transfer them to one or other part of the system (Heisenberg, 1930:3–6; Schrodinger, 1935:71–2). The decision among these strategies, as the decision among any strategies for coping with ambiguity, is inherently and inevitably indexical. It will depend on the context of the discussion and the purpose of the dialogue. Thus the survey researcher may decide that comparability of responses indicates that s/he impose a definition on the respondent. Such a position is defensible. It would not, however, be an appropriate strategy for a group discussion on techniques of safer sex.

In the SIGMA study we provide a definition of a sexual partner to respondents which forms the basis for questions about sexual behaviour: 'A sexual partner is any person with whom you had sexual contact, where the aim was orgasm for one or both of you.' It is probably impossible to provide a single intensive definition of a partner which is both clear and universally acceptable, and there are some problems with this definition. It was chosen as being relatively clear, consonant with a majority of self-definitions and comparable with other, ongoing research in this area. But what, for example, constitutes 'sexual contact'? When challenged on this, the interviewer was counselled to gloss this as 'physical, genital' contact. The overriding aim is to include any person with whom some physical contact has happened and with whom the respondent or the other person intended (even if this did not happen) to have an orgasm. This excludes sex over the telephone and voyeuristic sex, as well as sex which is not necessarily directed towards orgasm (such as in some SM sessions), as well as encouraging the respondent to speculate on the intentions of his partner, which, as generations of social science students know, is a process fraught with difficulty (see Searle, 1982). Thus some activities which some of our respondents may recognize as sex do not fit into our definition.

To distinguish between a sex partner and partners where penetration occurs, the project also asks about numbers of penetrative sexual partners (psp). A penetrative sexual partner is defined as: 'a sexual partner whom you fucked (either anally or vaginally) or were fucked by.' This definition explicitly excludes penetration of the mouth and implicitly excludes penetration of the anus or vagina by anything other than a penis.

The notion of a penetrative sexual partner (psp) is an extremely important and powerful one in understanding sexual behaviour in general and the epidemiology of HIV in particular. To illustrate its efficacy, consider the following. In a typical enquiry a man may be asked two questions: first, how many (male) sexual partners he has had, say in a year; second, how often he has engaged in anal intercourse. Further, let us assume he is asked these questions on two occasions a year apart. On the first occasion he states that he has had twenty partners and anal intercourse 'often'; on the second occasion he states that he has had ten partners and anal intercourse 'rarely'. Without the intervening notion of the number of psps, these responses can, without impugning the veracity of the respondent, refer to (at least) three states of affairs which are completely different from the point of view of assessing the degree of behaviour change that has occurred and predicting the effect of this change on the spread of HIV.

	Year 1	Year 2
Scenario 1	15 casual psps	2 casual psps
Scenario 2	1 regular psp	1 regular psp
Scenario 3	1 regular psp	3 casual psp

In the first scenario the man has reduced the number of his risk encounters. In the second he has lost a regular partner with whom he frequently had anal intercourse, but has had anal intercourse with one casual partner. His degree of risk will depend partly on his regular partner's behaviour. In the third scenario the man has increased his risk behaviour, even though he may have 'often' had anal intercourse in year 1 with his (one) regular partner. If one asks about psps directly, comparisons between different time periods are facilitated, and a clearer picture emerges of actual risk behaviours. Furthermore, comparisons can be more readily made with other studies, especially those of heterosexual behaviour. The numbers of partners heterosexuals have and homosexual men have are often referred to as though they indicate a similar set of acts. Studies of heterosexual behaviour do not distinguish between partners and psps. In our own work on the heterosexual behaviour of the (predominantly) gay cohort the majority (90 per cent) of female partners have been psps. The prospect of a large increase in the numbers with 'heterosexually' transmitted HIV in the next few years is thus supported by a study by Forman and Chilvers (1989) of heterosexual men in which a median lifetime number of female partners of five is reported. The figure of male lifetime partners of men in the SIGMA study is thirty-eight, yet the more equivalent comparison is probably of psps: for the SIGMA cohort the lifetime psp figure was just seven. Since the figures for risk encounters are very similar, it might be expected that the spread of HIV among heterosexuals in the next few years will mirror closely the spread among the gay community in the early years, unless there is major behavioural change.

Note

1 Project SIGMA is the *So*cio-sexual *I*nvestigations of *G*ay *M*en and *A*IDS, funded by the Medical Research Council and the Department of Health, with principal investigators Tony Coxon, Peter Davies and Tom McManus, and based at the South Bank Polytechnic, London.

References

ARABIE, P.A. (1972) 'Measures of Association for Partitions', in R.N. SHEPARD, S.B. NERLOVE and A.K. ROMNEY (Eds), *Multi-Dimensional Scaling: Theory and Applications in the Behavioural Sciences*, New York, Seminar.

BELL, A.P. and WEINBERG, M.S. (1978) *Homosexualities: A Study of Diversity in Men and Women*, New York, Summit Books.

COXON, A.P.M (1985) *The Gay Lifestyle and the Impact of AIDS*, Project SIGMA Working Paper No. 1.

COXON, A.P.M. (1988) 'The Numbers Game — Gay Lifestyles, Epidemiology of AIDS and Social Science', in P. AGGLETON and H. HOMANS (Eds), *Social Aspects of AIDS*, Lewes, Falmer Press.

CRIMP, D. (1989) (Ed.) *AIDS: Cultural Analysis, Cultural Activism*, Cambridge, Mass., MIT Press.

DAVIES, P.M., HUNT, A.J., MACOURT, M. and WEATHERBURN, P. (1990) *Longitudinal Study of the Sexual Behaviour of Homosexual Males under the Impact of AIDS: A Final Report to the Department of Health*, Project SIGMA.

DOUGLAS, M. (1960) *Purity and Danger*, Harmondsworth, Penguin Books.

FORMAN, D. and CHILVERS, C. (1989) 'Sexual Behaviour of Young and Middle Aged Men in England and Wales', *British Medical Journal*, 298, 1137–1142.

HEISENBERG, W. (1930) *The Physical Principles of the Quantum Theory*, Chicage, Ill., Cambridge University Press.

JOHNSON, A. (1988) 'Social and Behavioural Aspects of the HIV Epidemic — A Review', *Journal of the Royal Statistical Society*, A, 151.

KAUFMANN, A. (1975) *Introduction to the Theory of Fuzzy Subsets,* vol. 1, New York, Academic.

KINSEY, A.C., POMEROY, W.B. and MARTIN, M.S. (1948) *Sexual Behaviour in the Human Male*, London, Saunders.

MCMANUS, T.J. and MCEVOY, M. (1987) 'Some Aspects of male Homosexual Behaviour in the UK', *British Journal of Sexual Medicine*, 29, 110–120.

RICH, E. (1988) *Artificial Intelligence*, New York, McGraw-Hill.

SCHRODINGER, E. (1935) *Science and The Human Temperament*, New York,

SEARLE, J. (1982) *Intentionality: An Essay in the Philosophy of Mind*, Chicago, Ill., Cambridge University Press.

WELLINGS, K. (1989) 'Talking about Sex', paper presented at the Third Social Aspects of AIDS Conference, South Bank Polytechnic, London.

WITTGENSTEIN, L. (1973) *Philosophical Investigations*, Oxford, Blackwell.

ZADEH, L., FU, K., TANAHA, K. and SHIMURA, M. (Eds) (1975) *Fuzzy Sets and their Application to Cognitive and Decision Processes*, New York, Academic Press.

Chapter 4

Gay Men's Views and Experiences of the HIV Test

Jill Dawson, Ray Fitzpatrick, John McLean, Graham Hart and Mary Boulton

Since the test for antibody to human immunodeficiency virus (HIV) first became available in 1985, various controversies have arisen. While its use in screening blood supplies has been relatively unproblematic, other possible functions of the HIV test have caused concern. Early tests gave less accurate results and led to anxieties about the consequences of both false positive and false negative results (Mortimer, 1988). Technical problems of sensitivity and specificity, combined with growing concerns about loss of confidentiality and potential discrimination of individuals tested positive, have necessitated more deliberate appraisal of the purposes of the HIV test (Weiss and Thier, 1988).

Two functions have received particular attention. First, the HIV test has been considered an important means of facilitating behavioural change (Francis and Chin, 1987). The evidence for such effects is extremely difficult to interpret and appears to indicate at best modest effects upon behaviour of HIV testing with counselling (Cates and Handsfield, 1988). The second purpose of the HIV test is to monitor rates of change in HIV infection in total populations. Many of the data in Britain have come from those who voluntarily seek the HIV test, and it has always been difficult to determine how representative these samples are (Hull *et al.*, 1988; PHLS Working Group, 1989). Some early anonymous screening studies were conducted in genito-urinary medicine clinics (Carne *et al.*, 1987). A more extensive programme of unlinked anonymous testing, designed to provide more accurate estimates of the HIV epidemic, has been announced recently and has generated intense ethical and legal debate (Gill *et al.*, 1989).

One subject, with some notable exceptions (Welch *et al.*, 1986; Siegel, 1989), has been neglected in much of the research concerning the HIV test: that is, individuals' motives and decisions surrounding seeking or not seeking the test. One social group in particular — gay men — viewed the HIV test with grave suspicion as a potential source of homophobic discrimination or repression (Shilts, 1987). Early publicity in the gay press stressed the many potential costs to individuals of taking the HIV test (Siegel, 1989). Little is known of the impact of such debates upon gay men's views and actions about the test. One study in Pittsburgh (Lyter *et al.*, 1987) indicated that concerns about confidentiality and about psychological consequences of testing were important reasons for gay men not to want to be informed about the results of an HIV test. All of the men in this sample were participants in an AIDS cohort study, and it is difficult to draw inferences from such special circumstances of medical supervision to the views about, and patterns of use of, the test of gay men (Fitzpatrick *et al.*, 1989a).

This chapter considers the views and experiences of a sample of gay men in relation to the HIV test. Unlike studies such as the Pittsburgh cohort study, the HIV test was not part of the research protocol for recruiting and interviewing. Another limitation of much of the evidence to date is that views of men have been elicited at the time of attending for medical care (Welch *et al.*, 1986). Not only does this represent a potentially stressful moment at which views may be systematically distorted. It also means that the views of men not currently attending a clinic are not obtained. We hope to reflect the attitudes prevalent among gay men more generally during the period 1988–89, when the sample of men was interviewed.

Methods and Sample

The criterion for inclusion in this study was any man who had had sex with another man within the last five years. A sample of 502 men was recruited from a diverse range of sources: 283 (56 per cent) from gay pubs, clubs and gay organizations; 96 (19 per cent) by referrals from those already interviewed ('snowballing') and 123 (25 per cent) from departments of genito-urinary medicine. Four main towns and cities were used: London 228 (45 per cent), Manchester 145 (29 per cent), Oxford 65 (13 per cent) and Northampton 31 (6 per cent). A further 33 (7 per cent) of the sample were recruited from areas around these four centres. Three interviewers recruited and interviewed the sample.

Interviews focused on sexual behaviour in the previous month and previous year (Fitzpatrick *et al.*, 1990). A section of the interview focused on the HIV antibody test. This included more detailed questions for respondents who had been tested regarding circumstances of the test(s), and counselling. All respondents were asked a series of attitudinal questions about the test, presented in the Likert rating scale format. The tests of significance used were Chi Square test and Mann-Whitney.

The mean age of the sample was 31.6 (s.d. 10.4) with a range from 16 to 67. Eleven per cent of men were married, separated, divorced or widowed. Fifty-one men (10 per cent) described their sexual orientation as bisexual, 43 (9 per cent) as

Table 4.1   Attitudes to the HIV Antibody Test

Attitude	Strongly Agree/ Agree	Uncertain (percentages in brackets)	Strongly Disagree/Disagree
A positive test result reduces your chances of getting good medical and dental care.	246 (43)	11 (22)	144 (29)
There is nothing to be gained by knowing the results of the test.	108 (21)	41 (8)	353 (70)
I prefer/would have preferred not to know the results of the test.	91 (18)	30 (6)	381 (76)
I do not believe that records of the test result can be kept entirely confidential.	278 (55)	97 (19)	127 (25)
I worry that a positive test result would stop me getting life insurance or a mortgage.	370 (74)	44 (9)	87 (17)

homosexual and 392 (78 per cent) as 'gay'. A further 16 (3 per cent) preferred no designation or unique terms not included in the checklist such as 'transexual'. In terms of the Registrar General's classification of occupations, 85 per cent were in social classes I, II and III non-manual.

Results

Men were asked a number of questions about their views and attitudes in relation to the test (Table 4.1). First, questions were asked about discrimination and confidentiality. A majority of men (74 per cent) agreed with the proposition that a positive test result would 'stop an individual getting life insurance or a mortgage'; that records of the test result 'are not entirely confidential' (55 per cent); and that a positive test result 'reduces your chances of getting good medical and dental care' (43 per cent). A second set of questions asked about concerns about the personal consequences for individuals in terms of relationships and lifestyle. Forty-two per cent of men felt that 'a positive test result would ruin my sex life' and 29 per cent that 'I would worry about losing my friends because of a positive test result.'

Third, questions were asked about the value to the individual of information from the test. Far fewer men expressed negative views about the test in this respect. Only a minority of men (21 per cent) felt that 'there is nothing to be gained by knowing the results of the test' or that they would 'prefer not to know the results of the HIV test' (18 per cent). The sample was divided into three groups according to when they were interviewed: before July 1988 ($N = 237$); between 1 July and end of 1988 ($N = 121$); and any time during 1989 ($N = 144$). There were no significant differences in the proportions agreeing with any of the attitudes among the three groups, except that a decreasing proportion of men over the three periods agreed with the proposition that there was nothing to be gained from having the HIV test (23 per cent, 22 per cent, 18 per cent, chi square 22.3, df 8, $p < 0.005$).

Characteristics of men were examined in relation to views about the test. Men who described themselves as gay compared with other men were more likely to agree with the statement about the problem of confidentiality ($Z - 2.28$; $p < 0.005$). Similarly, this statement was more likely to be endorsed by men who described themselves as spending more than half their social lives with other gay men, compared with other men ($Z - 2.25$; $p < 0.05$); and also by men who said that more than half their friends were gay, compared with other men ($Z - 2.70$; $p < 0.01$). Men were more likely to agree with the statement about the implications for medical and dental care who spent more than half their social lives with other gay men ($Z - 2.03$; $p < 0.05$).

Thus men whose identities were gay and whose social world involved other gay men were much more likely to be concerned about discrimination and confidentiality. On the other hand, they were less concerned about some of the potential personal consequences of a possible positive test. Men who described themselves as gay compared with other men were less likely to say they would worry about losing friends because of a positive test result ($Z - 2.14$; $p < 0.05$). Concern about the impact of a positive test result on sex life was less frequently agreed with by gay men ($Z - 3.64$; $p < 0.001$); by men who spent more than half their social lives with other gay men ($Z - 2.50$; $p < 0.05$) and by men who said that more than half their friends were gay ($Z - 2.12$; $p < 0.05$). Finally, with regard to views about the value of the HIV test, younger men (under 25 years old) were more likely to disagree with the proposition that there is nothing to be gained from knowing the results of the test ($Z - 3.26$; $p < 0.005$).

Four hundred and thirty men (86 per cent) had *considered* having the HIV antibody test at some time, while 243 (48 per cent) reported having *had* the test. Two hundred and fifty-four men (51 per cent) had not had the test while five men (1 per cent) were unsure whether they had been tested in the context of other medical investigations. Those who had not been tested were invited to give their main reason for not seeking the test. The most common reasons given were either that the individual was concerned about the effects of the test result upon psychological well-being (101, 43 per cent) or that the individual regarded himself as being at low risk (89, 38 per cent). Fears about financial consequences (12, 5 per cent) or problems of confidentiality were cited by very few men (7, 3 per cent).

The relationship was considered between attitudes to the test (Table 4.1) and whether or not individuals had sought the test. Only two attitudes were related to actual use: men who had sought the test were more likely to disagree with the propositions: 'There is nothing to be gained by knowing the results of the test' (p < 0.005) and 'I prefer (would have preferred) not to know the results of the test' (p < 0.0001). Furthermore, men who had a positive test result were significantly less likely than men tested negative to agree with the view that a positive test result affected the individual's medical and dental care (p < 0.05).

Two hundred and forty-two men (48 per cent) reported being advised not to have the test. Such advice was more likely to have come from a partner or friend (186) rather than a health professional (51). Forty-six per cent of those ever advised against being tested had nevertheless been tested. There was no significant difference between those advised against testing by a health professional and those advised by anyone else in this respect; nor did the proportion receiving 'negative' advice alter significantly over the two years of interviewing.

Differences were examined between those who had and those who had not had the test. There were no significant differences with regard to age, sexual orientation, years of homosexual activity, marital status, or social class. Nor were there any significant differences between individuals recruited from different cities. Less highly educated men were more likely to have had the test (chi square 6.03; df 2, p < 0.05). Men recruited from genito-urinary medicine clinics were more likely than the rest of the sample to have been tested (92, 75 per cent vs 151 40 per cent; p < 0.0001).

One hundred and sixty-nine men (44 per cent) had a close friend, lover or former lover who had been tested HIV antibody positive. They were more likely than other men to have had the test (102, 61 per cent vs 141, 43 per cent; p < 0.005). Eighty-five men (17 per cent) had a close friend, lover or former lover who had died of AIDS. They too were more likely to have had the test than other men (53, 64 per cent vs 190, 46 per cent p < 0.005).

Experiences of the HIV test

In all, the sample had had 608 tests. The maximum number of tests reported by an individual was twenty and the median for those tested was two. We obtained more detailed information about the circumstances of the first test and, where appropriate, their second, penultimate and most recent test. Of the 483 tests for which more detailed information was obtained, 378 (78 per cent) were obtained from departments of genito-urinary medicine, 28 (6 per cent) from general practitioners, 16 (3 per cent) from either private practitioners or private clinics, and

61 (12 per cent) from a variety of other settings such as during in-patient care or in overseas clinics.

One hundred and fifty-five men (31 per cent of the sample as a whole), had received HIV test-related counselling from a health professional at some time, 9 men (2 per cent) had been offered counselling but declined the offer and 50 men (10 per cent) had not been offered counselling where, they felt, it might have been appropriate. Ninety-eight men (63 per cent of the 31 per cent ever counselled) had received counselling from a health adviser based in a genito-urinary (GU) medicine clinic, 47 (30 per cent) from a GU physician, 10 (2 per cent) from their general practitioner, a further 10 men (2 per cent) receiving counselling from another kind of doctor or health professional. Fifty-five men (11 per cent of the whole sample) had received HIV test-related counselling through a voluntary organization.

One hundred and thirty (54 per cent) received counselling at their first test. Respondents whose first test was obtained more recently (within one year of interview) were more likely to have received counselling than those tested earlier (64 per cent vs 49 per cent; $p < 0.05$). For the majority of men the decision to request the test had been their own (426, 85 per cent) or prompted by a current partner (45, 9 per cent). Forty-five men (9 per cent) felt that a general practitioner, or a doctor or health adviser based in a genito-urinary medicine clinic had also influenced them in deciding in favour of having the test.

Men reported the years in which they had their first test. Seventy-one men (29 per cent) were first tested in 1985, 68 (28 per cent) in 1986, 58 (24 per cent) in 1987, 40 (16 per cent) in 1988 and 10 (4 per cent) in 1989. Of those who were tested, at the time of interview 30 (12 per cent) were HIV positive; 201 (83 per cent) were negative and 12 (5 per cent) had not yet heard the result of a recent test.

Discussion

When the HIV antibody test first appeared in 1985, the responses of gay organizations focused upon the potential for the test to be used against gay men. Some arguments were to 'harden into an orthodoxy' (Bayer, 1989). The test could be used to identify, stigmatize and indeed segregate gay men with the virus; the test was technically flawed and would not provide information of benefit to the individual. Although reservations have diminished regarding the accuracy and predictive values of the test, the vital importance of confidentiality and the scope for abuse of information about HIV status, resulting in diminished access to work, life insurance, or to dental and medical care, have remained major concerns of gay organizations.

It is clear from our survey that such concerns remain and are reflected in a majority of men expressing anxieties about the confidentiality of information and risks of diminished access to life insurance and adequate medical and dental services that may arise from the HIV test. Men who identified themselves as gay and whose lives were more closely involved with other gay men were particularly likely to express such concerns. This is clear evidence of a heightened sense of vulnerability to social discrimination. It is significant that nearly half the sample had been advised by someone else, usually a friend or partner, not to take the test. Although enormous changes have occurred in gay sexual behaviour, potentially high risk sexual activities are still frequently reported by gay men (Fitzpatrick *et al.*, 1989b; Johnson and Gill, 1989). It remains essential that access to the HIV test for individuals who decide they need the test should not be impaired by fears of loss of confidentiality.

Only a minority of men expressed the view that the test did not provide the individual with useful information. This may reflect growing acceptance of the evidence of the accuracy of the test. Certainly, significantly fewer men held this view over the three periods covered in the survey. Further possible support for this interpretation is that younger men who may have been less influenced by the earlier evidence of the test's limitations were more likely to disagree with the view that nothing was to be gained from the test.

Despite many major concerns about the consequences of being tested, nearly half the sample had actively sought the test. To some extent this may have reflected the way in which men were recruited into the study. Men recruited through clinics were more likely to have sought the test. Nevertheless, 40 per cent of men recruited elsewhere had also been tested. It is difficult to assess the extent to which it is reasonable to generalize from this sample who volunteered to discuss matters regarding sexuality and HIV infection. Most studies of the acceptability of the HIV test to gay men have taken place in the context of clinics where men have been offered the test at some point in the course of their attendance for medical care. Such studies are largely used for the purposes of sero-prevalence research. It is not clear how much variation from clinic to clinic arises from differences in explaining such purposes or in pre-test counselling. The proportions of gay men accepting the test in these circumstances in the USA have varied from 61 per cent in Pittsburgh (Valdiserri *et al.*, 1988) and 66 per cent in Baltimore, Washington (Fox *et al.*, 1987) to 74 per cent in Boston (McCusker *et al.*, 1988) and 84 per cent in New Mexico (Hull *et al.*, 1988). In England proportions of gay and homosexual men offered the test for similar purposes and accepting it have varied from 70 per cent at one London teaching hospital (Welch *et al.*, 1986) to 92 per cent for a larger multi centred sero-prevalence survey (Collaborative Study Group, 1989). It is of interest that where acceptance rates of other social groups are available for comparison, it appears that either gay men have accepted at the same rate as other groups (Hull *et al.*, 1988) or in the case of the Collaborative Study Group's results (1989) were markedly more ready to have the test than heterosexual men.

However, such studies involve offering the test in the context of medical care and to individuals already motivated to seek some kind of medical attention. It is less clear how widespread is the use of the test by gay men generally. One community-based study of gay men early in the San Francisco AIDS epidemic found that only 27 per cent had been tested (Research and Decisions Corporation, 1986). A more recent survey found that by the end of 1986 41 per cent of a sample of San Francisco gay men had been tested (Coates *et al.*, 1987). A survey of gay men in Sydney carried out in late 1986 and early 1987 found that 67 per cent of men had been tested (Connell *et al.*, 1989), and consecutive studies of gay men in the Federal Republic of Germany for 1987 and 1988 found 52 per cent and 57 per cent respectively had been tested (Bochow, forthcoming). Overall the rate of men who have sought the test among those recruited other than through a clinic (40 per cent) is remarkably similar to that obtained by Project SIGMA's London and Wales community survey (41 per cent) (Coxon *et al.*, 1989). In the light of these results our figures are not so high, and cumulatively the different studies indicate widespread readiness for gay men to have the test, when it is felt necessary.

Concerns about confidentiality, about possible financial consequences and about loss of access to satisfactory medical and dental care did not appear to act as a deterrent to having the test. Such concerns were statistically unrelated to whether or not individuals sought the test and were not very often cited as the reasons why individuals had not sought the test. In the Pittsburgh study of gay men (Lyter *et al.*, 1987) only 1 per cent of those not wishing to know their HIV status cited concern about confidentiality as the main reason. As with other studies (Lyter *et al.*, 1987; Siegel, 1989), the main reason cited for not having the test was fear of the psychological consequences of knowing a positive result. Such results are also consistent with the evidence that greater perceived severity of AIDS as a disease is also associated with not seeking to find out one's test status (McCusker *et al.*, 1988). The other main reason individuals cited for not having the test was that they perceived themselves as being at low risk and that a test was therefore unnecessary. It is also important to note that men who identified themselves as gay were *less* concerned than other homosexually active men about one possible consequence of a positive test, namely loss of friends. Gay men in this sample enjoyed access to a wide social network of supportive social relationships (Hart *et al.*, 1990). It may be that the social costs, or at least *fear* of costs, surrounding the HIV test fall more severely on homosexually active men not involved in gay social relationships. However, much less is known about the experience of this group.

While fear of the consequences may inhibit men from seeking the test, having a close friend, lover or former lover who was HIV antibody positive or who had died of AIDS was associated with a greater likelihood of having the test. Similarly, McCusker *et al.* (1988) found that men with a lover with AIDS were more likely to seek their HIV status. As Siegel and colleagues observed among many of the men who had sought the test in their study of gay men: 'For many men, learning that past partners or close friends tested positive or were diagnosed with AIDS heightened their own sense of vulnerability and finally raised their anxiety to an intolerable level' (Siegel, 1989:375).

This study provides further evidence for the finding of Fox *et al.* (1987) that, among gay men, less well educated individuals are more likely to have had the HIV test. It is not clear why this should be the case. Generally, research studies of gay men tend to be biased towards recruitment of more highly educated men and effects of basic socio-economic variables remain poorly examined (Fitzpatrick *et al.*, 1989a; Ostrow, 1989).

The majority of tests and nearly all the HIV test-related counselling had been obtained from genito-urinary medicine (GUM) clinics. Many of these clinics, particularly in London, have long had a favourable reputation for non-judgmental care of sexually transmitted diseases. Some of the London clinics were long trusted by gay men prior to the HIV infecton. A possibly reassuring finding of this study was that men who were HIV positive were significantly less likely to feel a positive test result diminished access to good quality care.

Gay men with HIV regard the security and confidentiality of records at GUM clinics as much greater than, for example, would be the case if held by their general practitioner (GP), (King, 1988). This may be one key factor explaining the relative unimportance of issues of confidentiality in the decision whether to have the test. Alternatively, gay men may be less comfortable discussing sexual behaviour and HIV-related matters with their GP. One indication that this is the case is that only 46 per cent of men had revealed their sexuality to their GP. A very similar proportion — 39 per cent — of gay men with HIV infection had revealed their sexual orientation to their GP prior to becoming infected (King, 1988). On the GP's side, some surveys have also indicated a lack of confidence in counselling and related activities (Boyton and Scambler, 1988; Boyd *et al.*, 1990). Since there is also some evidence of more judgmental attitudes towards homosexuality in relation to HIV among GPs (Milne and Keen, 1988; Boyton and Scambler, 1988), it is likely that GUM clinics will continue to be the most important source of care for the majority of gay men in relation to HIV infection. More of the counselling provided for men from within GUM clinics came from health advisers. It is possible that this system may be overburdened by demands. Certainly, the large proportion of men reporting that they have had the HIV test without counselling is disturbing.

Lacking from this survey and from most other research to date is more direct evidence of men's experiences of the *processes* of care surrounding the HIV test. We have produced evidence that indicates that some potential barriers to care have been less damaging than might have been feared, particularly at the height of homophobic responses to the early phases of the UK AIDS epidemic. However, this could be more convincingly demonstrated if more evidence were available about the quality of care as perceived by recipients of the HIV test and related care.

References

BAYER, R. (1989) 'AIDS, Privacy and Responsibility', *Daedalus*, 118, 79–100.

BOCHOW, M. (forthcoming) 'AIDS and Gay Men: Individual Strategies and Collective Coping', *European Sociological Review*.

BOYD, J., KERR, S., MAW, R., *et al.* (1990) 'Knowledge of HIV Infection and AIDS and Attitudes to Testing and Counselling among General Practitioners in Northern Ireland', *British Journal of General Practitioners*, 40, 158–160.

BOYTON, R. and SCAMBLER, G. (1988) 'Survey of General Practitioners' Attitudes to AIDS in the North West Thames and East Anglia Regions', *British Medical Journal*, 296, 538–540.

CARNE, C., WELLER, I., JOHNSON, A., *et al.* (1987) 'Prevalence of Antibodies to Human Immunodeficiency Virus, Gonorrhoea Rates and Changed Sexual Behaviour in Homosexual Men in London', *Lancet*, 1, 656–658.

CATES, W. and HANDSFIELD, H. (1988) 'HIV Counseling and Testing: Does It Work?' *American Journal of Public Health*, 78, 1533–1534.

COATES, T., MORIN, S. and McKUSICK, L. (1987) 'Behavioural Consequences of AIDS Antibody Testing among Gay Men', *Journal of American Medical Association*, 258, 1889.

COLLABORATIVE STUDY GROUP (1989) 'HIV Infection in Patients Attending Clinics for Sexually Transmitted Disease in England and Wales', *British Medical Journal*, 298, 415–418.

CONNELL, R., CRAWFORD, J. KIPPAX, S., *et al.* (1989) Facing the Epidemic: Changes in the Sexual Lives of Gay and Bisexual Men in Australia and Their Implications for AIDS Prevention Strategies', *Social Problems*, 36, 384–401.

COXON, A., DAVIES, P., HUNT, A., *et al.* (1989) 'Factors Associated with HIV-1 Infection in a Non-Clinic Cohort of Homosexually Active Men', Project SIGMA Working Paper No. 15, Social Research Unit, Cardiff.

FITZPATRICK, R., BOULTON, M. and HART, G. (1989a) 'Gay Men's Sexual Behaviour in Response to AIDS: Insights and Problems', in P. AGGLETON, G. HART and P. DAVIES (Eds) *Social Representations, Social Practices*, Lewes, Falmer Press.

FITZPATRICK, R., BOULTON, M., HART, G., DAWSON, J. and McLEAN, J. (1989b) 'High Risk Sexual Behaviour and Condom Use in a Sample of Homosexual and Bisexual Men', *Health Trends*, 21, 76–79.

FITZPATRICK, R., McLEAN, J., BOULTON, M., *et al.* (1990) 'Variation in Sexual Behaviour in Gay Men', in P. AGGLETON, P. DAVIES and G. HART (Eds) *AIDS: Individual, Cultural and Policy Dimensions*, Lewes, Falmer Press.

FOX, R., ODAKA, N., BROOKMEYER, R. and POLK, F. (1987) 'Effect of HIV Antibody Disclosure on Subsequent Sexual Activity in Homosexual Men', *AIDS*, 1, 241–246.

FRANCIS, D. and CHIN, J. (1987) 'The Prevention of Acquired Immunodeficiency Syndrome in the United States', *Journal of American Medical Association*, 257, 1357–1366.

GILL, O., ADLER, M. and DAY, N. (1989) 'Monitoring the Prevalence of HIV', *British Medical Journal*, 299, 1295–1298.

HART, G., FITZPATRICK, R., McLEAN, J., *et al.* (1990) 'Gay Men, Social Support and HIV Disease: A Study of Social Support in the Gay Community', *AIDS Care*, 2, 2, 163–169.

HULL, H., BETTINGER, C., GALLAHER, M., *et al.* (1988) 'Comparison of HIV Antibody Testing in an STD Clinic', *Journal of American Medical Association*, 260, 935–938.

JOHNSON, A. and GILL, O. (1989) 'Evidence for Recent Changes in Sexual Behaviour in Homosexual Men in England and Wales', *Transactions of the Royal Philosophical Society, London*, B325, 153–161.

KING, M. (1988) 'AIDS and the General Practitioner: Views of Patients with HIV Infection and AIDS', *British Medical Journal*, 297, 182–184.

LYTER, D., VALDISERRI, R., KINGSLEY, L., *et al.* (1987) 'The HIV Antibody Test: Why Gay and Bisexual Men Want to Know Their Results', *Public Health Reports*, 102, 468–474.

McKusker, J., Stoddard, A., Mayer, K., et al. (1988) 'Effects of HIV Antibody Test Knowledge on Subsequent Sexual Behaviours in a Cohort of Homosexually Active Men', *American Journal of Public Health*, 78, 462–467.

Milne, R. and Keen, S. (1988) 'Are General Practitioners Ready to Prevent the Spread of HIV?' *British Medical Journal*, 296, 533–537.

Mortimer, P. (1988) 'Tests for Infection with HIV: Slandered Goods', *British Medical Journal*, 296, 1615–1616.

Ostrow, D. (1989) 'AIDS Prevention through Effective Education', *Daedalus*, 118, 229–254.

Public Health Laboratory Service Working Group (1989) 'Prevalence of HIV Antibody in High and Low Risk Groups in England', *British Medical Journal*, 298, 422–423.

Research and Decisions Corporaton (1986) 'Designing an Effective Prevention Campaign Strategy for San Francisco', San Francisco, San Francisco AIDS Foundation.

Siegel, K. (1989) 'The Motives of Gay Men for Taking or Not Taking the HIV Antibody Test', *Social Problems*, 36, 368–383.

Shilts, R. (1987) *And the Band Played On*, Harmondsworth, Penguin.

Valdiserri, R., Lyter, D., Leviton, L., et al. (1988) 'Variables Influencing Condom Use in a Cohort of Gay and Bisexual Men', *American Journal of Public Health*, 78, 801–805.

Weiss, R. and Thier, S. (1988) 'HIV Testing Is the Answer — What's the Question?' *New England Journal of Medicine*, 319, 1010–1012.

Welch, J., Palmer, S., Banatvala, J., et al. (1986) 'Willingness of Homosexual and Bisexual Men in London to Be Screened for Human Immunodeficiency Virus', *British Medical Journal*, 293, 924.

Chapter 5

Bisexual Men: Women, Safer Sex and HIV Transmission

Mary Boulton, Zoe Schramm Evans, Ray Fitzpatrick and Graham Hart

A recent report from the Working Party of the Public Health Laboratory Service has suggested that the AIDS epidemic in the United Kingdom is now entering a more complex phase (Public Health Laboratory Service Working Group, 1990). Since the mid-1980s, the incidence of HIV has declined markedly in the major exposure category of homosexually active men. The present epidemic is made up of a series of separate but interlinked epidemics in other exposure categories such as injecting drug users and heterosexual contacts of infected individuals. Drug users who share injecting equipment have long been a focus of research interest. Given this changing pattern, attention is now turning to those groups likely to transmit second-generation HIV infection within the heterosexual population through sexual contact. While intravenous drug users clearly play an important role in this, bisexual men have also been identified as potentially having a significant role.

It has proved difficult to assess the likely contribution of bisexual men to the spread of HIV in the general population, however, since little is known about their sexual behaviour or how it is changing in response to AIDS. Studies of bisexual men are few in number, and the findings they present are somewhat inconsistent. Two large-scale studies of homosexually active men report that patterns of homosexual behaviour among bisexual men are broadly similar to those among homosexual men, with only a minority of individuals continuing to engage in unprotected anal intercourse, more commonly with regular partners (about a third) than casual partners (a fifth to a third) (Connell *et al.*, 1989; Fitzpatrick *et al.*, 1990). However, these studies draw their samples largely from men who are active in the gay community. Bisexual men who identify as heterosexual and whose sexual activities with men are transient or secretive are rarely included. Such men may represent a significant proportion of behaviourally bisexual men, and may differ considerably from those who are involved in the gay community. Thus Palmer *et al.* (1989) found that married homosexual and bisexual men who called a telephone

65

counselling service in Melbourne, Australia displayed lower levels of knowledge of safer sex than was found within the local gay community. Similarly, Peterson *et al.* (1989) report that almost all of the fifty black bisexual men they studied continued to practise unsafe sex with both primary and other partners. At the other extreme Ekstrand *et al.* (1989) report that none of the fifty-eight bisexual men in the San Francisco Men's Health Study now engage in unprotected anal sex with men.

A question which has been particularly neglected in research on bisexual men, but which is of considerable importance in relation to their role in the transmission of HIV in the general population, is their sexual behaviour with their female partners. A number of the studies which include bisexual men in their samples are concerned primarily with the risks of HIV transmission among homosexually active men. They focus largely on homosexual behaviour and consider heterosexual behaviour only in passing (for example, Davies *et al.*, 1990). Some give no information at all on sexual behaviour with women (Connell *et al.*, 1989; Peterson *et al.*, 1989), while those that report their findings again present a contradictory picture. On the one hand, Fitzpatrick *et al.* (1989) and Bennett *et al.* (1989) report that unprotected vaginal sex continues to be common practice among bisexual men. On the other hand, Ekstrand *et al.* (1989) report that only a very small proportion (5 per cent) of bisexual men currently engage in unprotected vaginal sex. Only Bennett *et al.* (1989) consider sexual behaviour with both male and female partners, reporting that almost half the men in their sample were engaging in unsafe sexual practices with at least one male and one female partner. No studies, however, have considered explanations for this pattern of behaviour or the rationales offered by the men themselves. More detailed analyses of behaviour by type of relationship, and accounts of the beliefs and attitudes surrounding behaviour are almost entirely in relation to homosexual behaviour. Thus the persistence of high rates of unsafe sex with women has been documented, but the reasons for this remain largely unexplored.

This chapter presents the results of a study designed to investigate the sexual behaviour, and the social behaviour and experience more generally, of a diverse sample of bisexual men. The men's sexual behaviour with women and their perceptions and beliefs about it were central concerns of the study and are reported here.

Methods

One of the major challenges in investigating bisexual behaviour is in recruiting a sample of behaviourally bisexual men. While bisexual groups have recently been formed in some large cities, the organized bisexual community is very small and many bisexual men remain as isolated individuals, invisible within the gay community or the 'general population' (Wolf, 1987; MacDonald, 1981). Even more than homosexuality, bisexuality is stigmatized in Western societies, and bisexual men may take considerable trouble to hide aspects of their behaviour (Off Pink Publishing, 1988; Bennett *et al.*, 1989). Bisexual men are difficult to locate and identify and are often unwilling to become involved in research.

The approach to sampling adopted in this study was to use as many organizations, networks and locales as possible to try to recruit a wide range of men who have sexual contact with both men and women. Bisexual groups in several cities were approached and agreed to cooperate. These groups provide social and political organizations for self-identified bisexual men and women. Advertisements were placed in magazines likely to be read by bisexual men, and one response led to a number of other contacts. Men were also recruited in more traditional ways through an outpatient genito-urinary medicine clinic and through contacts in the gay community. Pubs frequented by 'rent boys' and organizations which provide community services for them were approached. The prison and probationary services were also contacted, although no men were recruited to the study through these routes.

A total of sixty-two men eventually agreed to take part in the study, although the data reported here concern only the first forty-nine men. All the men had had sexual contact with both men and women at some time during the previous five years. Five years was chosen as a period which was narrow enough to reflect recent behaviour but not so narrow as to exclude those whose bisexual behaviour was not always 'active'.

The men were interviewed by a female research officer (ZSE) using a structured interview schedule which included both open-ended questions and questions requiring fixed-choice answers. Most interviews were tape-recorded and the answers to open-ended questions were transcribed. Subjects covered included demographic information, sexual orientation, sexual history, recent sexual partners and sexual activities with each partner, attitudes to men and women as friends and sexual partners, knowledge of and attitudes to safer sex, experience of the HIV antibody test, attitudes to bisexuality, and personal and social networks. The interviews lasted between one and six hours.

Results

The demographic characteristics of the men in the sample are given in Table 5.1. The sample is on the whole young, middle-class and single, as is generally the case with studies of homosexually active men, although men from a wide range of ages, occupational statuses and living arrangements are also represented.

The diversity within the sample becomes more apparent when the men's private and public sexual identity and the social context in which they live are considered. Although all the men can be described as bisexual with regard to their behaviour, almost half describe their (private) sexual identity in other terms (Table 5.2). There is no straightforward relationship between sexual behaviour and sexual identity.

Over a third of the men were not open about their sexual identity and allowed a public identity of 'heterosexual' to prevail. These are the covert or 'closeted' bisexual men. They include over half the men who think of themselves as bisexual, but only a quarter of those who identify as gay. This difference may reflect the effect of the gay community in providing support for their sexual identity.

Gagnon (1989) has suggested that in looking at bisexual behaviour among adults a distinction can be made between bisexual men embedded in a heterosexual context and bisexual men embedded in a gay context. A third category, bisexual men embedded in a bisexual context, was added here, since a number of men were recruited through the organized bisexual community. Men were considered to be embedded in a heterosexual context if they were married or living with a female partner. The one man who thought of himself as heterosexual was also included in this group. Men were considered to be embedded in a gay context if they were significantly involved in the organized gay community, for example, by belonging to gay organizations or by regularly using gay pubs and clubs. The sample is fairly evenly divided among these three groups (Table 5.3). Three men could not be classified in this way: they were marginal to all social groups across a range of dimensions. In the subsequent analyses two are included in the group embedded in a heterosexual context and one in the group embedded in a gay context.

Current Sexual Partners

While all the men in the sample had had partners of both sexes in the previous five years, not all were behaviourally bisexual at the time of interview or in the previous year (Table 5.4). This reflects the different patterns of sexual history found among bisexual men (Boulton, 1989). Not all bisexual men have male and female partners through all periods of their lives: for some men, periods of homosexual activity alternate with periods of heterosexual activity; for others, these periods overlap; and for others, long periods of exclusively heterosexual (or homosexual) activity are broken by only occasional partners of the same (or opposite) sex. Looking only at men who currently have both male and female partners provides a limited picture of male bisexual behaviour. However, many of the questions considered in this chapter were asked in relation to *current* partners, and much of the subsequent analysis will use only those thirty-two men who have current female partners.

Numbers of male partners greatly exceeded numbers of female partners (Table 5.5). For those with male partners, the median number of partners was six (mean

Table 5.1 Sample Characteristics (percentages in brackets)

Age	Mean 30 years		
	Range 19 to 65 years		
Marital status	Single	35	(71)
	Divorced	1	(2)
	Married	13	(27)
Living arrangements	With female partner	17	(35)
	With male partner	2	(4)
	Other	30	(61)
Social class	Middle class	33	(67)
	Working class	4	(8)
	Students	7	(14)
	Unemployed	5	(10)

Table 5.2 Sexual Identity (percentages in brackets)

	Private identity	Public identity
Gay	11 (22)	8 (16)
Bisexual	29 (59)	13 (26)
Straight	1 (2)	20 (41)
Other	8 (16)	8 (16)
	Normal, unimportant, unrestrained, various	

Table 5.3 Social Context (percentages in brackets)

Predominantly heterosexual (Married or living with a female sexual partner)	16	(33)
Predominantly gay (Extensively involved in the gay community)	17	(35)
Predominantly bisexual (Involved with a bisexual group)	13	(27)
Other (No particular commitment)	3	(6)

Table 5.4 Sex of Partners (percentages in brackets)

	Last year		Current	
Male only	10	(20)	14	(28)
Male and female	30	(61)	26	(53)
Female only	7	(14)	6	(12)
None	2	(4)	3	(6)

Table 5.5 Numbers of Partners in Last Year (percentages in brackets)

Males			Females	
0	9	(18)	12	(24)
1	7	(14)	20	(41)
2+	33	(67)	17	(35)

20); for those with female partners, the median number was one (mean 2). This pattern is similar to that reported by other studies of bisexual men (Fulford *et al.*, 1983; Boulton and Coxon, submitted for publication). The mean number of female partners is lower than that of the 'general population' (Turner *et al.*, 1989), though a higher proportion have multiple female partners (DHSS, 1987). The mean number of male partners is higher than that of gay men, but a smaller proportion have multiple male partners (Davies *et al.*, 1990).

Current Sexual Activities

Table 5.6 shows the proportion of men who engage in penetrative sex, with and without condoms, according to the sex of their partners. A strikingly high proportion no longer have any kind of penetrative sex with their male partners, a third of the sample compared to a quarter of the sample in studies of gay men (Davies *et al.*, 1990; Fitzpatrick *et al.*, 1990). The proportion who always use condoms is also high and twice that reported among gay men (Fitzpatrick *et al.*, 1990). Overall, less than a third of the men currently engage in unprotected penetrative sex with male partners.

By contrast, all but one of the men who had female partners engaged in

Table 5.6   High Risk Sexual Activities (percentages in brackets)

	With male partners (N = 40)		With female partners (N = 32)	
No penetrative sex	13	(33)	1	(3)
Always used condom	16	(40)	12	(38)
Sometimes/never used condom	11	(28)	19	(59)

penetrative sex, including nine men (26 per cent) who practised anal intercourse with their female partners. It has been suggested from heterosexual transmission studies that bisexual men may be more likely than men in other risk groups to engage in anal intercourse with their female partners (Padian *et al.*, 1987). The proportion of men in this study who reported anal intercourse with female partners is similar to that in the study of bisexual men by Bennett *et al.* (1989), but higher than that in general population surveys (DHSS, 1987) and in studies of women attending a genito-urinary medicine clinic (Evans *et al.*, 1988).

The proportion of men reporting that they always use condoms with female partners is markedly higher than among the 'general population', where less than 10 per cent of men always use condoms (Sonnex *et al.*, 1989). Nevertheless, almost two-thirds of the men currently engage in unprotected penetrative sex with female partners. There are no differences in patterns of behaviour with regular and casual partners.

One factor which appears to be important in whether or not they continue to have high risk sex with female partners is the social context in which the men live. Of those who have current female partners, almost all the men in the 'heterosexual' context (13/15, 87 per cent) have unprotected sex with them. An example is Allan, a 40-year-old lecturer with one male and four female partners in the last year. No one knows anything about his homosexual activities, and he continues to have unprotected sex with his female partners in the same way as he has for about twenty years. Only half the men in the 'gay' context who have current female partners (4/8, 50 per cent) have unprotected sex with them. An example is Brian, a 21-year-old administrative officer with one regular female and five male partners in the last year, who always intends to use condoms but does not always manage to do so. By contrast, the majority of the men in the 'bisexual' context (7/9, 78 per cent) always use condoms with their female partners. An example is Charlie, a 29-year-old trade union official with five male and four female partners in the last year. All his female partners are themselves bisexual, and both they and he implicitly assume that condoms will always be used in penetrative sex.

Table 5.7 shows 'bisexual behaviour', that is, sexual behaviour with both male and female partners. Of the twenty-six men who had current partners of both

Table 5.7   Safe and Unsafe Sex with Male and Female Partners
(percentages in brackets)

No partners			3	(6)
Either male or female partners but not both			20	(41)
only safe sex with everyone	9	(45)		
unsafe sex with male *or* female partners	11	(55)		
Male and female partners			26	(53)
only safe sex with everyone	11	(42)		
unsafe sex with male *or* female partners	15	(58)		
unsafe sex with male *and* female partners	4	(15)		
Total			49	(100)

sexes, less than half (eleven, 42 per cent) had safer sex with all partners. However, only four (15 per cent) had unprotected penetrative sex with all partners. This contrasts with the high proportion, 44 per cent, in Bennett *et al.*'s (1989) study of actively bisexual men who used 'beats' in the Western suburbs of Sydney, Australia. The marked difference may be due to a combination of cultural differences and differences in sampling: almost all the men in the Sydney sample were covert bisexual men, with little contact with either the gay community or organized bisexual groups. About half the men in both studies had unprotected intercourse with at least one male or one female partner. If a longer period were considered, it is likely that a much larger proportion of the men in this study would have had unprotected sex with both men and women.

The influence of the social context in which the men live is also clear with regard to their pattern of 'bisexual behaviour' (Table 5.8). Among men who live in a bisexual context, the single most common pattern (6/13, 46 per cent) is to have safe sex with both male and female partners. Among men who live in a heterosexual context, the most common pattern of behaviour (11/18, 61 per cent) is to continue to have unprotected intercourse with women and to have no male partners or only safer sex with male partners. For men who live in a gay context, the most common pattern is to have safer sex with male partners (10/17, 59 per cent) regardless of their activities with women.

Perceptions of Risk of Acquiring HIV from Female Partners

In reporting that men continue to engage in unprotected vaginal sex, Ekstrand *et al.* (1989) note that this may be because they perceive it to be less risky than

Table 5.8   Bisexual Behaviour and Social Context (percentages in brackets)

	Heterosexual		Social Context Homosexual		Bisexual		Total
No male partners (including no partners)	5	(28)	1	(6)	3	(23)	9
No female partners	3	(17)	9	(50)	2	(15)	14
Safe sex with both male and female partners	2	(11)	4	(22)	6	(46)	12
Safe sex with men, unsafe sex with women	6	(33)	2	(11)	2	(15)	10
Unsafe sex with both male and female partners	2	(11)	2	(11)	—		4
Total	18	(100)	18	(100)	13	(100)	49

unprotected sex with men. This appears to be the case for the men in this sample. Of the thirty-two men who have a current female partner, only one felt that he was at risk of HIV infection from his female partners. This was a 41-year-old company director, married, with 100 male and four female partners in the last year. He said, 'I'm as likely to get it from a woman as a man because the type of sex I'm liable to have with women, with the exception of my wife, is "fantasy" sex with women who are part of that scene. And they are more likely than most women to have HIV.' Three other men acknowledged the theoretical possibility of infection from female partners, but felt it was remote in real terms. For example, Michael, a 59-year-old surveyor with sixty male and two female partners, said, 'It's less likely than from a man as there are fewer women who are HIV positive but it's still a physical possibility.'

The other thirty men, however, felt that they were *not* at risk of infection from their female partners. Most said this was because very few women were HIV positive; others indicated that whatever the prevalence of HIV among women in the area, *their* partners were not the sort to be positive. For example, Gregory, a 32-year-old computer programmer with one male and two female partners, said, 'Even in Edinburgh, the kind of women I would sleep with, I wouldn't expect to sleep with any drug addicted women. I suppose there's the assumption on my part that I'm sleeping with low risk women compared to some of the women in Edinburgh.' Some also added that female to male transmission was less efficient than male to female transmission.

Perceptions of Risk of Transmitting HIV to Female Partners

Only one of the men in the sample felt that their female partners were at risk of HIV infection from them, although this was less clearly articulated. Some were aware that the issues surrounding risks were different in relation to female and male partners, and made comments such as, 'With men, the risks are equal. With women, the risks are very one-sided.' However, what they generally saw as significant in this was not that their partners were at risk from them but that they were not at risk from their partners. Although some acknowledged a 'potential' or 'theoretical' risk to women, virtually all the men felt that they personally were not putting their female partners at any real risk of HIV infection.

The main reasons offered for this view concerned the men's perceptions of their own risks of having or contracting HIV infection. Only one of the men who currently had female partners thought that there was a significant possibility that he was HIV positive. He always intended to use condoms with women but sometimes did not, which he was aware put them at potential risk of infection. The other thirty-one men who had current female partners felt that the likelihood of their being HIV positive was negligible. Twenty-one continued to have unprotected sex with women but felt that, since they were very unlikely to be HIV positive, the question of risk to their partners was simply not relevant. This perception that they are not particularly at risk is a common finding in studies of homosexually active men (Joseph et al., 1987; Fitzpatrick et al., 1989). However, such studies also report that there is little association between levels of perceived risk and actual high risk sexual behaviour. Perceptions of risk may be a poor basis on which to make decisions about continuing unprotected intercourse with women.

Female Partners' Perceptions of Risk

According to the men's accounts, their female partners were less sanguine than they were about their risks of becoming infected with HIV through sexual contact with them. Almost half (14, 44 per cent) reported that these women felt at significant personal risk of infection and voiced anxieties about it. For example, George, a 31-year-old carpenter with four male partners and two female partners, said, 'My wife is very concerned. With Sharon it's a personal thing because she knows I've slept with men in the past. So with her it's a personal concern and a general concern because we know a lot of gay men.' Some women expressed their concern by insisting on only safer sex. For example, John, a 28-year-old clerical officer with fifteen male and two female partners, said, 'They are quite concerned. We talk about it sometimes. They are definitely concerned that we always have safer sex.' A few women made monogamy and a negative HIV test a condition for continuing the relationship. For example, Harry, a 27-year-old engineer, married, with one female partner, said, 'We've discussed this and that's why I don't have sex with men any more, because we do see it as a problem. My wife was very worried about me and about herself. She wanted me to have an HIV test, which I did.'

About half (14, 44 per cent) of the men reported that their female partners did not appear to feel at any significant personal risk of HIV infection. A few indicated that women were concerned about HIV infection in general terms but acted in a way which they took to mean they did not feel at personal risk. For example, Ken, a 33-year-old labourer with one male and two female partners, said, 'Women are generally warier now than they were before because they know about risk groups, but they don't demand condoms. They are less concerned than men are and they're prepared to let me take responsibility.' The majority, however, reported that their partners were concerned about AIDS but not in a personal way. For example, Lawrence, a 44-year-old administrative officer with eight male and one female partners, said, 'The talk is only general. She knows about AIDS but she is not personally concerned.' Similarly, Martin, a 61-year-old college lecturer with twenty male and twenty-four female partners, said, 'They feel a public concern but not a private concern. They don't see it has anything to do with them.' The other four (13 per cent) men had 'no idea' about their partners' sense of personal risk of HIV infection.

The women's perceptions of their risks of HIV infection, as reported by the men in the study, appear to play a role in whether or not the couples engage in unprotected sex. Less than half (6/14, 43 per cent) of the men whose partners felt at significant personal risk engaged in unprotected sex, while three-quarters (13/18, 72 per cent) of those who said that their partners felt no particular personal risk continued to engage in unprotected intercourse.

An important question, then, is why so many women do not perceive themselves to be at *personal* risk of HIV infection. One reason may be that they do not know that their partners have sex with men and may be putting them at increased risk of HIV infection. Of the eighteen men who reported that their female partners appear to perceive no personal risk of infection, two-thirds (12, 67 per cent) said the women did not know that they also had sex with men. Of the fourteen men who also continued to have unprotected sex with their female partners, over half (8) said their female partners did not know of their activities with men. As Richardson (1990) points out, while the assumption in much health education literature is that the negotiation of safer sex takes place between equals, this is rarely the case. In particular, female partners of bisexual men may be at a marked disadvantage in such negotiations due both to their subordinate position in gender relations generally and to their reliance on their partners' openness about possible risks of infection.

Discussion

This chapter provides an account of the sexual behaviour of a category of men about whom very little is known. The sample is not statistically representative of behaviourally bisexual men, but does include a range of men encompassed within the epidemiological category 'bisexual'. While the numerical results need to be interpreted with caution, the findings of the study indicate the different patterns of behaviour found among behaviourally bisexual men.

Overall, the findings of this study suggest that bisexual men are no longer putting themselves or their male partners at risk of acquiring HIV infection: only a small minority of the sample now have unprotected intercourse with their male partners, and a significant minority no longer have penetrative sex of any kind with other men. However, the great majority of those with female partners continue to have unprotected intercourse with them and so potentially put them at risk of infection.

The study also has important implications for health education. First, it suggests the need for further educational efforts about the risk of HIV infection and the relevance of safer sex for 'heterosexual' couples. The men in the study continue to have high risk sex with women in the context of a set of beliefs and attitudes that it is 'safe' for them and their partners to do so. The men felt that they were neither at risk of acquiring HIV from women nor that they were at risk of passing HIV to women. It was largely when their female partners felt at personal risk of infection that they regularly used condoms in heterosexual sex. However, a number of men reported that their female partners did not perceive any personal risk of HIV infection, particularly those who were unaware of the men's homosexual activities. For these couples, there was little incentive to adopt safer sex practices. As many men pointed out, this contrasts with the situation with their male partners. The majority indicated that their male partners recognize the potential risks in their sexual encounters and now expect or insist on safer sex. Women who do not perceive a personal risk of HIV infection in their sexual encounters do not expect safer sex and, indeed, do not even appear to be conscious of it as an issue for consideration.

Second, the study suggests that health education campaigns directed at bisexual men need to be very specifically targeted. Bisexual men who live in different social contexts manage their bisexuality differently and have developed different strategies with regard to safer sex. Men who live in a bisexual context are most likely to have only safer sex with both male and female partners. This probably reflects the influence of the bisexual community both in facilitating the men's openness to women about their homosexual activities and in making them aware of the importance of safer sex in both homosexual and heterosexual sex. Among these men and their partners, safer sex appears to have become the normative practice in *all* sexual encounters. Among men who live in a gay context, safer sex is expected and accepted in homosexual encounters, particularly with casual partners. Men who are *openly* gay may also feel at ease in having safer sex with women, while women who are aware that they are gay may also find it easier to discuss or insist on safer sex with them. However, gay men appear to see safer sex as relevant primarily in homosexual encounters (where they perceive a possible risk to themselves) and, when there is no instigation from women, do not bother to use condoms in heterosexual encounters. Men who live in a heterosexual context have safer sex with men but continue to have unsafe sex with women. This appears to be an explicit strategy which they have adopted in relation to the AIDS epidemic. That is, they take the view that as long as they have safer sex with men, it is acceptable to continue to have unsafe sex with women. Since the homosexual activities of men who live in a heterosexual context are largely covert and hidden from public view, most of their female partners are unaware that they are behaviourally bisexual and are at a particular disadvantage in negotiating safer sex. It is for this group of men that AIDS education and preventive campaigns are particularly urgently required.

References

BENNETT, G., CHAPMAN, S. and BRAY, F. (1989) 'A Potential Source for the Transmission of the Human Immunodeficiency Virus into the Heterosexual Population: Bisexual Men Who Frequent "Beats" ', *Medical Journal of Australia*, 151, 314–318.

BOULTON, M. (1989) 'Bisexual Men: Identity and Behaviour in Sexual Encounters', paper presented at the Twenty-first Annual Conference of the Medical Sociology Group of the British Sociological Association, Manchester, 15–17 September.

BOULTON, M. and COXON, T. (submitted for publication) *Bisexuality in the United Kingdom*.

CONNELL, R., CRAWFORD, J., DOWSETT, G., *et al.* (1989) 'Unsafe Anal Sexual Practice among Homosexual and Bisexual Men', Social Aspects of the Prevention of AIDS Study: Report No. 6, Macquarie University, Australia.

DAVIES, P., HUNT, A., MACOURT, M. and WEATHERBURN, P. (1990) *Longitudinal Study of Sexual Behaviour of Homosexual Males under the Impact of AIDS*, Final Report to the Department of Health, London, South Bank Polytechnic.

DEPARTMENT OF HEALTH AND SOCIAL SECURITY (1987) *AIDS: Monitoring Response to the Public Education Campaign February 1986–February 1987*, London, HMSO.

EKSTRAND, M., COATES, T., LANG, S. and GUYDISH, J. (1989) 'Prevalence and Change of AIDS High Risk Sexual Behaviour among Bisexual Men in San Francisco: The San Francisco Men's Health Study', Abstract MDP31, Fifth International Conference on AIDS, Montreal, Canada, June 1989.

EVANS, B., MCCORMACK, S., BOND. R., *et al.* (1988) 'Human Immunodeficiency Virus Infection, Hepatitis B Virus Infection and Sexual Behaviour of Women Attending a Genito-urinary Medicine Clinic, *British Medical Journal*, 296, 473–475.

FITZPATRICK, R., HART, G., BOULTON, M., *et al.* (1989) 'Heterosexual Sexual Behaviour in a Sample of Homosexually Active Men', *Genito-Urinary Medicine*, 65, 259–262.

FITZPATRICK, R., MCLEAN, J., DAWSON, J., BOULTON, M. and HART, G. (1990) 'Factors Influencing Condom Use in a Sample of Homosexually Active Men', *Genito-urinary Medicine*, 66, 346–350.

FULFORD, K., CATTERALL, R., HOINVILLE, E., *et al.* (1983) 'Social and Psychological Factors in the Distribution of STD in Male Clinic Attenders III: Sexual Activity', *British Journal of Venereal Disease*, 59, 386–393.

GAGNON, J. (1989) 'The Management of Erotic Relations with Both Genders', paper presented at the CDC Workshop on Bisexuality and AIDS, Atlanta, Ga., USA.

JOSEPH, J., MONTGOMERY, S., EMMONS, S., *et al.* (1987) 'Magnitude and Determinants of Behavioural Risk Reduction: Longitudinal Analysis of a Cohort at Risk for AIDS', *Psychology and Health*, 1, 73–95.

MACDONALD, A. (1981) 'Bisexuality: Some Comments on Research and Theory', *Journal of Homosexuality*, 6, 21–36.

OFF PINK PUBLISHING (1988) *Bisexual Lives*, London, Off Pink Publishing.

PADIAN, N., MARQUIS, L., *et al.* (1987) 'Male to Female Transmission of Human Immuno-deficiency Virus', *Journal of American Medical Association*, 258, 788–790.

PALMER, W., *et al.* (1989) 'Accessing, Educating and Researching Married Homosexual and Bisexual Men', Abstract MEP 43, Fifth International Conference on AIDS, Montreal, Canada, June 1989.

PETERSON, J., FULLILOVE, R., CATANIA, J. and COATES, T. (1989) 'Close Encounters of an Unsafe Kind: Risky Sexual Behaviours and Predictors among Black Gay and Bisexual Men', Abstract WDP 27, Fifth International Conference on AIDS, Montreal, Canada, June 1989.

PUBLIC HEALTH LABORATORY SERVICE WORKING GROUP (1990) 'Acquired Immune Deficiency Syndrome in England and Wales to End 1993', *Communicable Disease Report*, January 1990.

RICHARDSON, D. (1990) 'AIDS Education and Women: Sexual and Reproductive Issues', in P. AGGLETON, P. DAVIES and G. HART (Eds), *AIDS: Individual, Cultural and Policy Dimensions*, Lewes, Falmer Press.

TURNER, C., MILLER, H. and MOSES, L. (1989) *AIDS: Sexual Behaviour and Intravenous Drug Use*, Washington, D.C., National Academy Press.

SONNEX, C., HART, G., WILLIAMS, P. and ADLER, M. (1989) 'Condom Use by Heterosexuals Attending a Department of Genito-Urinary Medicine: Attitudes and Behaviour in the Light of HIV infection', *Genito-Urinary Medicine*, 65, 248–51.

WOLF, T. (1987) 'Group Counselling for Bisexual Men', *Journal for Specialists in Group Work*, November, 162–165.

Chapter 6

Prostitutes' Perceptions or Risk and Factors Related to Risk-taking

Hilary Kinnell

Prostitutes have been the focus of social control in sexually transmitted epidemics since at least the sixteenth century (Bullough and Bullough, 1987). In this century the historian Allan Brandt (1985) has chronicled the perception of prostitutes as 'pools of infection' for sexually transmitted diseases in the United States. It is hardly surprising, then, that the identification of HIV and its categorization as sexually transmitted should again focus attention on the prostitute as a source of infection. Early studies of prostitutes with respect to HIV and AIDS were primarily concerned to discover rates of HIV infection, to assess the 'threat' posed by prostitutes. Davies and Simpson (1990) have commented with regard to male prostitutes on this deplorable tendency to regard prostitutes as a vector of disease and a threat to the monogamous pretensions of their clients, rather than as workers whose work puts them at risk of coming into contact with HIV.

At the time the work reported in this chapter began, there were few published studies relating to HIV and prostitution, and those available reported widely varying HIV prevalence rates. In Nevada (Padian *et al.*, 1987) zero infection was found among 535 brothel workers, although 7 per cent had injected drugs within the previous five years. In Kigali, Rwanda (Van de Perre *et al.*, 1985) twenty-nine of thirty-three (88 per cent) female prostitutes were found to have HIV antibody. In Jersey City, USA (MMWR, 1987) 57 per cent were reported HIV positive, while in 1985 in Paris (Brenky-Fanudeux and Fribourg-Blanc, 1985) none of a group of fifty-six was found to be infected. In London in 1985 (Barton *et al.*, 1985) none of a group of female prostitutes attending a London STD clinic was found to be infected. By 1987 a cohort of prostitutes attending this same clinic had been followed up over a longer period, and two (< 2 per cent) had been found to have HIV infection, both of these women reporting injecting drug use.[1] In contrast to this low-profile, health-oriented work, there have been press reports claiming that HIV infected, drug using prostitutes in Edinburgh commonly practised unsafe sex with their clients (see, for example, Sarler, 1987). The conclusion from these studies that HIV sero-prevalence was relatively low may in some senses be regarded as reassuring, but unsafe sexual practices between prostitutes and their clients continued to place many women at risk as the general level of HIV continued to increase.

Studies of prostitutes elsewhere appeared to indicate that in Europe and in North America HIV infection was very strongly associated with injecting drug use, but that in Africa, where condom use had not been a traditional feature of prostitutes' working practices, prostitution itself constituted a strong risk factor for HIV infection.

In 1987 Central Birmingham Health Authority's Department of Public Health Medicine began to investigate local prostitution as a possible current or future element in the transmission of HIV within the city's population. Street prostitution has been a visible aspect of community life in parts of Birmingham for many years,[2] eliciting a variety of institutional responses from the police and local authority which have focused upon the amenity and public order aspects of this branch of the sex industry.[3] The neighbourhood most characterized by street soliciting in recent years, Balsall Heath, lies largely within the area covered by Central Birmingham Health Authority.

Central Birmingham's Department of Public Health Medicine set out to discover the extent of injecting drug use among prostitutes; their sexual practices including condom use; their numbers and age and the numbers and age of their clients, in order to assess the importance of commercial sexual activity in the local population. The Department of Public Health Medicine also sought information regarding prostitutes' health behaviour, including use of genito-urinary medicine (GUM) services and contraceptive practices, and asked subjects questions relating to their knowledge of and attitudes towards AIDS and HIV. The purpose of this study was both to assess if and to what extent commercial sex was a risk factor for HIV transmission in Birmingham, and to inform the development of an HIV prevention outreach project about the practices, concerns and beliefs of women sex workers.

The Study

Advice was sought from women with experience of prostitution on the issues to be addressed, approaches that might prove successful, and on the organization of the local sex industry. After some months of preparatory work, it was decided that a survey of knowledge, attitudes and behaviour was feasible. An interview schedule was drawn up with advice from sex workers and with assistance from the University of Birmingham Department of Social Medicine. This schedule was designed to be readily understood by sex workers, so that it could be either self-

Table 6.1 Sample: Location of Interviews
(N = 258)

Street outreach	79
Magistrates' court	56
Home of respondent	52
Place of interview not recorded	45
Drop-in centre	21
Home of interviewer	5

completed or filled in with the assistance of an interviewer. Questions covered prostitutes' working practices, including numbers of clients and type of sexual service given; health behaviour; condom use; effect of policing on working practices; and knowledge of and attitudes to AIDS and HIV.

With Regional Health Authority funding to investigate the percentage of prostitutes who inject and the percentage of injectors who are prostitutes, three women were employed as part-time interviewers in early 1988. Two hundred and fifty-eight interview schedules were collected between February and November 1988.

Sample

It is not possible to obtain a random sample of prostitutes, since their identities, locations and numbers are unknown. In this study women were contacted at the magistrates' court, at a 'drop-in' centre in the red-light areas and on the street. Snow-balling methods were used to obtain interviews with less 'visible' women, i.e. those working in hotels, saunas, massage parlours, through contact magazines and through escort agencies (see Table 6.1). Women who solicit on the street are the most visible sex industry workers, and the most liable to arrest. Police figures for 1987 showed 898 individual women arrested for street prostitution offences.[4] This figure varies year by year, depending on policing policies. However, police figures can give no assistance in trying to estimate numbers of off-street sex workers. An earlier study of prostitution in Birmingham (McLeod, 1982) estimated a total of 800 prostitutes in the city, of whom only one-quarter would be working on the street at any one time. McLeod's assessment of the distribution of workers in different locations is shown in Table 6.2.

While McLeod's estimates are lower than recent police figures, her estimates of the proportions working in different locations at any one time may be more helpful than an annual total of street arrests, since sex workers in Birmingham tend to move between different locations and work settings, possibly adopting several different methods of meeting clients in the course of the week.

Table 6.2   *McLeod's Estimate of Prostitution in Birmingham, 1989*
(N = 800)

Street	200
Indoor contact	300
Saunas/massage parlours	130
Escort agencies/clubs	70
Hotels	100

Table 6.3   *Methods of Meeting Clients*
(N = 258)

Method	Number	Percentage
Street only	109	42.2
Street and other	104	40.2
Off-street only	45	17.5

The sample which was obtained in this present study comprised over 80 per cent who solicited either solely or partly on the street (see below). However, half of these also used other methods of soliciting. Relating our sample characteristics to police figures and to McLeod's work, we believe our sample to be a good representation of street working prostitutes, and a good indication of the characteristics of off-street prostitution.

Findings

Methods of Meeting Clients

Forty-two per cent of the study group reported meeting clients exclusively on the street. Forty per cent used several methods of meeting clients, including street soliciting; 17 per cent did not use the streets, but met clients in other ways (see Table 6.3). Off-street methods of meeting clients are shown in Table 6.4. Prostitutes using exclusively off-street methods were very unlikely to use only one method of meeting clients.

Number of Clients

The mean number of clients per woman in the week prior to interview was twenty-two (range 0–70). There was no significant difference in numbers of clients

Table 6.4   *'Off-street' Methods of Meeting Clients*
(*N* = 149)

Method of meeting clients	Number	Number using this method only
Hotels	55	0
Contact magazine/ visiting massage	49	6
Escort agency	36	3
Sauna/massage parlour	32	2
Own home	25	0
Public bars/clubs	22	0
Cafes	6	0
Other	19	0

Table 6.5   *Numbers of Clients over Previous Week*

Method	Mean
Street soliciting only	22
Street and other	23
Off-street only	19

in relation to the style of soliciting. This was an unexpected result, as it is often assumed that street workers service many more clients than off-street workers (see Table 6.5).

Sexual Services to Clients

Respondents were asked to record the sexual services given to each client on the last day they worked and to indicate condom use or condom breakages. Data were recorded on a total of 1157 prostitute-client contacts. Fifty-six per cent of these contacts involved vaginal sex, 20 per cent oral sex (fellatio) and 12 per cent masturbation. Six per cent of interactions involved other forms of sexual activity, and for 5 per cent no information was recorded about the details of the sexual service given (Table 6.6).

The predominance of vaginal sex calls into question the myths that commercial sex caters mainly to minority sexual interests. However, it also em-

Table 6.6   Sexual Services to Clients: Prostitute/Client Contacts

Type of service	Number	Percentage
Vaginal sex	649	56.0
Oral (fellatio)	237	20.5
Masturbation	141	12.0
Other	72	6.5
Missing information	58	5.0
Total	1157	100.0

phasizes the importance of condom use to prevent transmission of sexually transmitted diseases, including HIV.

Condom Use and Condom Breakage

Prostitutes reported that condoms were used satisfactorily for 91 per cent of instances of vaginal sex. In 1 per cent of cases condoms broke, and they were not used at all in 8 per cent of the occurrence of vaginal sex. Condoms were also used in 84 per cent of the oral sex encounters, and in 24 per cent of cases of masturbation. These results show that our respondents were well aware of the importance of condom use and well motivated to avoid contact with their clients' semen. The low rate of condom breakage was also encouraging.

Injecting Drug Use

A quarter of the study group ($N = 64$) had either injected drugs in the previous five years, or had a non-commercial sex partner who injected. Injectors and their partners came from a similar age range as their non-injecting counterparts. Both injectors and other prostitutes had an average age of 25. Women in both groups reported a similar number of clients, those in the injecting group reporting an average of twenty-three clients per week, while the non-injectors had an average of twenty-one.

The injecting group was slightly less likely to meet clients on the street, although this was the most frequent style of soliciting in both groups — 76 per cent of the injecting group compared with 84 per cent of the non-injectors. However, as the exclusive method of soliciting, there was a marked difference between the two groups. Only 25 per cent of the injectors met clients exclusively on the street, compared with 47 per cent of non-injectors. This result was highly significant ($p < .003$).

Table 6.7   Prostitutes Reporting Risk-Taking with Clients (CBHA Prostitute Survey)
N = 258

Subsample	Prostitutes reporting a 'risk event' with a client		
	Subsample	Number	Percentage
All	258	70	27
'Injecting group'[1]	64	26	40.6
Sauna workers	32	17	53
Escort agency workers	36	15	41.6
No street work[2]	45	20	44.4

Notes: 1 'Injecting group' refers to prostitutes who had themselves injected since 1983, or who had a non-commercial partner who injected.
2 'No street work' refers to prostitutes who solicited exclusively through off-street methods. Of the twenty (44 per cent) reporting a risk event, ten were in the injecting group and ten did not report any involvement with injecting.

Sexual Risk Events

For the purposes of this study, possible 'risk events' were defined as anal sex with or without condoms, unprotected vaginal or oral sex, experience of condom failure or client-prostitute contacts in which the type of sexual activity was unspecified. Fourteen per cent of all client-prostitute interactions were 'possible risk events', and 27 per cent of respondents recorded one or more such events on the last day worked.

Those involved with injecting drug use ($N = 64$) were more likely to record a possible 'risk event' with a client than women not reporting any involvement with injecting ($N = 172$); 40.6 per cent of the former ($N = 26$) and 23.8 per cent of the latter ($N = 41$) reported risk-taking with clients (chi square (Yates) 5.67; $p = 0.017$).

Sexual risk-taking with clients was also associated with off-street forms of prostitution. Women who never solicited on the street were significantly more likely to report a possible risk event with a client than were street workers (44 per cent compared with 20 per cent; $p < .006$ — see Table 6.7).

In addition, women aged 25 or over were marginally more likely to record a possible risk event than younger women. It is not clear why *older* women should take more risks, except that this study shows women over 25 were also less well-informed about HIV than younger women. Neither of these differences was statistically significant, but the trend is an interesting challenge to those who assume that younger women are the most vulnerable and least 'professional' (see Table 6.8).

Table 6.8   *Age and Possible Risk Events Reported*

Age	Risk event reported		No risk event reported	All
Teens	11	(22%)	39	50
20–29	41	(28.5%)	103	144
30–39	16	(29%)	39	55
40+	2	(22%)	7	9
Total	70	(27%)	188	258

The association between injecting, off-street working and risk-taking is easier to understand. Off-street working (saunas, hotels, escort agencies, etc.) attracts much higher earnings than street work, and where more money changes hands, it is more difficult for the woman to insist on condom use. Unprotected sex universally attracts a higher tariff than sex with condoms. There may also be management pressure undermining condom use; for example, sauna managers who do not allow their workers to keep sufficient condom supplies on the premises lest, in the event of a police raid, the condoms provide evidence that sexual services are being offered. It is also likely that the more lucrative end of the market attracts women whose financial requirements are high due to their own or their partner's drug use.

Knowledge and Attitudes about AIDS and HIV

Forty-eight per cent of respondents either failed to identify blood, semen, vaginal fluid and injecting equipment as capable of transmitting HIV, or failed to classify unprotected vaginal sex and anal sex for both men and women as presenting a high risk for HIV. These respondents were classified as misinformed. No blame attaches to this classification, since sections of the media have conducted an unrelenting campaign of misinformation about the routes of HIV transmission. Nor can any direct comparisons be made with women not working in the sex industry, since no control group was similarly interviewed. However, a 1987 survey of 352 Birmingham University medical students found that 15.7 per cent believed HIV could be caught by *donating* blood, while only 49.1 per cent described vaginal intercourse as high risk for 'catching AIDS' (Nicholl, 1988). Birmingham's prostitutes, therefore, are not necessarily less well informed than the general population. Nevertheless, it was felt to be important to find out whether accuracy of information related to sources of information, risk behaviour or any other variables.

Risk-taking *was* related to misinformation, 58 per cent of risk takers being misinformed, compared to 44 per cent of women not reporting a possible 'risk-event' (p < .60). This relationship is stronger when one compares specific elements of misinformation. For example, 34 per cent of risk-takers did not classify unprotected vaginal sex as high risk for HIV, compared to 9.6 per cent of non risk-takers (chi square (Yates) = 21.08; p < 0.000001). Overall, only 16 per cent of prostitutes did not recognize unprotected vaginal sex as high risk, compared to 51.9 per cent of medical students.

The proportion of female prostitutes who did not rate anal sex for women as high risk for HIV was considerably higher than those not recognizing vaginal sex as high risk; 48.6 per cent of risk-takers, compared to 27.6 per cent of non-risk-takers was significant (chi square (Yates) = 9.12; p < .001).

The extent of misinformation about heterosexual anal sex was one of the most striking results, since it had been assumed that the risks of anal sex would be common knowledge. Only 4 per cent failed to rate anal sex for men as high risk, but 33 per cent overall did not classify anal sex as high risk for women. Although anal sex was only reported as a service given to clients in five instances out of the 1157 client contacts recorded, anecdotal reports in the course of outreach work to prostitutes lead us to suspect that anal sex occurs more frequently than these results show. However, the taboo against reporting or discussing heterosexual anal sex does not seem to be related to a clear recognition of its HIV risk. In a parallel survey of prostitutes' clients (N = 126), 36 per cent did not classify heterosexual anal sex as high risk for transmission of HIV. Only one client specified anal sex as a service he sought from prostitutes. This man also recorded that he thought condom use 'not relevant' to his situation.

Unprotected oral sex (fellatio) was classified as a 'possible risk event' when estimating the proportion of commercial sex which might transmit HIV. While there is little epidemiological evidence for the oral transmission of HIV, this route is an efficient transmitter of other sexually transmitted diseases. The study group appears to err on the side of caution — as already mentioned, condom use was reported for 84 per cent of instances of oral sex. We did not, however, include women's estimates of the riskiness of oral sex in our classification of the proportion 'misinformed', since there was felt to be no definitive right answer. However, women not recording a possible risk event (N = 92) were significantly more likely to rate oral sex as high risk: 49 per cent (N = 92), compared to 34 per cent (N = 24) of 'risk-takers' (chi square (Yates) = 3.85; p = 0.0049).

Twenty-two women (9 per cent) classified oral sex as high risk for HIV, while also rating heterosexual anal sex as not high risk. Thirty-five women (13.5 per cent) perceived hand relief (masturbation) as being a high or medium risk activity. These particular misconceptions were shared by similar proportions of risk-takers and non-risk-takers.

It is reassuring that the majority of women surveyed were able to make an accurate assessment of the risks involved in various sexual activities, but the extent of misinformation, and the association between misinformation and risk-taking,

Figure 6.1 Sources of Information about HIV/Misinformed RE HIV (N = 258)

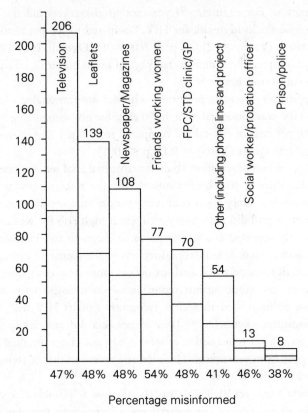

underlines that importance of making reliable information available to sex industry workers.

Sources of Information/Contact with 'Helping Agencies'

There were no significant correlations between misinformation and stated sources of information (Figure 6.1). We have instead tried to relate knowledge to contact with 'helping agencies'.

This survey was undertaken when the outreach project was at an early stage of its development; in many cases the interview formed the first contact of the respondent with the project. However, many prostitute women had been contacted at the magistrates' court over five months before the start of the survey, and approximately forty had visited the drop-in centre. Of the small number of women who completed the questionnaire at this drop-in centre (N = 27), only six (28.5

Figure 6.2   *Where Questionnaire Completed/Misinformed RE HIV (N = 258)*

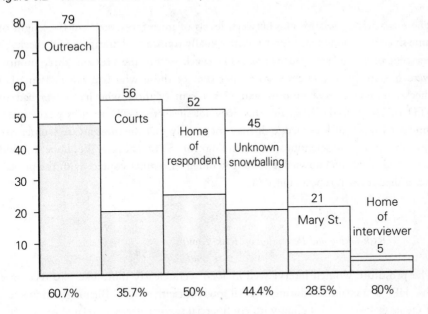

Percentage misinformed

per cent) were misinformed, compared to 48 per cent overall (see Figure 6.2). Similarly, women interviewed at the court, where many 'regulars' had had contact with the outreach project for some months, showed lower levels of misinformation than average. The numbers involved are too small to test statistically, but they give some encouragement nonetheless.

If the court's interviews are combined with the project base interviews and compared to all others, there is a significant difference: fewer (33.8 per cent) of those with presumed previous contact with the project were misinformed than those with no presumed previous contact (54.1 per cent misinformed) (chi square (Yates) = 8.19; p = 0.0042).

This does not mean that our outreach work was the *cause* of better levels of information. It is possible that the better informed women were the first to take advantage of the services that were offered, or that the previous contact with the courts had improved women's knowledge of HIV. It is difficult, however, to see how the latter could be the case since no HIV education was at that time attempted by other agencies at the court. We did find that women who cited police and prisons as their main sources of information about HIV were relatively well-informed, but as only eight women (3 per cent) were involved, police and prisons cannot be regarded as useful avenues of communication with prostitute women.

Levels of Knowledge/Contact with STD Services

There is a strong relationship between levels of misinformation and the length of time since the respondent's most recent sexually transmitted disease (STD) check: 39 per cent of those who had had an STD check within the previous three months were misinformed, compared to 66 per cent of those who had not had an STD check for over twelve months, and 77 per cent of those who had never had an STD check (p < 0.03). Again, this does not mean the STD services were *causing* improved levels of knowledge: it may mean only that the most aware women are also the most conscientious in attending for STD checks. We hope to find improved levels of knowledge among women in regular contact with the project when the survey is repeated in 1990.

Risk-taking and Perception of 'Risk-Groups'

The prostitute women interviewed in 1988 were clearly more likely to recognize that HIV is transmitted during vaginal intercourse than were Birmingham medical students in 1987. Risk-taking with commercial sex partners was related to injecting and to more 'up-market' settings. Both these variables are likely to reflect the financial incentives offered by clients for unsafe sex.

The findings relating misinformation to risk behaviour are two-edged. On the one hand, we can hope that providing accurate information will lead to reduction in risk-taking; on the other, it may be that women who failed to rate vaginal sex as high risk for HIV did so not only because they had received poor information, but because they did not *believe* that vaginal sex *could* be a high risk. Beliefs and attitudes influence behaviour. We found this reflected in a small proportion of responses to our open-ended question, 'How can we stop AIDS spreading?' Only seven respondents made comments specifically defining AIDS/HIV as a problem only for gays and injectors. Six of these had themselves reported risk-taking with clients. For example:

> Try to stop young teenagers becoming gay.... Try to stop people using needles to inject drugs. Explain about what you have to do to get AIDS. (I'm not really sure I know too much even though I don't need to as I'm not queer and only smoke drugs and have the odd drink). (aged 23 at risk)

> All this fuss is probably to frighten people into stop sleeping around. I still think it affects queers and junkies more than anyone else. (aged 21 at risk)

Similarly, of the women agreeing with the statement, 'Only gays and junkies get AIDS', 44 per cent were at risk, compared to 22 per cent of those who disagreed (chi square (Yates) 9.67 per cent; p = 0.0018).

Discussion

This study was carried out by recruiting former prostitutes to use their 'street credibility', their personal friendship networks, and their expert knowledge of the local sex industry to contact and interview working women. This method of peer group contact was found to be successful, as it has been in many other places throughout the world (Ngugi *et al.*, 1988; Overs, 1989; Monny-Lobe, 1989; Cohen *et al.*, 1988). This can be contrasted with other approaches. For example, Phillips' (1989) study of eight prostitutes in Rochdale concluded that 'the difficulties involved in identifying prostitute women greatly hinder the implementation and effectiveness of a health education programme about AIDS/HIV specifically targeted at them.' The Central Birmingham initiative, beginning with respect for the expertise of sex workers, succeeded in interviewing 258 women within eleven months. The contacts thus made assisted the development of an outreach HIV prevention project which, by April 1989, had contacted over 600 individual female sex workers and had made over 3000 contacts with them in the previous year.

Neither the study reported here nor the experience of nearly three years of outreach work have indicated as high levels of injecting drug use among prostitutes in Birmingham as have been found elsewhere; for example, in Glasgow 60 per cent were thought to be injecting (McKeganny *et al.*, 1990), and in the USA a multicentre study of prostitutes reported that half gave a history of injecting (MMWR, 1987). It is likely that both styles of prostitution and methods of using drugs vary greatly in different cities and different countries; for example, a report of drug use among female patients at an STD clinic in Sydney (Ross Philpot *et al.*, 1989) showed that prostitutes reported injecting less often than non-prostitutes. In Birmingham 15 per cent reported having ever injected and a further 10 per cent, while not having injected, had an injecting non-paying sex partner. This group (N = 64) were significantly more likely to record a possible 'risk event' with a client than women not reporting any involvement with injecting drug use (N = 194): 40.6 per cent of the former (N = 26) and 23.6 per cent of the latter (N = 41) reported risk-taking with clients (chi square (Yates) = 5.67, p = 0.017).

Sexual risk-taking with clients was also associated with off-street forms of prostitution. Women who never solicited on the street were significantly more likely to report a possible risk event with a client than were street workers. It was also found that off-street working was more frequent among women who reported involvement with injecting drug use than among those who did not. While it may be that women who are financing their own or their partner's drug consumption may be drawn to off-street work because the pay is higher than for street work, it was also evident that off-street workers who reported no involvement with injecting were also more likely to report risk-taking with clients. This indicates that the setting for sex work, and the concomitant financial pressure from clients to offer unsafe sex, are important factors related to risk-taking by sex workers. The association that has been found between off-street working, injecting drug use and risk-taking with clients has led our project to commit a large proportion of its resources to working with injectors and off-street sex workers.

This study also found that 'risk-takers' were more likely to have serious misconceptions about the relative dangers of different sex practices: over a third of risk-takers did not classify unprotected vaginal sex as high risk for HIV transmission, compared to less than 10 per cent of those not reporting any risk-taking with clients, while nearly half the risk-takers did not recognize heterosexual anal sex as high risk for HIV, compared to just over a quarter of non-risk-takers. Of the very few ($N = 7$) respondents who expressed views associating AIDS solely with gays or injectors, six were 'risk-takers'.

The majority of women interviewed did not report unsafe sex, but nearly half had worrying levels of misinformation about the transmission of HIV. A realistic assessment of personal risk factors is clearly important for the development of strategies for risk reduction, as well as access to the paraphernalia of protection — condoms, spermicides, lubricants and sterile injecting equipment.

The following responses to the final question on our schedule, 'How can we stop AIDS spreading?', articulate graphically the concerns and attitudes of the women interviewed:

> Find out real facts and all doctors be in agreement as to what ways people can get it, then try to explain it clearly to everyone so they can understand the risks. Get everyone to carry a rubber just in case they fancy a fuck if they meet someone new. Most people get tempted especially if a bit drunk and at least if you carried a rubber you would 'be prepared!' (aged 20)

> I don't think the message about AIDS is getting across because lots of my friends laugh and make jokes about it. It's more serious than people realize. I don't know how we can stop it spreading. (aged 22)

> Tell them freaky gal don't fuck out. Stay with your man and him with you. The AIDS sick people could be on TV looking ill and warn people off. My man saw a picture of AIDS person and don't fuck out a street no more, neither me.

Keep up campaign. Regular advertisements on TV and in newspapers. Get across message that AIDS knows no bounds, anyone who practises risky sex or shares works can get it. Have needle exchanges and free condoms in most large cities. Put condom machines in all public loos and in secondary schools.

I don't know much about AIDS. There should be more knowledge available for a working girl. (aged 38)

A lot of people I know wouldn't know what to do or where to go if they did find out they had AIDS (neither would I, come to think of it). (aged 37)

Stop people panicking...new book out last week said you could get it from toilet seats and restaurants.

These quotes show that prostitutes are at least as likely to come up with the best answers to the question, 'How can we stop AIDS spreading?' as the professional health educators. They are experts on human sexual behaviour, and on safe sex techniques; as such, they deserve to be listened to.

Acknowledgments

With thanks to the SAFE Research and Administrative Officer, Andy Stackhouse, for his help in extracting and interpreting data, and to my secretary, Jennie Lowdell.

Notes

1 S. Day and H. Ward, personal communication.
2 See E. McLeod (1982) *Women Working: Prostitution Now*, London, Croom Helm.
3 *Balsall Health and North Moseley Inner Area Study* (1986) City of Birmingham.
4 Report of the Chief Constable of the West Midlands Constabulary, 1987.

References

BARTON, S.E., UNDERHILL, G.S., GILCRIST, C., JEFFERIES, D.J. and HARRIS, J.R.W. (1985) 'HTLV III Antibody in Prostitutes', *Lancet*, 2, 1424.
BRANDT, A. (1985) *No Magic Bullet: A Social History of Venereal Disease in the United States since 1880*, New York, Oxford University Press.

BRENKY-FANUDEUX, D. and FRIBOURG-BLANC, A. (1985) 'HTLV-III Antibody in Prostitutes' [letter], *Lancet*, 2, 424.

BULLOUGH, V. and BULLOUGH, B. (1987) *Women and Prostitution: A Social History*, New York, Prometheus.

COHEN, J., *et al.* (1988) 'Sexual Behaviour and HIV Infection Risk among 354 Sex Industry Women in a Participant Based Research and Prevention Program', paper given to the Fourth International Conference on AIDS, Stockholm.

DAVIES, P. and SIMPSON, P. (1990) 'On Male Homosexual Prostitution and HIV', in P. AGGLETON, P. DAVIES and G. HART (Eds) *AIDS: Individual, Cultural and Policy Dimensions*, Lewes, Falmer Press.

KINNELL, H. (1989) 'Prostitutes, Their Clients, and Risks of HIV Infection in Birmingham', *Occasional Paper*, Department of Public Health Medicine, Central Birmingham Health Authority.

MCKEGANNEY, N., BARNARD, M. and BLOOR, M. (1990) 'A Comparison of HIV Related Risk Behaviour and Risk in Reduction between Female Street Working Prostitutes and Male Rent Boys in Glasgow', *Sociology of Health and Illness*, 12, 274–292.

MCLEOD, E. (1982) *Women Working: Prostitution Now*, London, Croom Helm.

MMWR (1987) 'Antibody to Human Immunodeficiency Virus in Female Prostitutes', *Morbidity and Mortality Weekly Reports*, 36, ii.

MONNY-LOBE, M. (1989) 'Prostitutes as Health Educators for Their Peers in Yaoundé: Changes in Knowledge, Attitudes and Practices', Abstract No. WGO 21, paper given to the Fifth International Conference on AIDS, Montreal.

NGUGI, E.N., SIMONSEN, J.N., *et al.* (1988) 'Prevention of Transmission of HIV in Africa: Effectiveness of Condom Promotion and Health Education among Prostitutes', *Lancet*, 2, 887–890.

NICHOLL, D. (1988) *Sexual Attitudes and Behaviour in Medical Students — Has AIDS Led to Any Changes?* University of Birmingham Medical School, Fourth Year Social Medicine Project.

OVERS, C. (1989) 'Prostitution and AIDS', *Lighthouse News*, December, 4.

PADIAN, N., CARBON, J., BROWNING, R., NELSON, L., GRIMES, J. and MARQUES, I. (1987) 'HIV Infection amongst Prostitutes in Nevada', paper presented at the Third International Conference on AIDS, Washington.

PHILLIPS, R. (1988) 'AIDS Awareness of Prostitute Women', unpublished paper, Manchester Polytechnic, Health Education Certificate Course.

PHILLIPS, R. (1989) 'AIDS and Prostitute Women: Exploring Effective Methods of Education', *Health Education Journal*, 48, 1, 26–27.

ROSS PHILPOT, C., HARCOURT, C.I. and EDWARDS, J.M. (1989) 'Drug Use by Prostitutes in Sydney', *British Journal of Addiction*, 84, 499–505.

SARLER, C. (1987) 'A City at Risk', *The Sunday Times Magazine*, 21 June, 24–28.

VAN DE PERRE P., CARAEL, M., ROBERT-GUROFF, M., FREYENES, P., GALLO, R.C., CLUMECK, N., NZABIHIMANA, E., DE MOL, P., BUTZLER, J.P. and KANYAMUPIRA, J.P. (1985) 'Female Prostitutes: A Risk Group for Infection with Human T-Cell Lymphotropic Virus Type III', *Lancet*, 2, 424.

Chapter 7

London's Homosexual Male Prostitutes; Power, Peer Groups and HIV

Tim Robinson and Peter Davies

The study of male homosexual prostitutes is bedevilled by sensationalism and academic myopia. For example, the titles of two well-known papers on the subject, 'Dollars Take Priority over Love' (Humphreys, 1972) and 'The Meat Rack' (Ginsburg, 1967), are without doubt spicier and more enticing than the average sociology article but employ imagery which is almost Dickensian in its evocation of an iniquitous white slave trade. The cost of such intellectual laxity, always considerable for the male prostitute, has substantially increased with the emergence of AIDS, when the dilemmas of the individuals involved require more imaginative understanding than has so far been commonplace.

The first step towards an understanding of homosexual male prostitution is to recognize its many manifestations (Davies and Simpson, 1990). This entails a consideration of more than just the prostitute types traditionally described by sociologists and the press. The dominant images are of two convergent types: the straight male hustler, as described in Reiss (1962), and the teenage runaway prostitute as described by Harris (1973). In Reiss' seminal article, the prostitute emerges as a heterosexual with a distaste for homosexual sex, propelled into this work by economic necessity and heavily preoccupied in preserving his sense of masculinity. This dilemma is partially resolved by the individual concerned always adopting the role of insertor in homosexual sex — a role which is ascribed dominant, masculine values. Harris's more moralistic account imbues the homosexual male prostitute with the same qualities, but adds two other important elements: his homelessness and the role of the client as seducer and corruptor, trading on the prostitute's innocence and powerlessness. Here the prostitute, again heterosexual by inclination, is presented as the passive object of the client's perverting will. Although these two writers, and other (Butts, 1946; Caukins and Coombs, 1976; Coombs, 1974; Craft, 1966; Ginsburg, 1967; Hoffman, 1972; Humphreys, 1972; MacNamara, 1965), have not claimed to describe homosexual male prostitution in *all* its forms, a uniform picture of the male homosexual prostitute has nevertheless been the result.

Coombs (1974: 784) sums this up as follows.

> [The male homosexual prostitute] is a drifter, has a poor work history, possesses no vocational skill, is of low to average intelligence, comes from a deprived socioeconomic background, and is below the average of educational attainment. He is a drop-out and comes from a broken home or a home in which his parents were poor models. His was a shattered family in which there was a dearth of warmth and an excess of violence and rejection. He was the victim of indifferent mothering. Most hustlers have been found to be irresponsible, immature, unstable and neurotic, with a strong dislike for authority.

As this chapter will demonstrate, these theories and portrayals not only hide the diversity of types within those homosexual male prostitutes who meet clients in bars or outdoor trading places ('streetworking prostitutes') but also ignore those prostitutes who meet their customers through advertisements carrying a telephone contact number. Referred to as 'call-boys' in American vernacular, these other prostitutes advertize themselves by the title of 'escort', 'masseur', or 'model', most usually in the gay press (Davies and Simpson, 1990).

A second intention here is to challenge the status of child sexual abuse in accounts of the process by which some become male homosexual prostitutes (Coleman, 1989). Sexual abuse at an early age is often presented as a factor central to the character type of some young men who sell sex. This theory has been advanced at length by McMullen (1988: 40), for instance.

> A boy victim of sexual abuse...may commit himself more fully to the previously and reliably known quantity of the self-legitimating process which tells him that he enjoyed, wanted and is responsible for that which took place in his earlier years. This tried and tested psychological survival system now acts as a viable motivating agent which allows him to abuse others and/or set himself up for further abuse. If, in those early experiences of abuse, he had been given gifts or money it is not too difficult to see a logical process into prostitution.

This link between sexual abuse and homosexual male prostitution has been echoed by many other writers. For instance, Search (1988: 31) writes, 'The statistics present a horrifying picture...almost all male prostitutes were sexually abused as children.' So confident is she of this claim that she omits any reference to the source of these exceedingly interesting 'statistics'.

This line of argument has two important corollaries. First, sexual abuse (inevitably within the context of a 'problem' family) is presented as the ultimate explicatory factor. As a result, one object of fear (same-sex child abuse) is conveniently imbued with a sense of 'otherness' residing in the make-up of obvious social deviants, namely rentboys. Conversely, the 'alien' nature of homosexual male prostitution is affirmed via its essential link to child abuse. This theory — with its comforting circular method of abstraction — is clearly an attractive way of isolating two problems and placing them outside the quotidian. From this follow distinctive patterns of interaction, borrowed from child-abuse relations, and inherent in popular representations of the relationship between 'rentboy' and 'punter': the 'boy' is a disturbed, vindicative, but in the last instance powerless individual; the punter is a proto-abusive manipulator in whom ultimate power always rests. The boy's claim to power is evidence of self-delusion, and so further confirms his profoundly powerless position. This approach has implications for the manner in which clients respond to male prostitutes. As McMullen (1987) pointed out, courts tend to fine women prostitutes but recommend psychological reports on rentboys.

Second, and more importantly, most literature on male prostitutes, with the notable exception of Luckenbill (1985, 1986) and Reiss (1962), depicts the occupation as the last resort of the utterly powerless. In the tradition of classical criminology, a long list of variables, mixing the psychological and socio-economic, is offered to explain the irresistible forces which have confronted the subjects with prostitution as the only option. It is clear from many accounts that the authors cannot conceive of prostitution as a rationally chosen occupation, with the writers making a series of normative judgments about the 'real' interests of the prostitute, of which he is not necessarily aware, in order to explain his behaviour. He is *really* fighting for position, not money (Ginsburg, 1977); he is *really* directing anger against his father (Coombs, 1974); or he is *really* seeking a victory over his childhood abuser (McMullen, 1987). Since the prostitute has no power over himself, it is scarcely surprising that these writers perceive the homosexual male prostitute to be powerless in other ways. There can be no *real* power battles in the life of the homosexual male prostitute, because, by very virtue of what he is doing, he has lost all ability to fight. As Caukins and Coombs (1976: 441) write: 'To be successful in the profession, a prostitute must be... willing to do anything sexually that the customer wants.'

From the viewpoint of HIV/AIDS health promotion these stereotypes are important. A powerless individual is presumably incapable of changing his behaviour, and if this is the case, notions of health education might usefully be forsaken in favour of a mass round-up of clients and prostitutes. This chapter therefore attempts to describe the diverse knowledge and lifestyles of London's male prostitutes in those aspects relevant to epidemiology and HIV/AIDS health education and health promotion.

The Study

The investigation which is reported here was funded by the AIDS Education and Research Trust (AVERT) and carried out as part of Project SIGMA, an investigation into aspects of the social behaviour of gay men under the impact of AIDS. As noted above, there are two main types of male homosexual prostitutes, streetworking prostitutes and non-streetworking prostitutes, and given the nature of their employment, different methods were used to investigate each group. The term 'non-streetworking prostitute' will be used interchangeably with the term 'call-men', a more accurate title than call-boy given that the median age of the non-streetworkers in this study was 25.

Non-streetworking prostitutes and their clients were contacted by placing advertisements in some of the publications that the prostitutes themselves use to advertise their services, namely *Capital Gay, Gay Times* and *Him*. Our advertisement called for those willing to participate in this research to come forward. From those who responded, a 'snowballing' to friends and acquaintances was also undertaken.

This group cannot be claimed to be representative of all non-streetworking prostitutes, principally because the features of the population are not known. What is certain is that there are extreme variations in the prostitutes' levels of engagement in their trade, from those who see one client every one or two months to those who meet four or five a day. What is significant about the interviewed group is that they or their friends volunteered for interview, thus introducing a particular response bias. By way of contrast, the majority of streetworkers contacted in their trading places were initially suspicious and uncomprehending about the aims and function of this research.

Taped unstructured interviews of two and a half hours' duration were conducted initially with five non-streetworking prostitutes and two of their clients. These interviews served as a pilot for subsequent more structured interviews and provided information about the appropriate terminology, structure and range of topics. Field notes made subsequent to these initial meetings were also used to inform the administration of the final schedule. The final structured two and a half hour interviews dealt with the same subject areas as the earlier unstructured interviews, and used a mixture of pre-coded and post-coded questions. Twenty non-streetworkers and two of their clients were interviewed using this latter schedule, making a total of twenty-five non-streetworkers and four clients in all.

Participant observation in the places of contact was undertaken with streetworkers accompanied by ethnographic and semi-structured interviews with twenty-eight prostitutes and five clients. Many streetworking prostitutes consume amounts of alcohol and drugs while at the trading places, and therefore some of the interviews conducted have been less coherent than was perhaps desirable, and of necessity the questioning and recording were less standardized.

Demography

In contrast to the dominant images of the male homosexual prostitute earlier discussed, the backgrounds of respondents were far from uniform. Concentrating first on the twenty-five call-men, it is difficult to identify any generalities which support the notion that prostitution is the product of 'unstable' backgrounds. They were not 'runaways' or 'throwaways', but had left their parents' homes on reasonably amicable terms (nine were indigenous to London); twenty-one had two living parents, about a fifth of whom were divorced or separated; and twenty-two described a close relationship with at least one parent, usually the mother. Ties were, in general, maintained with at least one sibling; and perhaps most significantly, at least one 'close' relative knew that the respondent was gay. The traditional account of the heterosexual prostitute, most famously presented in Reiss's (1962) work, but universalized by others (Butts, 1947; Coombs, 1973; Harris, 1973; Ginsburg, 1967; MacNamara, 1965), does not gain support from our research. All but two respondents felt themselves to be 'exclusively homosexual', the exceptions labelling themselves 'mainly homosexual but a degree of heterosexual'.

Perhaps predictably, the 'disorderly background' tag is more easily pinned on the streetworking prostitutes: four had been in children's homes; five came from 'problem' backgrounds involving alcohol abuse or physical abuse; the parents of eleven were divorced or separated (as opposed to six of the non-streetworkers), and where the boy identified as gay, his parents were less likely to know. Importantly, about a quarter identified themselves as heterosexual. For eight streetworkers, all links with family were severed, and a flight to London searching for fortune but leading to prostitution was a more common scenario for the streetworkers (twelve as opposed to two non-streetworkers). Even where this was so, however, nineteen of the respondents had previously engaged in other, but less profitable, forms of prostitution in their home town. The 'corrupted' provincial innocent seems to be a minority character, with only three respondents recognizable in such terms.

Accounts which explain male homosexual prostitution in terms of child sexual abuse are not supported by evidence collected in this study. Only two of the call-men reported having experienced sexual abuse, and this had been in their late teens. Although extremely upsetting, the incidents had not marked any changing point in their sexuality. While the others reported genital experiences with a partner from as young as 11, all of the reported incidents were consensual in any meaningful use of the term. For the streetworkers, the picture was less clear, and because of its sensitivity, sexual abuse was an extremely difficult topic to raise in the public contexts in which the data were collected. Five out of thirteen respondents questioned on the matter reported incidents of abuse, and in three of these cases the abuser had paid the boy, perhaps in an attempt to make the non-consensual appear voluntary (McMullen, 1987). Those rentboys concerned interpreted the experience as one in which an economic opportunity has become apparent to them, rather than the beginning of some psychological spiral descent.

Explaining Male Homosexual Prostitution

One explanation for male prostitution which was explicitly advanced by every male prostitute interviewed is financial. Most rentboys depict themselves as being (within limits) free agents, rationally responding to economic deprivation — or in the cases of the wealthier call-men the desire for monetary accumulation. When the streetworkers and the non-streetworkers were asked why, principally, they became involved in their work and why they remained so, their replies were without exception variants on the theme: 'Money, of course', or 'I wouldn't do it if it wasn't for the money, would I?' Indeed, to enquire into such matters is to be perceived as asking 'stupid questions', so obvious was the answer in the respondents' minds. It is astonishing that so simple a rationale has been given so little credence by previous researchers.

Even a crudely materialist analysis of this kind certainly makes more sense of the data than a psychological one, and where the most consistent distinctions between the two types of rentboy become apparent is in the socio-economic demography of background and present situation. Succinctly, the non-street-workers tend to come from more affluent, educated backgrounds, and to have obtained higher educational qualifications. Their prostitutional work thereby presupposes some degree of material stability, in that they must have access to a telephone and a residence in which to receive telephone calls. This financial outlay is unnecessary for the streetworkers. Non-streetworking prostitution involves skills which are commonly associated with 'middle-class' occupations (see Coxon and Davies, 1986), such as the ability to engage in diverting conversation and the ability to act as a casual counsellor. Predictably, therefore, this form of prostitution is more lucrative than streetwork, and the prostitutes involved tend to be more professional, both objectively in that their work is far more likely to entail specializations such as sado-masochistic practices involving relatively sophisticated technology, and subjectively in that they are more ready to identify as prostitutes or sex workers.

The importance of the conversational and 'counselling' role of the non-streetworker was corroborated by the men themselves and their clients. Almost all call-men, when asked to compare their jobs with another, named 'social worker', and all said that conversation was a vital part of their jobs. Conversely, most streetworkers were at a loss to think of any job by way of comparison, but a few saw companionship or conversation as vital. Similarly, the punters who saw call-men all emphasized the conversational skills of the boy as important. 'You can have a nice, pleasant chat with most of the boys I see', said Keith; but he also remarked, comparing his earlier experiences with streetboys: 'These middle-class boys may be much nicer, but they do tend to be rather (sexually) inhibited.' Another client, Mr Humphries, whose preference was exclusively for streetworkers, particularly those who identified themselves as heterosexual, described call-men as 'extremely boring', emphasizing that his desire was for quick, unfettered sex. Throughout our meeting he bemoaned the passing of the days when one could engage in quick, easy encounters with guardsmen, often in the foliage of London's parks. Richard, on the other hand, another client, succinctly articulated his preference for call-men above streetworkers thus: 'I want an escort, not a whore.'

The call-men's fee started at £25 per hour, with the majority charging £35 to £40 per hour. Clients pay one-third on top of this if their prostitutes work for an agency. In general, call-men travelled to clients' houses, and this tended to be more lucrative than having an 'in-call', although as services are frequently required at post-London Underground hours, an additional £10 or £15 was often paid by the punter for taxi fares. Streetworkers' income was less predictable, and there was a tendency for many of them, when asked about the financial side of their occupation, to relate anecdotes which tell of dubiously high sums of money (i.e. £150) paid for occasions in which they were required to do 'hardly anything' — a phrase which on closer scrutiny usually acts as a euphemism for masturbating the client to orgasm. Tales about the prices charged by others are often more revealing. One boy pointed at various rentboys, saying, 'He'll do it for a tenner', or 'He usually gets £30.' The market price is far more volatile, but it seems that most expect to receive £20 to £25 for a 'session'. The younger, more attractive and assertive ones report an occasional rise to £50. However, many at the end of the evening will go home with a client for £10, or nothing at all so long as accommodation is provided. It is interesting to note that all the call-men as well as their clients denied that the amount paid varies according to sexual acts.

Streetworkers were reluctant to identify themselves either as prostitutes or as rentboys. On the first visit to a rent pub, for example, a tall, broad skinhead asked what I did for a living. I replied: 'I'm doing research into gay male prostitutes.' He replied: I'm not a prostitute and if my girlfriend heard you call me gay, she'd glass you in the face.' Whether or not this was pure hyperbole I did not wait to find out. On a subsequent occasion the question: 'Are you a rentboy' met this response: 'I'm not a rentboy, but I do punters, understand?' Henceforth, I did. On the other hand, all the call-men accepted 'prostitute' as a title, although most said that they preferred the term 'escort' or 'masseur' or some other more euphemistic description.

What emerges from this preliminary work is a picture of the homosexual male prostitute, subject to the same socio-economic forces as any other person. Male homosexual prostitution can, thus, be seen as job, rather than a psychological condition — in direct contradiction to the pathological models advanced by much of the existing literature.

Support Networks

The support networks used by prostitutes were also informed by the socio-economic status of the individual concerned. In particular, they were related to value systems characteristic of the prostitutes' social location. Thus to the simple question, 'Whom do you turn to when you feel down', Tim, a masseur, replied: 'Family, friends and the boyfriend, of course — like anyone else.' This affirmation of a lifestyle consisting of conventional support components was common to almost all the non-streetworkers and, as described earlier, family links remained intact for most of this group. It is significant that the call-men identified themselves as gay — in fact nearly three-quarters (18) said they were 'exclusively homosexual', the other quarter saying they were 'mainly homosexual but with a degree of heterosexuality'. As might be expected, this meant that they were all well integrated into the 'gay community': most of their friends were other gay men, all but one knew other call-men, and with the exception of one person all had become knowledgeable of this kind of prostitution because friends involved had suggested it to them. For all respondents, close friends knew of their work, although over half (14) also had friends who were ignorant of this. Only a third (8) had regular boyfriends, all but two of whom were similarly employed. One of these knew, but the relationship with his partner had ceased to be sexual, while the other remained in blissful ignorance. Kevin, an escort, commented: 'It puts an unbearable strain on a relationship if one of you is on the game, and the other one isn't — I just don't think you can have a relationship unless you're both doing it.' While relationships with clients rarely developed beyond the professional, over three-quarters of the non-streetworking prostitutes had at one time seen a client on the level of a non-sexual friendship.

Given the very different social organization of the streetworkers, it should come as no surprise to learn that their support networks were very different. In both the pubs and the outdoor pick-up places there exists a 'hard-core' of regulars who tend to socialize together. In the outdoor trading-places, however, they generally stand apart from one another with the intention of attracting the attention of clients, regrouping after a period of, say, 15 minutes if none has been successful. Triads or pairs will eventually leave the scene of work together if individuals have not already departed with a client. In the bars this 'hard-core' also socialize together, moving to different bars and clubs in groups. Individuals new to the scene stand alone, although eventually become integrated if they appear often enough. On the basis of group conversations it seems (as in many a pub conversation) that the participants mislead, brag and hector one another. They jokingly accuse one another of being 'slags', the jokes sometimes erupting into open hostility. One conversation, typical of many that I have witnessed, ran thus: 'So d'you want to suck my cock, like you do all the old men', said one boy to another, simultaneously thrusting his hand towards his companion's groin. 'Fuck off, fuck off', replied the accosted boy, attempting to push his assailant from him. The aggressor was eventually repulsed by a blow to the arm, accompanied by this verbal ejaculation: 'I never fucking suck anyone's cock, right?'[1]

The other principal support relations which exist for streetworkers are with the clients themselves, although, as might be predicted, these relationships are often more problematic. In the bar, for example, regular clients will frequently chat with prostitutes whom they have previously paid for sex, although they are never allowed into rentboys' conversations. Similarly, boys will appear with customers who are temporarily providing them with accommodation and funds. Often the boys will depart with another client, although they may reappear in the bar with their 'sugardaddy' the next day.[2]

These support networks have a double function in relation to HIV/AIDS health education and health promotion: they are both possible and actual conduits for the acquisition of HIV-related knowledge, as well as contexts for empowerment through collective decision-making, or the simple exercise of group pressure. Non-streetworkers' knowledge about safer sex, and their punters', was extremely comprehensive relative to that of the streetworkers. This was ascertained when respondents were asked to place different sexual acts into three different categories — 'high risk', 'low risk' and 'no risk' — rated using the Terrence Higgins Trust (THT) guidelines (1989) on 'safer sex'. All the call-men (accurately) saw receptive and insertive anal sex as high risk activities. The 'no-risk' activities (masturbation, body rubbing, dry kissing, use of non-shared sex toys) were also correctly categorized by all the call-men. There was a tendency, however, to overestimate the risks involved in 'low risk' activities. About three-quarters (17) of this group classified active sucking to orgasm and active rimming as 'high risk'. All, on the other hand, viewed insertive and receptive anal sex with a condom as 'low risk'. Here their evaluations differed from those of the THT which argues that penetrative sex with a condom is the most dangerous activity after unprotected penetrative sex.

Streetworkers have as yet been subjected to less detailed scrutiny, but with the exception of the more educated streetworkers mentioned earlier (who exhibit very similar understandings to the call-men, stressing body fluids as well as condoms) the emphasis here is entirely on condoms. For streetworkers, 'safe sex' (note the omission of the 'r') is synonymous with condom use, pure and simple, of any brand or strength, with or without lubricants. Representative of many an enquiry about safer sex made in the course of conversing with streetworkers is this exchange, which took place in a pub: 'I've only been fucked once, and then fully protected', said a prostitute, who had earlier claimed never to have been the receiving partner in anal intercourse. 'Yes, what condoms did you use?', I asked. 'I don't know.' Did you use a lubricant?' 'Well, spit, but anyway I was fully protected.' The possibility of a condom failure, especially when non-water-based lubricants are used, makes this a dangerous approach to adopt.

The Negotiation of Sex: Circumstances and Outcome

The client will bring certain desires and expectations to an encounter with a homosexual male prostitute. Whether or not these are realized is largely dependent on his ability to negotiate with the prostitute. This ability is, in turn, dependent on the desires, power and skills of the prostitute. For the call-men, the rules of negotiation are rigid relative to those of streetworkers. Their nature varies between masseurs and escorts since the former advertize independently, while the latter use an agency which places advertisements. Accordingly, the masseur has immediate direct telephone contact with the client, which he will generally use to speak of price, duration and 'if pushed' the services provided. The agency, on the other hand, will act as a broker, relating information about the escorts to the clients and vice versa. The behaviour of the agency is not within the control of the escort, and can sometimes result in a less than accidental mismatching of prostitute with client. Escort Mark complained about occasions when his agency had sent him to clients who had, he felt sure, desired a different physical type, citing one example:

> I went to see this Arab guy — and I quite fancied him, because I really like Arabs — but as soon as he opened the door I could see that he didn't like me. He said: 'You're late' and I was a bit late, but I got this feeling that he wanted someone a bit more, you know, boyish. I could just tell when he looked at me that I wasn't what he was expecting. So he just gave me the taxi fare home.

Tim experienced a great amount of difficulty with the negotiating process, with the result that he acquiesced frequently in clients' requests which other prostitutes refused. There were, it seems, two principal reasons for this. First, his agency had offered him few guidelines on how to act with the clients; second, he know no- one else who was on the game. For instance, asked if he normally found it difficult to terminate a meeting with a client, he replied:

> I'm given no guidelines about how long to spend. I think it would be nice in a way to say 'look you've got one hour' and the person knows they've got one hour, then you've got something to fall back on. But when you haven't you — it's very difficult....I don't get much feedback from the agency. I don't get any feedback at all.

As a result, Tim admitted that he often spent two or three hours with a client, as opposed to the one to one and a half hour sessions common to other escorts. After asking me what I knew about other escorts, he was surprised to learn how little it was possible to 'get away with'. This was particularly evident when it came to anal sex. Tim was not merely the only call-man without other call-men for friends, but also the only one currently having regular penetrative sex with his clients (although always with condoms). Asked how confident he felt about the services he provides, he answered: 'I don't think I'm very good. I don't think I'm giving them very much.'

Most of the other call-men said they had felt this way at the beginning of their careers as prostitutes, and it was comparing their experiences with others who were similarly employed that made them less worried about the limitations of the service they offered. Escort Kevin said: 'At the beginning, before I'd really talked about things with other escorts, I'd thought, you had to fuck and everything, but now I feel fine about just sticking to a hand-job.' Masseur Gerry also remarked: 'You go and meet people in a bar, and talk about the punters — the gorgeous one you had, the ugly one you had, the weird one — and if someone, for instance, says they've been fucked, then everyone else will say "You must be mad to do that", so I think that does make a difference.'

Length of time 'on the game' was perceived by all the prostitutes as a chief determining factor on the ability to negotiate. All said they felt more confident and assertive now than they had done when they had first engaged in prostitution. Although only one of the non-streetworkers now had anal sex with clients, just over a third (9) had done so in their prostitutional careers. Three of these had been fucked without protection at least once, and for only one of them had this predated knowledge of HIV safer sex. Mark recalled his one experience of prostitutional penetration: 'He was lying on top of me, and I really didn't realize that he slid it in, and then — I know it was really stupid — I didn't feel I could stop him.'

When asked who they felt was in control of an encounter, all the call men named themselves. However, so also did the clients, leading to the suggestion that it may be necessary for both parties to share this belief if the situation is to be negotiated well. It is interesting to note how those who have been longest on the game describe their roles: 'I'm always completely in control, I can usually see things about their sexuality that they can't even see themselves — I can make them want what I want them to do', said Derek, a masseur, who claims now never to fuck or to suck with clients. Instead, he always adopts a 'dominant' role in a sado-masochistic scenario with most of the session being taken up with insulting, beating or whipping; with direct physical contact, and genital contact in particular, being kept to a minimum. Gerry, a masseur with a seven-year prostitutional career, also specialized in similar skills, saying: 'In some ways, you know, AIDS hasn't been such a bad thing for us — there's a lot more demand for the kinky things, which are much more pleasant to do than fucking.' Such activities may be particularly important in the context of HIV since they provide pleasure without the exchange of body fluids. Younger prostitutes, on the other hand, especially streetworkers, are less likely to have knowledge of or use these specialities and are accordingly forced back into a more limited repertoire of sexual activities which may include the exchange of body fluids.

Non-streetworkers and their clients were asked in detail about their sexual activities over the last month: specifically how many times (if at all) they had actively or passively wanked, sucked, fucked, rimmed, fingered, fisted, scatted, douched, body-rubbed, thigh-fucked, massaged, deeply kissed and engaged in water-sports or corporal punishment. These questions were asked of activities both off and on the game. On the game, only one prostitute had engaged in fucking — three times as the receiving partner — while one client had been similarly engaged, twice, also as the receiving partner. Only one of the call-men had not sucked in the last month, receptive and (to a slightly lesser degree) insertive sucking being an almost routine part of the occasion. None of the respondents (prostitutes or clients) had used condoms for oral sex, but none reported ejaculation in the mouth. None of the call-men had rimmed — in fact, most expressed aversion at the idea — although just over a third had been rimmed by their clients. There were only three instances of scat and watersports, two involving the same boy and the other involving a client, and one act of douching. Only three call-men admitted to any deep kissing, although all the clients said that they had deep kissed their boys. All prostitutes reported having wanked a client to orgasm and all clients reported having been wanked, and apart from the exceptional cases of fucking reported, this was the commonest cause of orgasm. Mutual wanking was almost ubiquitous, but the prostitute was far less likely to climax than the client. All the call-men said they had never and would never engage in unprotected anal sex, even for an unusually large fee.

Far more worrying among the non-streetworkers interviewed were their sexual activities off the game. Unprotected anal sex, although not common, was far more likely than in prostitutional sex. Protected fucking was also more common, and condom failure — breakages and incidents of slipping off — were reported. Escort Paul articulated succinctly what many of the prostitutes were saying about the relative riskiness of their non-prostitutional sex: 'When it's real sex, I want to do something different from what you do with the punters — some of those things you can't do.' This reaction indicates that rigid adherence to safer sex guidelines within paid relations may increase the desire for riskier practices outside. This conclusion is paralleled by findings from Day's (1989) research into prostitute women and HIV. She found that while most of her respondents always used condoms with paying partners, they did not usually do so with non-paying partners. Many other respondents explained this by distinguishing between sex with lovers and the sex involved in their work.

Streetworkers had very different ways of meeting clients, and these altered the rules of negotiation. Considering many pick-ups take place in bars, an important factor which influences the ability to negotiate here is the consumption of alcohol and, occasionally, illegal drugs. Participant observation has suggested that most of the rentboys tend to reach a fairly severe degree of inebriation before the bars they work in close. Also bars and clubs tend to be foci for the distribution of illegal drugs, and many of the prostitutes will take either hash or barbiturates in the course of an evening.

Both in the bar and outdoors approaches are sometimes made by the boys and sometimes by the clients: there is no fixed rule about this. Outdoors the punters tend to stand relatively still, while the boys circle around them. Eyes will meet and an approach will be made. They will negotiate for maybe a minute, and then leave. In the bar the client will sometimes buy the boy a drink, over which they will negotiate further, before leaving the venue. In both these situations negotiation is relatively informal compared with that between call-men and their clients.

Lack of accommodation is another factor that can place streetworkers in a weaker bargaining position than the call-men. Asked where they live, about a third of those spoken to replied: 'with friends', 'round and about', and similar phrases indicative of the fact they have no fixed address. Some will stay for periods with a particular punter, moving on to another one after some time, or leaving on the request of the client. Few seem to sleep outdoors regularly, although over half of those spoken to said that they had done this on occasion. Hostels are available in London, but demand for beds exceeds the supply and there are limits to the length of time that people are allowed to stay. Thus for many streetworkers, the cost of refusing clients' demands is greater, and their power to resist the requests of the client, including a possible desire for high risk sex, is substantially reduced.

This is corroborated by the reports from streetworkers and their confidants. John, who is now 24 and a streetworker since 16, knows many of the regulars in a particular bar. He claimed that all the boys, whether or not they admitted it, engaged in active and passive oral sex. He also claimed that at least half sometimes engaged in anal sex: 'They're going to tell you that they don't do it, but I know for a fact that a lot do and they're not always that careful either, especially if they're pissed out of their brains!' The search for accommodation, he argued, was often the overriding reason why boys accompanied clients home where the younger or weaker ones, he maintained, often found it difficult to resist demands for unprotected anal sex. John himself claimed that he now rarely fucked with punters. He asked a fee of at least £70 for an active fuck, while he always refused to be the receiving partner. However, until about two years ago he had engaged in unprotected fucking, actively and passively.

Those streetworkers who were not integrated in the core of regulars (about a third) maintained that they never fucked on the game — 'I save that for the boyfriend', said one. The rest maintained that they always used condoms. None of the regulars would admit to engaging in anal sex, but when a 'friend' was not present, they often accused the absent person of such behaviour, the accused frequently returning the compliment at a later time.

Both the clients of streetworkers who were interviewed in depth about their sexual practices claimed to (actively) fuck regularly with protection, although one of them had not done so in the last month. The other, who had fucked, had used condoms. However, both admitted to having fucked without a condom in the last year. Of the punters spoken to in or at a trading-place, most claimed to fuck or be fucked by prostitutes, although they did not always demand it. Again the need for condoms was acknowledged, but so also with many was the resigned recognition that high risk sex was in some cases almost unavoidable.

Off the game the rentboys' sexual activities exhibited similar trends to those of the call-men. Both the 'heterosexuals' and the 'bisexuals' had unprotected sex with their wives or girlfriends, and reacted aggressively to the suggestion that they should do otherwise: 'Do you think I'm fucking well going to give her AIDS?' was one reply. The bisexuals acknowledged participating in non-prostitutional homosexual activities, and most claimed to 'nearly always' use condoms during anal sex. The openly gay prostitutes also said that they sometimes had unprotected anal sex with boyfriends, and justified this by explaining the need to depro-fessionalize non-prostitutional sex as a prerequisite to pleasure.

Conclusions

On the basis of this research it is difficult to corroborate the views and conclusions which can be found in the canon of literature on the subject of homosexual male prostitution. Where the dominant voices seek to present the fundamental innocence, naiveté and powerlessness of the male prostitute, this research finds otherwise. It is less than accurate to think in terms of a single character type which represents all homosexual male prostitutes. Most obviously in the distinction between call-men and streetworkers, there are different social and economic factors working on actors from different social, economic and educational backgrounds. Among the streetworkers, who hitherto have been the virtually exclusive focus of academic or journalistic interest, we find a variety of different backgrounds, sexual identities, reasons for working as prostitutes and attitudes towards work. Of course, it is possible to look to child abuse as the single factor which explains a still morally uncomfortable form of behaviour from individuals who appear to share few common characteristics. Unfortunately, our evidence from this study does not support this theory.

Thus we are compelled to examine different kinds of homosexual male prostitute in their specificity, and to look to financial and educational status, combined with knowledge of life on the game, as the principal factors determining the power of the prostitute. This way it becomes clear that the prostitute is not by nature or character a powerless victim, but a person whose ability to make and carry out considered decisions about his life depends on factors such as whether he can afford to rent a place to live; whether he can afford telephone installation; whether he has the kind of educational background which enables him to organize himself as a small businessman; whether he has a set of supportive friends, family or acquaintances; whether he knows other people similarly employed with whom he can discuss his experiences and make collective decisions about the sexual acts he will or will not perform with clients; whether or not he is comfortable with his sexual identity; whether or not he is integrated in the gay scene and therefore more likely to be exposed to explicit debate around HIV and safer sex; how experienced he is at negotiating with the client; whether he has specialized sexual skills to offer which can be substituted for practices which involve the exchange of body fluids; and whether or not he consumes alcohol and drugs which alter his ability or desire to negotiate safer sex. The amount of knowledge a prostitute has about HIV and ways of reducing risk is dependent on many of these factors, as is his ability to act upon that knowledge.

Homosexual male prostitutes must ultimately be seen as an amorphous group or set of subgroups containing individuals who have been subject to, and are still influenced by, the same forces which emanate from the (albeit shifting) social structures of our society. Given such understanding, no magical explanation or essential factor buried in the substratum of the prostitute's character need be sought to 'explain' prostitutes' actions and behaviour. Instead, practical assistance is needed by a set of people with concrete, material problems.

Notes

1   This encounter brought into play certain preoccupations that many of the streetworkers have concerning their gender. The effect is to make honest discussion about their prostitutional sexual practices problematic, both among themselves and with a researcher. These complications seem to be singular to the streetworkers; the 'out' gay self-identification of the call-men neutralizes the problem to a large extent. About half the streetworkers ($N = 13$) were prepared to identify themselves as gay, another quarter ($N = 7$) as bisexual, the remainder ($N = 8$) as heterosexual. However, it is significant that the assailed boy in question identifies as gay, yet partakes in the dogma which sees certain 'passive' sexual activities as shameful. Of those who identify as bisexual, a large number took pains to speak firstly and — unless directed away from the topic — exclusively of their sexual relations with their girlfriends. All the 'bisexuals' and 'heterosexuals' — and many of the others — questioned me at an early stage about my sexual preferences. This was rarely a topic raised by non-streetworkers, their assumption being that it would inevitably transpire that I, too, was gay.

Doing fieldwork accompanied by a woman has, in both the cases in which this has been undertaken, resulted in an ostentatious degree of attention being paid to the women by the rentboys, myself being called upon to corroborate their opinions on the sexual desirability of the women in question. This is reminiscent of Reiss's (1962) argument that hustlers' anxiety about their masculinity resulted in excessive displays of behaviour denoting heterosexuality. However, the 'bisexuals', in conversation with me — and having perceived, after much questioning, my own uncomplicated treatment of my homosexuality — have eventually spoken more relaxedly of their homosexual experiences. Statements have ensued which contradict earlier affirmations designed to establish perceived limitations to the subject's homosexual potential. (This is of utmost importance in regard to the discussion of sexual practices and will be dealt with later.)

Interestingly, though, there are no barriers to the social integration of the 'gays', 'bisexuals' and 'heterosexuals' within the pub/club environment.

2   A 'sugardaddy' may be defined as an older man who gives a younger one regular financial or other material supplements in return for his company and some sexual favours.

References

Butts, W.M. (1947) 'Boy Prostitutes of the Metropolis', *Journal of Clinical Psychopathology*, 8, 673–681.

Caukins, S.E. and Coombs, N.R. (1976) 'The Psychodynamics of Male Prostitution', *American Journal of Psychotherapy*, 30, 441–451.

Churchill, W. (1967) *Homosexual Behaviour among Males*, New York, Hawthorn Books.

Coleman, E. (1989) 'The Development of Male Prostitution Activity among Gay and Bisexual Adolescents' in G. Herdt, (Ed.) *Gay and Lesbian Youth*, New York, Haworth Press.

Coombs, N.R. (1974) 'Male Prostitution: A Psychosocial View of Behaviour', *American Journal of Orthopsychiatry*, 44, 782–789.

Coxon, A.P.M. and Davies, P.M. with Jones, C.L. (1986) *Images of Social Stratification: Occupation, Status and Class*, London, Sage.

Craft, M. (1966) 'Boy Prostitutes and Their Fate', *British Journal of Psychiatry*, 112, 1111–1114.

Davies, P. and Simpson, P. (1990) 'On Male Homosexual Prostitution and HIV', in P. Aggleton, P. Davies and G. Hart (Eds) *AIDS: Individual, Cultural and Policy Dimensions*, Lewes, Falmer Press.

Day, S. (1989) 'Prostitute Women and the Ideology of Work in London', unpublished paper presented at the Third Conference on Social Aspects of AIDS, South Bank Polytechnic, London.

Ginsburg, K.N. (1967) 'The Meat Rack: A Study of the Male Homosexual Prostitute', *American Journal of Psychotherapy*, 21, 170–185.

Harris, M. (1973) *The Dilly Boy: The Game of Male Prostitution in Piccadilly*, London, Croom Helm.

Hoffman, M. (1972) 'The Male Prostitute', *Sexual Behaviour*, 2, 19–21.

Humphreys, L. (1972) 'Dollars Take Priority over Love', *Sexual Behaviour*, 2, 19.

Luckenbill, D.F. (1985) 'Entering Male Prostitution', *Urban Life*, 14, 131–153.

Luckenbill, D.F. (1986) 'Deviant Career Mobility: The Case of Male Prostitutes', *Social Problems*, 33, 283–298.

McMullen, R. (1988) 'Youth Prostitution: A Balance of Power', *Journal of Adolescence*, 10, 35–43.

MacNamara, D.E.J. (1965) 'Male Prostitution in American Cities: A Socioeconomic or Pathological Phenomenon?' *American Journal of Orthopsychiatry*, 35, 204.

Reiss, A.J. (1962) 'The Social Problems of Queers and Peers', *Social Problems*, 9, 102–119.

Search, G. (1988) *The Last Taboo: Sexual Taboo of Children*, Harmondsworth, Penguin.

Chapter 8

Towards a General Model of Sexual Negotiation

Peter Davies and Peter Weatherburn

In the preamble to a paper in the second volume of this series we read,

> It has...been a strange experience over the last few years, to hear in conferences throughout the world, scientists from many disciplines addressing large and growing audiences on the intricate and intimate details of male homosexual practice. (Davies, 1989)

This process, which Michel Pollak (1988) has termed the *banalisation* of homosexuality, has not only inured those of us on the conference circuit to discussions of sex[1] but has validated — or, more accurately, revalidated — a particular discourse of sex and sexuality (see Watney's comments, Ch. 1, this volume), which is empirical, epidemiological and atomistic.

It would be otiose to list all those conference papers, journal articles and chapters which claim to increase our knowledge about the factors associated with the practice of unsafe sex among homosexually active men (from here on, any reference to sexual behaviour not otherwise qualified will be to male homosexual practice). As we will seek to explain, we have become disenchanted with and distrustful of the search for such factors and believe that part of the reason for the stultification of research in this area is a failure of the imagination: specifically, the failure to see through the assumptions that lie deeply embedded in the medicalized discourse of AIDS research. In the first part of this chapter we examine some of these assumptions; in the second we sketch a preliminary attempt at a more informed and, we hope, productive understanding of sexual behaviour.

Take One? Take Two

We begin with the problem of causality, a central debate in the social sciences and despite the number of contributions a seemingly intractable one.[2] The problem, and that of inductive knowledge to which it is closely linked, revolves around the leap of faith that is required to move from the observation that *x* is related to or correlated with *y* to the statement that *x* causes *y*. Statistical tests allow us to say with an exact certitude whether a particular relationship exists; they do not allow us to draw any conclusions about the causal status of that relationship. Thus we might discover that unsafe sex is correlated with, say, perceived HIV status, but to move from that observation to the assertion that the one causes the other is not straightforward. Such a statement is possible only after a theoretical link is established between the two phenomena. Epidemiology (the medics' social science) and, it has to be said, much contemporary American sociology have always relied heavily on statistical techniques, but ridden relatively lightly on the theory which allows such techniques to inform statements about cause. The emergence of the computer and the consequent wide availability of powerful statistical techniques have ensured that any data set will be beaten into submission by multiple logistic regression, log-linear analysis or whatever the preferred instrument is. Unfortunately, this automatic recourse to number crunching can all too easily take the place of sustained critical thought. Thus papers report that such and such a list of variables is associated with unsafe sex (or HIV antibody status or progression to AIDS), with the implication that these are in some sense causal. This may or may not be the case.

We do not suggest that such data dredging is without utility. Such techniques can, in principle, throw up hitherto unsuspected relationships which further investigation and theorization may reveal as important. We have performed such analyses ourselves, hoping for such a lead, only to be disappointed. For example, one such analysis (Davies *et al.*, in press) isolated those variables associated with the practice of anal intercourse among our cohort of 930 men. These were (gay) relationship status; their wish that they had been given a pill at birth that would make them heterosexual; a reported attempt at suicide; self-assessed sex appeal; perceived HIV antibody status; and educational level. What, precisely, are we to make of such information? We might use these data to assemble an identikit of the man likely to have unsafe sex. He would have a current regular sexual relationship, wish that he had been born heterosexual (but not regret the fact that he was gay, as another question asked), have made an attempt at suicide and regard himself as of above average sex appeal. It is far from clear what utility such a portrait has. We do not assume that only those who share all the characteristics above are the only ones to have unsafe sex, nor is it the case (we can conclude from the statistical model used) that the more variables on which an individual scores, the more likely it is that he will have unsafe sex. Thus we must conclude that any one of these qualifications puts an individual at risk — and which of us does not qualify under one or other of these headings?

Here the researcher is faced with an exquisite dilemma. The first temptation is to 'publish and be damned': to increase the number of publications on the subject by one; to bolster the curriculum vitae and enhance one's reputation among the 'never mind the quality, feel the width' school of academic advancement, which is more concerned with the length of a publication list than the contribution to knowledge or to an understanding of the social context of AIDS that the list represents. Alternatively, one can fall prey to the brooding fear that the data that have occupied years in collection and months in analysis are nonsense because of incompetence at questionnaire construction or data analysis or perhaps the respondents' truculence or sense of humour in misanswering lovingly constructed questions. Our preferred option is to publish the results of our investigations, being as honest as possible about their shortcomings and then to consider their import and implications.

We begin by examining some of the assumptions that lie behind these approaches to data and knowledge (see also Cohen, Ch. 2, this volume). Implicit in the analysis is the assumption that the cause of unsafe sexual behaviour is to be found in the characteristics of the individual. More specifically, those who engage in unsafe sex are presented as, in some sense, pathological: driven to this behaviour by malfunctions of the intellect or the emotions. The terminology is indicative: recidivism or relapse are the favoured terms for those who engage in unsafe sex after a period of safer activity, with implicit analogies to models of addictive behaviour.[3] The search in multivariate space for individuals who are in some sense disturbed, depressed, angry, or unable to realize their true desires is thus continued.

An allied assumption is that unsafe sex is irrational behaviour: a loss of control in the heat of the moment, a surrender by the intellect to the animal passions. As Prieur's (1990) important work has emphasized, this is simplistic. Penetration in our culture is paramount as an expression of power, the ultimate violation of self. The penetration of the anus carries a particularly potent charge and lies at the basis of much homophobia. The act of anal intercourse, therefore, imparts not only physical but symbolic pleasure: a pleasure that is essentially dangerous. It is dangerous because it blurs the boundaries of so many social categories. To add to the thrill of this ambiguity the danger of life-threatening infection only increases the statement of trust that accepting a man into your body makes.

These assumptions, which focus the search for the causes of unsafe sex in the characteristics of the individual, are one aspect of the atomism of social science. The roots of atomism — the individualistic fallacy — in Western social sciences are deep and far too tangled to excavate in this chapter (see, for example, Galtung, 1967:3ff). Attempts to move beyond statements about collectivities of individuals have come from the anthropologists (Parker, 1987; Kochems, 1987, for example) and what we might loosely term the post-modern critical theorists (Watney, 1987; Patton, 1985; Altman, 1986). This attention has focused, rightly — and in some cases with subsequent illumination — on the meanings implicit in sexual actions or discourses about sexuality and control. But there remains a tantalizing gap in the centre of our discussions, around the notion of the dyad: the couple who communicate sexually. Despite the rhetoric about interaction that permeates the social sciences, the dyad remains relatively unexamined. Discussions of dyadic interaction usually concentrate on the characteristics of individuals who form the dyads, while social psychology becomes interesting only at the level of the triad. Even the social network analysis, which claims the dyad as the logical primitive of its theorems, describes three formal properties of the dyad and moves on to consider patterns in the wider network (see Berkowitz, 1982). Attempts seriously to theorize the dyad are scarce.

One early attempt comes from the Jewish scholar Martin Buber. In his best-known work, *I and Thou* (1970), Buber is concerned with what he calls the 'realm of the between': what we, more prosaically, have termed the dyad. He distinguishes two modalities of the dyadic experience which he terms I-You (or I-Thou) and I-It, two fundamental forms of relation, the first of which tends to a totalizing, loving relationship, the latter towards a superficial, uninvolving objectification.[4] In one light, Buber does little more than restate and render an epithalamion on the distinction between sacred and profane love that has been the subject of literary endeavour for centuries. But it is particularly interesting from our current, restricted focus of attention. It is assumed that the individual will want to have safer, non-penetrative sex as an expression of love for the other. But this tendency is contradicted by the deeply rooted symbolic meaning of penetration as an expression of the same love. It is this contradiction that lies at the heart of the problem of safer sex.

It has become something of a commonplace to state that safer sex in particular, and sex in general, is the result of negotiation; for example, Fitzpatrick *et al.* state:

> One potential limitation of the Health Belief Model with regard to sexual behaviour is that it focuses upon individuals' perceptions in isolation, whereas most sex is social action. Sex involves at least two individuals and some form of relationship. (1990:122)

Quite so, though having stated the weakness at the heart of the approach, the remainder of the chapter concentrates on just those individual characteristics. What this most potently illustrates is the strength of atomism as a constraint on research: an example of a set of methods dictating the questions asked, rather than vice versa. One important outcome of this blinkered approach is the rather naive notion of negotiation which it all too often presents: a notion which restricts negotiation to the explicit and verbal and ignores the implicit and paralinguistic. It sees the negotiation of safer sex as a once and for all contract made verbally before or at the start of a sexual encounter and mediated only by the negotiating individuals' propensities, deficiencies and desires. By contrast, and as we will seek to make clear, we prefer a notion of negotiation which is continuous throughout the encounter, verbal and non-verbal and situated in a real physical and social context.

The restriction of attention to the explicit and verbal also obscures a number of the germane features of negotiation. First, the process of communication in general and the process of negotiation in particular are notoriously difficult to quantify. This is at least partly due to the unhelpful dichotomy, which also underlies conversation analysis and sociolinguistics, between the content of communication and the structures (both semantic and social) which underlie it. The distinction is generally unhelpful, but particularly so in the case of sexual communication because the content (particular sexual acts) forms part of the ramifying structure of the encounter and, conversely, the structural pattern of the session is at least part of the 'information' content.

This prefigures perhaps the most important point in this overlong preamble and one which is often paid lip-service, though rarely given prolonged consideration. Sex is communication. This is true in two senses. Externally, as it were, the decision agreement to have sex forms part of the ongoing dialogue between two or more individuals. This dialogue might be brief and predicated upon the expectation of sex — the casual pick-up — or part of a long, subtle and multistranded discussion — the long-term relationship. Within either of these dialogues the sexual encounter may have any number of specific meanings, often more than one in any one encounter: I love you; I hate you; I forgive you; do you love me; you are special, etc. Internally, the structure of the encounter will have its own internal logic or grammar which will carry certain other messages which may confirm or confuse the main message of the encounter. It is the protean nature of this relationship which has ensured its avoidance by the analyst. The imperatives of AIDS urge its understanding.

In conclusion, then, let us summarize. The tendency in discussions of the continuation or re-emergence of unsafe sexual behaviour has been to isolate the characteristics of those individuals who engage in unsafe sex. Recently, attempts have been made to elicit and explain the symbolic meanings of sexual acts, particularly unsafe acts. This leaves the path open for a theory of sexual behaviour in an epidemic which emphasizes the rational aspects of individuals' choices. Our contention is that this theory requires a sustained and serious examination of dyadic sexual communication in order to succeed in moulding together what are now very disparate bits of information. It is to the beginning of such an examination that we now turn.

The General Model

It is relatively straightforward to write down the general form of the model which underlies sexual behaviour in general, and safer sex in particular: it is much more difficult accurately to operationalize the model into a persuasive and usable form. A sexual relationship is a sequence of sessions or sexual encounters between two people (we recognize the popularity of sexual encounters between three or more, but for simplicity, we restrict attention to the pair). Clearly, the number of sessions in any one relationship may range from one in the case of a casual pick-up to some very large number in the case of a long-term sexual relationship.

Each of these sessions may, in turn, be described as a combination of five logically distinct factors. First, it involves two individuals, each with his own character, background, desires, needs, etc. These two are involved in an interaction which itself has certain identifiable features, and which forms the major focus of this discussion. This interaction takes place in a particular physical context, which also imposes constraints and imparts meaning to the encounter and, finally, the session occurs in a particular scenario — or psychic context.

We propose that the 'cause' of unsafe sexual behaviour is more profitably sought in the interaction of the encounter than in the characteristics of the individuals involved. In the rest of this section we will develop an outline of the processes involved in this interaction, while in Appendix A we present a formal description of the model. We specifically discuss the operation of power in the sexual interaction and propose a partial explanation of unsafe sex in those terms. While this explanation is tentative, our belief that the correct focus of interest is the interaction would not be negated should the specific explanation we propose be disproven.

One of the main difficulties in this approach is the fact that each session or situation is dynamically constructed by the individuals involved. From moment to moment, the shared definition of the situation, the perception of the roles in that situation of self and other will change. It is this sense of protean construction and reconstruction that makes unlikely the notion that an individual's ability to 'negotiate' safer sex can be assessed by the answering of carefully worded questions in the anodyne context of an interview or group discussion. What it also allows us to appreciate is the notion of sex as a process of insistent negotiation, agreement and compromise, and the occurrence of unsafe sex, our particular focus, as the result of decisions made by individuals in specific, real circumstances.

Let us consider the elements of the model in turn. As we have noted above, studies have traditionally looked at the individual engaging in unsafe sex for signs of irrationality or incipient pathology. While it may be the case that those who display such traits do indeed engage in unsafe sex, it is our contention that the majority of those who so engage are neither mad nor bad — and may be dangerous to know only in particular circumstances. We suggest that the relevant features of the individual's psyche will include: past sexual experience, preference for particular sexual acts, notions of masculinity, feelings about penetration, self-esteem, etc., but that these features are not fixed items in the individual's manifest. They will vary with mood, crucially with circumstance and, no doubt, other factors also.

As our preamble has suggested, we believe that the core of the model is the interaction. A sexual relationship, of whatever duration, begins before the sex itself begins. It will, perhaps, begin as the person decides to go out to look for a sexual partner, deciding what to wear, where to go, when to do so. The diversity of the sexual marketplace that comprises gay culture encourages specialization of this sort, though it clearly presupposes knowledge of this diversity. The specialization has strict norms, whose infringement causes social sanction. Who has not been amused by the appearance of the disco bunny in the leather bar, or the wrinkled clone at the agape of the body beautiful? This is a decision to look for someone who will be attracted to the image I am presenting, and a decision to present an image that the type of person I wish to attract will find appealing.

It is worth noting at this point that the confluences of desire that coalesce into the notion of preference are time-specific. I may, for example, today prefer the notion of sex with a disco bunny, tomorrow I may prefer a wrinkled clone. While there are those who are strongly attracted to a fixed 'type', there are many more, we vouch, whose (manifest if not avowed) preferences are more fluid.

The next stage is the pre-contract, where eye contact is made and reciprocated. This is the mutual agreement to engage in further (verbal or non-verbal) negotiation. But even at this stage a choice has been made, which involves the grounding of abstract desire in the individual. Standard data theory (deriving from Coombs, 1964) encourages us to think of individuals having a notion of the ideal sexual partner, from which they measure actual individuals, with the assumption that the closer one comes to this ideal, the more likely it is, *ceteris paribus*, that he will be preferred as a partner. It is particularly important to note that the distance from the ideal of the actual that I am willing to contemplate is itself a function of time. The man deemed acceptable a quarter of an hour before the club shuts might have been dismissed as quite unacceptable when the night was yet young.

The feeling of desire for the other and its reciprocation may seem a mystic process, not amenable to scientific description; but the problem is a practical one, not one of principle. *Ex post facto* I will be able to say, 'I liked his eyes/build/cock/...' or, less specifically, 'there was something about him....' In principle, therefore, the basis of attraction may, at least retrospectively, be established. Indeed, the statement, 'I like such-and-such a type' is an induced generalization from a number of such past experiences.

The important point in this concerning safer and unsafe sex is that the basis of the attraction may have important consequences. The psychoanalysts suggest, and their arguments are too complex to state at length here, that because our sexuality is mediated at the Oedipal crisis, which is the point at which our powerlessness within the nexus of relationships which constitute the family is recognized, we experience sexual desire in terms of power. The experience of sexual desire involves, centrally, a desire to be powerful or powerless. The expectations which are set up in the negotiation are, therefore, expectations about the expression of that power in sexual terms. The matrix of transformation which is the sexual encounter begins to be limited as soon as the first eye contact is made. When that contact is made, even as it is made, expectations about the type of sexual behaviour are formed. These are often crudely expressed as 'what I would like to do to him/have him do to me'.

We suggest that it is useful to distinguish the attraction of like to like and the attraction of the unlike. The latter may be in the grossest terms — the attraction of the so-called opposites which perpetuates the misguided 'butch-femme' distinction — or in more subtle foci of desire: dark and fair, hairy and smooth, tall and short, etc. We further suggest that the attraction of the unlike invests one of the partners with the role of the powerful and the other with that of the powerless, while the attraction of the like makes those roles ambiguous.

Let us be quite clear that we are not merely reinventing or restating the hoary old chestnut about gay men falling into either 'masculine' or 'feminine' types, with all that that implies about roles in the sexual encounter. On the other hand, we do not deny that sexual attraction between men is partly moulded in terms of gender difference. Indeed, it would be curious were this not so in a patriarchal and heterosexist culture. If the psychoanalysts are right and we experience our sexuality as the play of power, then the power differential between men and women must be central. Equally, however, gay men challenge that simple dichotomy, and it is not the case that many men adopt exclusively 'masculine' or 'feminine' roles; nor, as we shall see, is this dichotomy the only way to experience sexuality and sex. In some cases the emergent probability is that I will be one or the other in these encounters. In others it will be that I wish that particular person to be something particular with me. Second, of course, I can always be wrong. The urban folk-tale of the hunk who turns over at the crucial moment is mythical in the true sense of that word.

Crucially, therefore, the pre-contact stage sets up in the two individuals concerned a set of *expectations* about the sexual encounter to come. Evaluations of risk are made also at this point, sometimes based, as research has shown (Gold, 1989) on misguided notions of cleanliness and other cues. These expectations may be the subject of explicit negotiation if verbal interaction now intervenes. It is worth noting that the pre-contract stage may end before or after the contract to have sex is made. For example, in a club or pub the verbal interaction — the chat-up — will be part of the pre-contract, a 'sussing out' of the other before agreeing to have sex. In the case of a pick-up at a cottage or a cruising ground such talk may be eschewed altogether but, when it takes place, may come after the implicit contract is made and the partners to the contract are going off to some other place to carry it out.

It is at this verbal substage that the subject of safer sex can be raised explicitly. In this context it is worth noting that a standard conversational gambit for the case of the cottage/cruising ground pick-up, which long pre-dates AIDS: 'What do you like doing, then?', gives a perfect opportunity for adherence to safer sexual practices to be averred. What must be stressed, however, is that such a commitment does not preclude unsafe sex in the encounter. The process of negotiation is incessant and complex. When such verbal interaction does not intrude between the striking of the contract and its pay-off, non-verbal strategies are used to indicate preferences, dislikes and 'oh, all right if you insist'.

After this verbal stage the expectations will be confirmed or altered. This set of expectations draws on each individual's sense of his own desire, knowledge of and attachment to the precepts of safer sex, but is situated in the precise context of interaction between those individuals. When a relationship moves from its first sexual encounter to its second and subsequent, other considerations come into play — in two senses. First, subsequent sexual encounters refer to previous ones, either in the ritualization of past acts and patterns of acts, or in the exploration of new modes of pleasure. Second, these encounters occur in circumstances where different meanings are implicit. In the first encounter the bulk of the message is 'I desire you', in subsequent ones it can say that 'I love you', 'I forgive you', 'I hate you' and many other more subtle messages and combinations of messages.

The context in which sex takes place will have an effect on the sort of sex that takes place and on the meaning of that sexual session to the participants. In the most obvious case, sex in a semi-public place will not only be restricted to those acts which are possible while allowing the fast return to a posture of legitimacy if an intrusion takes place, but will also carry for the participants a charge of danger and transgression that would not obtain if the same sequence of acts took place in private. In the same way a sexual session on the kitchen table or the stairs may carry a weight of novelty in challenging norms of privacy. By context, therefore, we mean physical context which imposes certain constraints on activity. The context itself may also carry information about unsafe sex. 'Jack-off parties', etc. are attempts to provide contexts where safer sex is explicitly condoned and encouraged. These developments have immense implications. As Michel Pollak has noted, they embody reactions to HIV infection that celebrate an orgiastic sexuality.

> Mais, contrairement aux orgies traditionelles — la connotation religieuse de transgression — la ritualisation du 'safer sex' s'accompagne d'une desacralisation du sexe. Développé par la conscience du risque, le 'safer sex' introduit le concept de prudence. (1988: 81)

It is also possible, though, to consider the psychic context in which activity takes place, the scenario. In one sense this is the combination of mood and meaning that we mentioned earlier. The session will mean what the participants want it to mean at that juncture of the relationship, and that meaning can change in the course of a session. In a casual pick-up one or other of the partners may become bored with the other, may find that the emergent meanings of the sex do not measure up to the expectations that he had of the other. Within a longer-term relationship these feelings may also occur, but so can others: of habituation as a session unfolds in a totally predictable way; of annoyance at a partner's wish to do something that you dislike; of suspicion as a partner springs on you some novel practice or mode of behaviour, etc. More specifically, the scenario of an encounter can be explicitly negotiated, in terms of role playing or of game playing. Clearly, the agreement to play, say trucker and hitchhiker or construction workers, will create roles which rigidly channel the shape of the session. This explicit negotiation of role and scenario is most highly developed in the sado-masochistic (SM) scene, where rigid roles, explicit power negotiation and ritualized activity are the norm. Less explicit negotiation may also occur. For example, consider a sexual encounter in a long-term relationship after one partner has come off worse in an argument with the other. The 'winner' may consolidate his 'victory' (the terms are instructive) by symbolically dominating the 'loser' sexually, or the 'loser' may reassert himself by dominating the 'winner'. Alternatively, they may choose not to play such games and celebrate the restored mutuality of their relationship.

We argue, therefore, that each session begins with a set of expectations in the mind of each of the participants, a set of expectations about the probability of occurrence of particular acts, about the type of pleasure that is to be forthcoming, about the 'risk status' of his partner and so on. These expectations are multivalent and based on the simultaneous weighing of a number of different pieces of diverse information. They are also fuzzy in the sense that for each expected probability there is an associated uncertainty. It is these expectations that are negotiated in the sexual encounter.

The Sexual Encounter

These, then, are the independent variables: those factors which we believe influence sexual activity in general and unsafe sex in particular. We are left with the dependents. What is it that we are seeking to predict with this long list of variables? In the traditional approach the search is for the individual who engages, at least once in a given period, in unsafe sex. Since we have argued that the search for individual factors is at best a partial account, at worst highly misleading, so also we believe that the focus of attention should be on the session in which unsafe sex occurs. If we take seriously the indexicality of sexual activity, then we are bound to consider the effect of different contexts on the activity of individuals and of couples. Having said that, there is no doubt that couples of moderately long acquaintance will fall into patterns: habits of sexual communication.

What is it in the session that we are trying to predict? Clearly, it is not merely the occurrence/non-occurrence of unsafe sex. What the factors we have so far outlined do is to create in each of the participants a set of expectations about the occurrence of sexual acts. Each will, therefore, have a high or a low expectation that a particular act will occur or not occur. The important thing to note is that these individual expectations may be concordant or discordant. The likelihood of an act occurring is, in the simplest model, highest if both participants expect it to happen, low if they both expect it not to happen. If, however, there is discordance, the likelihood of occurrence will be negotiated. One way in which this negotiation can be resolved is to invoke a rule that any act not wanted by one of the participants does not occur: a form of veto. Otherwise, it might be that the wishes of the powerful partner will predominate: a form of tyranny. It is unlikely that one form of decision-making always obtains. What we wish to argue is that there are underlying patterns of sexual activity which carry their own logic, and that anal intercourse plays a particularly crucial — and different — symbolic role in these patterns.

We have elsewhere argued that we should look at the grammar of sexual activity (Davies, 1989). This begins with the observation that the occurrence of sexual acts in sessions is not random. Certain acts always follow rather than precede others. More generally, we believe that underlying the diversity of sexual activity are certain regularities without which such activity would be rendered unpredictable and therefore disconcerting and meaningless. Using information from detailed accounts of sexual activity kept by men in the form of sexual diaries (Coxon, 1988), we think that some of these patterns are now apparent (Davies, 1990). These patterns, we argue, are the result of a negotiation of sexual pleasure.

Let us begin by recognizing two central aspects of male sexual pleasure in our culture. First, such pleasure is primarily and predominantly concentrated on the genitals. Second, as we have already remarked, that pleasure is also contructed as penetrative. Most importantly, the pleasure to be gained from penetrating and from being penetrated is essentially and absolutely distinct. In the former case the penetrator violates the body and by extension the self of the other, thus asserting his (sic) powerfulness. It is, ultimately, an assertion of self. To be penetrated is, conversely, a giving up of self. When this is involuntary, as in rape, the harm is not merely physical, and rape is rightly regarded as among the most heinous of crimes for this reason. When penetration occurs by consent, the experience can be profound, because the individual at the same time abrogates and celebrates selfhood.

In the heterosexual hegemony, of course, the roles of penetrator and penetrated are invested absolutely in the male and the female partner respectively. The challenge that lesbians present to this hegemony is to assert that penetration is not a necessary part of sexual pleasure. Male homosexuality, and gay culture in particular, challenge the heterosexual paradigm by asserting the penetrability of the male. This profound threat, which underlies the hysterical blatherings of the anti-gay claques, is all the more potent since the threat of penetration centres on the anus with its associated complex of symbolisms: (self-)control, retention, integrity, etc. Thus men having sex with men have available at least two distinct forms of sexual pleasure, that of penetrating and that of being penetrated. The decision to enjoy one pleasure or the other, or both or neither, is the result of an implicit or explicit choice and negotiation, since both men are, at least in principle, able to take either part.

A similar distinction can be made concerning the second principle of male sexual pleasure in this culture, the primacy of penile stimulation. While there are those who have prostatic orgasms, for most of us, direct stimulation of the penis is necessary for orgasm. But when men have sex together, once again an implicit choice is made either to stimulate your partner's penis, or to seek to be stimulated, or both or neither. It is important to note that in some cases, though not all, penile stimulation is the dual of penetration, as in fucking and sucking. In other cases this is not so: wanking, fingering, body-rubbing. But to penetrate and to be stimulated carry distinct forms of pleasure from being penetrated and stimulating another's penis.

In any encounter, therefore, both partners negotiate the distribution of these several pleasures. Broadly, the choices are that one person does all the stimulating and gets penetrated, while the other gets stimulated and penetrates. Otherwise, they can share these two roles, either by alternating — an 'if you do it to me, I'll do it to you' protocol — or by engaging in acts simultaneously. The third alternative is to eschew these notions completely and go for non-penetrative, non-penis-centred sex.

Our analysis of data from the sexual diaries of gay and bisexual men has suggested that sexual sessions fall into two types which we have termed respectively role-specific and reciprocal. In the former the role of penetrator/stimulatee is vested in one of the partners for the whole of the session, whereas in the reciprocal case this role is alternated between the partners in the course of the session. The distinction is important because it turns out that reciprocal sessions are less likely to feature anal intercourse as part of the repertoire, and when it does occur, it is less likely to lead to ejaculation. To that extent the reciprocal mode is the safer from the point of view of HIV transmission.

The point is that as the session develops, a logic emerges which makes certain acts, certain modalities of acts, more or less likely. For example, there is in the role-specific case, a clear tendency for masturbation to be followed by fellatio to be followed by anal intercourse. This protocol, which is recognized in the discussions of sex by our respondents (see Hunt and Davies, Ch. 3, this volume) and has psychoanalytic overtones, would seem to make anal intercourse more likely, simply because it seems the right thing to do next. It is much more difficult to negotiate the omission of anal intercourse from a sequence whose 'natural' end it is, than it is from a sequence where it is an optional act. It must be stressed that the reciprocal mode does not exclude anal intercourse; but it is less likely and it features much less often as the final orgasmic act in that mode of relation than in the role-specific.

The equation is appealing. It would seem that unsafe sex occurs when desire is articulated through a rehearsal of domination rather than a celebration of equality. We may conclude that the maximization of mutual pleasure — creating, in Buber's terminology, an 'I-Thou' relationship — satisfies the demands of excitement and prudence more completely than the interaction which creates dominant and submissive partners. The question remains, however, at what point in the sexual encounter is the predisposition to reciprocal or role-specific sex formed? *A posteriori* it is impossible to decide whether a session is one or the other until the second act in the session, since it is only at that point that it becomes clear whether the role of insertor is to remain vested in one of the partners or to alternate between them. It is likely, however, that the disposition is formed early in the negotiation, when desire is evoked by, and focused on, an individual. There is some evidence that domination sexual encounters follow social lines of inequality. For example, in our data it is the case that where there is an age difference between the partners, the older man tends to be the insertive partner in anal intercourse. But the negotiation is not a simple one and will involve not only age but class, education, masculinity, the state of the relationship and many other contingent factors which require further investigation.

Summary

Our general contention is that the factors which cause unsafe sexual behaviour are to be found not by examination of the characteristics of individuals, but in the dyad — with features of the interaction. We have suggested that interpersonal attraction, the physical context of the encounter and its psychic scenario all influence the eventual content of the sexual session.

Our specific contention is that the session is predisposed to reciprocal or role-specific form in the pre-sexual interaction and that predisposition is located in the negotiation of desire that occurs between individuals. While we would expect a greater likelihood for the attraction of opposites to produce role-specific sex, the influence of other factors cannot simply be ignored, as we have tried to show.

The implications of this approach for research into sexual behaviour are profound in that they entail a complete realignment of focus. For health education, too, the implications are not trivial. We suggest that we need to concentrate more on the processes of verbal and particularly non-verbal communication, less on the dissemination of information. Education programmes which directly address the patterning of behaviour within the sexual session seem appropriate, concentrating not on saying no and disrupting the flow of the encounter but in constructing it in such a way as to make the occurrence of safer sex more likely, more logical and more consonant with the emergent logic of the session.

Finally, if this analysis is correct, and unsafe sex is more likely in role-specific than reciprocal sessions, then the campaign within gay liberation to jettison the 'butch-femme' distinction is not mere shibboleth, but an urgent necessity.

Notes

1 One of my colleagues was heard the other day to comment that theorizing about sex seemed to have taken the place of the practical in his life at the moment.
2 Any discussion must begin with Hume (1974), and take in the debate between Winch (1958) and Macintyre (1973). A conc̈se and erudite discussion can be found in Galtung (1967:469–476).
3 The search for alternatives continues. My francophone colleagues, Michel Pollak and Jean-Blaise Masur, prefer the term *rupture*, signifying a breaking out of imposed bounds. Attempts within the project to popularize the term 'backsliding' have the dual disadvantage of retaining the notion of pathology while suggesting a novel sexual practice.
4 Powell (1986) has recently suggested, intriguingly, that Buber's notion of the 'between' is a secular version of the female immanent aspect of the Jewish godhead, the Shekinah, who has been traditionally ignored in favour of the male transcendant aspect, Yahweh.

References

ALTMAN, D. (1986) *AIDS and the New Puritanism*, London, Pluto.
BERKOWITZ, S.D. (1982) *An Introduction to Structural Analysis*, London, Butterworth.
BUBER, M. (1970) *I and Thou*, EDINBURGH, T. and T. CLARK.
COOMBS, C.H. (1964) *A Theory of Data*, New York, Wiley.
COXON, A.P.M. (1988) '"Something Sensational..."; The Sexual Diary as a Tool for Mapping Detailed Sexual Behaviour,' *Sociological Review*, 36, 2, 353–367.
DAVIES, P.M. (1989) 'Some Notes on the Structure of Sexual Acts', in P. AGGLETON, G. HART and P. DAVIES (Eds), *AIDS: Individual, Cultural and Policy Dimensions*, Lewes, Falmer Press.
DAVIES, P.M. and COXON, A.P.M. (1990) 'Patterns in Homosexual Relations: The Use of the Diary Method', in M. HUBERT, (Ed.) *Sexual Behaviour and Risks of HIV Infection*, Brussels, Facultés Universitaires, St. Louis.
DAVIES, P.M., WEATHERBURN, P., HUNT, A.J., HICKSON, F., COXON, A.P.M. and McMANUS, T.J. (in press) 'Factors Associated with Unsafe Sex in a Large Cohort of Homosexuals Active Men in England', *Journal of Social Behaviour*.
FITZPATRICK, R., *et al.* (1990) 'Variation in Sexual Behaviour in Gay Men', in P. AGGLETON, P. DAVIES and G. HART (Eds), *AIDS: Individual, Cultural and Policy Dimensions*, Lewes, Falmer Press.
GALTUNG, J. (1967) *Theory and Methods of Social Research*, London, Allen and Unwin.
GOLD, R., SKINNER, M., GRANT, P. and PLUMMER, D. (1989) 'Situational Factors Associated with and Rationalizations Employed to Justify Unprotected Intercourse in Gay Men', Paper presented at the fifth international conference on AIDS, Montreal.
HUME, D. (1974) *A Treatise on Human Nature*, Vol. 1, London, Everyman.
KOCHEMS, L.M. (1987) 'Meanings and Health Implications: Gay Men's Sexuality', paper presented at American Anthropological Association.
MACINTYRE, A. (1973) 'The Idea of a Social Science', in A. RYAN (Ed.), *The Philosophy of Social Explanation*, Oxford, Oxford University Press.
PARKER, R. (1987) 'Acquired Immunodeficiency Syndrome in Urban Brazil', *Medical Anthropology Quarterly*, 1, 2, 155–175.
PATTON, C. (1985) *Sex and Germs: The Politics of AIDS*, Boston, Mass., South End Press.
POLLAK, M. (1988) *Les Homosexuels et le SIDA: Sociologie d'une Epidemie*, Paris, A.M. Metailie.

Powell, E.J. (1986) 'The Influence of the Feminine upon the Intellectual Development of Martin Buber', unpublished PhD thesis, University of Wales.

Prieur, A. (1990) 'Gay Men: Reasons for Continued Practice of Unsafe Sex', *AIDS Education and Prevention*, 2, 2, 110–117.

Watney, S. (1987) *Policing Desire*: Pornography, AIDS and the Media, London, Comedia.

Winch, P. (1958) *The Idea of a Social Science*, London, Routledge and Kegan Paul.

Appendix A

We define a set

$$\mathbf{A} = \{a_j\} \qquad j = 1, \ldots, p$$

of sexual acts with proper subsets

$$\mathbf{A}' \subset \mathbf{A}$$

and

$$\mathbf{A}'' \subset \mathbf{A}$$

with

$$\mathbf{A}' \cap \mathbf{A}'' = \phi$$

of insertive and receptive acts respectively.

The matrix

$$\mathbf{E} = \{e_{ij}\} \qquad \begin{matrix} i = 1, 2 \\ j = 1, \ldots, p \end{matrix}$$

is a matrix of expectations for the two individuals involved in a sexual encounter for the acts in arbitrary but fixed order.

We further define a diagonal context matrix whose diagonal elements record the probability of occurrence of each act in the given context

$$\mathbf{C} = \{c_{jk}\} \qquad j, k = 1, \ldots, p$$

The likelihood of occurrence of acts in the encounter is given by the pre-multiplication of $\mathbf{E}$ by a unit agreement vector $\mathbf{1}$ and its postmultiplication by $\mathbf{C}$. Thus the general model is:

$$\mathbf{1} = \mathbf{1EC}$$

The sequence of acts in a given session is generated by the operation of one of two stochastic matrices. In the first case the transition probabilities are high for acts within $\mathbf{A}'$ or $\mathbf{A}''$ and low between, while in the other case, transition probabilities are low within and high between the two subsets. While stochastic, the matrices are unlikely to describe a Markov process.

Chapter 9

Between Embarrassment and Trust: Young Women and the Diversity of Condom Use

Janet Holland, Caroline Ramazanoglu, Sue Scott,
Sue Sharpe and Rachel Thomson

A: If I don't die of ignorance I will die of embarrassment instead.

Q: Do you think that's a real issue?

A: Yes I think it's embarrassment.

Q: Embarrassment about what? Talking about it?

A: Yes, just talking about sex is a very embarrassing thing to do.
(Young woman interviewed in Manchester, 1989)

Two major assumptions underlie the attempts by state agencies in the UK to manage the AIDS crisis by advocating the use of condoms as a simple and practical solution to the sexual transmission of HIV (Weeks, 1989): first, that heterosexual sexual intercourse is a factor in the spread of HIV; second, that using condoms is a rational strategy which people can discuss and decide about prior to sexual intercourse. These assumptions, however, are not straightforward as they seem to hide two major areas of ideological tension: between those who consider that heterosexuals are not at risk and those who consider that they are; and between the notion of individual responsibility and the recognition of social constraints on individual behaviour. There have been public statements that AIDS is not an immediate threat to heterosexuals in the UK and USA based on a particular interpretation of official statistics (see, for example, Lord Kilbracken; Fitzpatrick and Milligan, 1990; Fumento, 1990). In opposition to these claims, Britain's Chief Medical Officer, doctors and epidemiologists are concerned about the likely spread of HIV in the population. They support the current Health Education Authority (HEA) campaigns which advocate condoms and are aimed specifically at young heterosexuals. The second area of ideological tension is between the policy of individual responsibility for safe sex, and the social pressures and relationships which constrain people's talk and behaviour in sexual encounters. In this chapter we are assuming that a threat to the heterosexual population does exist, and are primarily exploring the complexities of condom use in the experience of young women.

On a global scale AIDS is increasingly recognized as an issue for those who engage in heterosexual sex (Panos Institute, 1988; Rieder and Ruppelt, 1989; Holland *et al.*, 1990a, 1990b), and the World Health Organisation (WHO) announced in July 1990 that AIDS had become the leading cause of death for women aged between 20 and 40 in major cities of the sub-Sahara, Western Europe and America (*Guardian*, 28 July 1990). WHO statistics in early 1990 report that three million women worldwide are infected with HIV, and Clarke *et al.* (1990) conclude from the UK HIV and AIDS statistics that 'young women account for a high proportion of infections in the 15–24 year age group, particularly of infections through heterosexual contact and drug use'. Factors which are now known to contribute to the spread of HIV make it seem that complacency in the UK would be misguided (Gross, 1987; Padian, 1987; Heyward and Curran, 1988; Johnson, 1988, Pye *et al.*, 1989). The spread of HIV into the heterosexual population is still limited, but the ways in which young women understand the risks, negotiate their sexual relationships and reach agreement on strategies for safer sex will play a significant part in the spread or limitation of AIDS in the UK.

In the official campaigns which encourage condom use and disparage complacency about the risks of spreading HIV through heterosexual intercourse, condoms are represented as a means of self-help in which the individual takes responsibility for safer sex. Campaign advertisements represent young women as well as young men as bearing responsibility for sexual safety, and now recognize some of the problems that young women face in introducing a condom into a sexual encounter. One advertisement comments, '. . . and she's too embarrassed to ask him to use a condom . . . wouldn't it have been easier to talk about it earlier . . . ?' We are arguing here that embarrassment over using condoms is not simply a question of bad timing, but indicates a very complex process of negotiation.

The Women, Risk and AIDS Project (WRAP) currently has questionnaire data from 500 young women aged between 16 and 21, and qualitative interview data from 150 of these respondents.[1] These data are beginning to provide knowledge of the social situations in which condoms are used or are rejected, and of the symbolic significance of condoms as young women negotiate their sexual relationships. A major focus of our study is the negotiation of safe sex among young heterosexuals. We intend that our findings will feed into public education and debate and will, therefore, make some contribution to the limitation of HIV infection.

In this chapter we both illustrate and conceptualize the contradictions which have arisen around condoms for many of the young women we have interviewed. We will examine condom use in heterosexual encounters and argue first, that the issue cannot be understood without taking account of the gendered power relations which construct and constrain choices and decisions, and second, that condom use must be understood in the context of the contradictions and tensions of heterosexual relationships. We have drawn on our data to illustrate the importance of men's power in sexual encounters and their control of sexual pleasure; women's opposition to condoms; the ways in which women can demand safer sex; the complications of love in unequal relationships; and the contradictions of asking young men to use condoms.

AIDS, Young Women and the Negotiation of Sexual Encounters

AIDS has presented us with an opportunity to reassess and redefine sexuality (Watney, 1987; Coward, 1987). Exploring the social construction of AIDS sharpens the mind and focuses the attention on how little we know about sexuality. AIDS has given us the space (if not the time) to explore the meanings which we attribute to sexual practices, and to rethink our knowledge and language of sexuality and the forms of its social construction. The threat of death has made change imperative, but, for change to be effected, the processes through which sexuality is socially constructed must be identified. AIDS has given us an opportunity to understand how sexuality takes on the appearance of being natural rather than social. In the negotiation of sexual relationships, the discourse of romance widely available to young women (McRobbie, 1978) does not necessarily prepare them for the contradictions of sexual encounters.

Our data suggest that the HEA campaigns have been very successful at the level of information and ideas as, almost without exception, the young women we have spoken to equate 'safer sex' with condom use (see also Scott, Aldridge and Temple, 1990). There is ample evidence, though, to suggest that while public education may be able to affect what people think, the acquisition of information does not necessarily affect behaviour (Gatherer, *et al.*, 1979; Azjen and Fishbein, 1980; Hanson *et al.*, 1987). Condoms are not neutral objects about which a straightforward decision can be made on health grounds (COI-DHSS, 1987; Freeman, 1990). The idea that women are free to choose the most rational form of protection ignores the nature of systematic inequalities in the social relationships between women and men. The linking of sex and health is in itself problematic in a cultural context which endows sex with meanings which are far from healthy. It is in the light of the social character of sexual relationships, and the weight of meanings carried by condoms, that we will analyze young women's accounts of condom use.

Our data illustrate the complexity and contradictions of the processes of negotiation over condoms and indicate a range of potential outcomes. We will explore these processes and the relationship between knowledge of risk and safer sex practices through an analysis of our respondents' reported experiences of condom use for contraception and prophylaxis. We make the case that condoms carry symbolic meanings which can differ for each sexual partner and for individuals over time, and that these meanings are illustrative of the gendered nature of responsibility and what is considered 'appropriate' behaviour in contraception and safer sex. These meanings cannot simply be swept away and replaced by public education.

Asking Him to Use a Condom: The Social Context

The social context of condom use is the gendered relationships within which sexual encounters occur. In feminist social theory, sexual intercourse in Western societies has been identified not only as a social relationship, but also as an unequal relationship in which men exercise power over women (Shulman, 1971; Millett, 1977; Dworkin, 1987; Hite, 1989a). The institutionalization of heterosexuality (Rich, 1983) means that sexual intercourse is socially located in gendered power relationships. This helps to explain the tensions and embarrassment of condom use and also the risk taken where condoms or other forms of protection are not used. From a feminist perspective, using or not using a condom is not a simple, practical question about dealing rationally with risk; it is the outcome of negotiation between potentially unequal partners. Sexual encounters are sites of struggle between the exercise and acceptance of male power and male definitions of sexuality, and of women's ambivalence and resistance.

The physical intimacy which can lead to orgasm, pregnancy or sexually transmitted disease is potentially an experience of both pleasure and danger (Vance, 1984), but it is also unknown social territory. Even for the sexually experienced, encounters with new sexual partners are not wholly predictable, yet sexual intercourse entails trusting our bodies, our identities, our self-respect to others and, not uncommonly, to strangers. Sexual practice in Western society is heavy with moral meanings, but while the English education system may equip pupils with some knowledge of the mechanics of vaginal intercourse, many of the dangers and virtually all the pleasures of sexuality are an embarrassed area of silence.

In many sexual encounters women have little choice about whether or how to engage in sexual activity with men, the options being physical injury or more subtle forms of sanction. The accounts given by the young women in our sample support Liz Kelly's conception of a continuum of sexual violence, from sexism to mild pressure to have unwanted intercourse, to more overtly coerced sex, child abuse and rape (Kelly, 1988). Women, though, are not simply helpless victims in the face of male control of sexuality. Male power in sexual relationships is both embraced and resisted by young women in the course of negotiating sexual encounters. The same woman can negotiate very different sexual encounters with different men or at different points in her sexual career.

The social context of condom use may or may not be problematic for young women, depending on their priorities in a particular relationship, the degree of trust between partners and other factors which we discuss below, but condom use remains the focus of a number of social tensions. Male sexual power, the privileging of men's sexual pleasure and the dominance of men over women can be challenged by a woman's insistence on her need for safety being met. Asking him to use a condom is embarrassing when it is a potentially subversive demand. The spontaneity of passion can be undermined by recognition of risk and responsibility (see also Gross and Bellew-Smith, 1983). If coming to orgasm means losing control, being taken over by sensation, then condoms symbolize control and a curb on passion and spontaneity. Sexual fulfilment and sexual safety pull against each other when they are defined in terms of men's fulfilment.

There is more than one way in which men can express their masculinity (Morgan, 1987), but it takes a special combination of circumstances for young women to gain sufficient control in sexual encounters to ensure both safety and their own sexual pleasure. Hite (1989b:529) concludes from her survey of predominantly well educated American women that women are tired 'of the old mechanical pattern of sexual relations, which revolves around male erection, male penetration and male orgasm.' We have found that much, if not most, of young women's sexual experience is not particularly pleasurable. Sometimes it seems that what is valued is the social relationship with a partner rather than the sexual activity. Young women are not without the ability to choose and to act for themselves, but they are heavily socially constrained. Young men are much better placed socially to gain sexual pleasure for themselves. When a young woman insists on the use of a condom for her own safety, she is going against the construction of sexual intercourse as man's natural pleasure and woman's natural duty.

Asking Him to Use a Condom: Young Women's Experiences

Health educators and policy-makers want to know who uses condoms, and this information can be produced. Of the 500 respondents to our questionnaire, 82 (16 per cent) said that they had used condoms without any other form of protection, 62 (12 per cent) had used condoms while they were taking a contraceptive pill, 2 (0.5 per cent) had used condoms with spermicide[2] and 3 (1 per cent) had used a condom and a cap at the same time. We can, therefore, say that 30 per cent of our sample had used condoms, but we know from our interview data that this statement is of limited value because it tells us nothing about the circumstances of condom use.

The fact that a young woman uses a condom on one occasion does not necessarily mean that she will be able to negotiate the continuation of this practice even if she wants to.

Power, Control and Pleasure

In our study general aspects of men's power over women and their control of sexual relationships emerge from young women's accounts of situations in which they have or have not felt able to ask for, or insist on, condom use. These accounts illustrate the contradictions through which young women often have to negotiate their way. In our data we have found a wide spectrum of behaviour and experience, from the active negotiation of condom use in a situation of trust to rape.

One problem in asking for accounts of sexual encounters is the lack of an agreed language in the UK for talking about sex (Spencer *et al.*, 1988). Much of our sexual vocabulary, and particularly that relating to female sexuality, doubles as obscenities, or is too technical for everyday use. There is no language for women's ambivalence about male sexuality, or for concepts which fall between 'sex' and 'rape' for identifying pressures to have sexual intercourse, or women's ambivalence in situations where they are reluctant to have sexual intercourse, but also reluctant to refuse it. 'Sex' covers a range of ideas and practices.

We have taken the young women's own definitions of what constitutes a sexual encounter or relationship, and some of these include events and relationships which did not include sexual intercourse. The 500 respondents to our questionnaire, for example, reported 491 instances of sexual relationships or encounters which did not include sexual intercourse, and 590 which did. But, when asked in the interview what sex meant for them, most of the young women accepted the prevailing construction of sex as heterosexual sex with male penetration, whether they are sexually active themselves or not.

Q: You only count it as a sexual relationship if you actually. . . .
A: Having sex I think.

'Sex' was very generally associated with vaginal intercourse:

A: Yeah, most of the time when I think about sex it is actually sexual intercourse.
Q: Yeah. And other sorts of things might not be, wouldn't be included, like we've been talking about masturbation and oral sex. I mean, do you think of those as being sex?
A: It comes in as part of sex, yes, but when I think about sex, those things don't come to my mind.

In general, young women saw this association between sex and intercourse as obvious.

> A: When anyone ever said 'sex' before, all I ever thought was sexual intercourse. That's what it is, isn't it?

Recent publicity about safe sex had given young women some reason for thinking about the possibilities of 'having sex' without penetration:

> A: I know that safe sex can be just touching each other and anything else except for intercourse, but it always seems to me ultimately all sex always leads up to intercourse, so I always just think of safe sex as just using condoms.

But even when they had some knowledge of safer sex, the idea of sex as intercourse seemed to dominate.

> A: ... I think if they say sex they mean going the whole way.
> Q: So sex actually means penetration —
> A: I think that's basically what it means now ... which maybe isn't quite fair because there's lots of other things that go on before you get there, sort of part of the same game as it were, but at the end of the line that's what you're talking about. That's how I would see it anyway.

It was much more uncommon to find young women who had thought of the possibility of sexual pleasure without sexual intercourse.

> A: I don't think that, you know, men feel that they have to actually be inside somebody before they can feel as if they've had any pleasure.

It also became clear in the interviews that for many, vaginal intercourse was something they did not particularly enjoy, although they assumed that it was what men wanted. A number said that they never experienced orgasm through penetrative sex and that they much preferred other sexual activities in which they engaged. One felt that if she stopped short of intercourse, she would be labelled a tease:

> A: Actually, seeing as you asked me earlier, 'did you find it enjoyable or pleasurable?' I find everything enjoyable and pleasurable except for the actual penetration, so I mean, why bother? I think really if you're with a guy and you are going to do everything but, it's obviously a big tease.

Behind this definition of sex as the need to fulfil male sexual desires in a specific way lies the notion of men's uncontrollable sexual drive which cannot be interrupted or diverted. While this idea implies that women must take responsibility for moral standards and contraception, it can also lead to failure to use contraception, particularly condoms where these have connotations of breaking the flow and destroying the passion.

Some women showed a limited sense of the potential for their own sexual pleasure, particularly when this was something which they had not experienced. One young woman, when asked why she didn't like using a condom, responded, 'because it was like having a bath with your clothes on.' She said later that sex had been very painful at first but that after the third time it got better. This turned out to mean that intercourse had stopped hurting. This comment was made well into the interview, and it seems it had been easier initially to draw on the public/male discourse of condoms as pleasure killers than to admit to personal pain which could indicate personal failure. She went on to say that she and her boyfriend did not talk about sex and she felt unable to tell him what she liked sexually. Even where couples did experiment sexually, they did not necessarily discuss what was pleasurable. One young woman said that she could not tell her boyfriend what she wanted, but she could indicate acceptance or rejection of his suggestions for their shared sexual repertoire. Even where women had high expectations of sexual pleasure, they were often prepared to settle for less:

Q: Have you found the sexual relationship satisfactory, satisfying, pleasurable?
A: Yes. Yes.
Q: You sound a bit doubtful.
A: Well, I'm not — I've never, in all the sexual relationships I've had I've never — it's never been like it is in the books, I've never, you know — I'm sure it could be a lot better but — yeah, it was okay, yeah.

The meanings associated with a heterosexual encounter, which are accepted or assimilated by young women, help to reinforce male power. These are located in a discourse which positions young men as knowing sexual actors vis-à-vis young women who are constructed as lacking knowledge and expertise in relation to sex. This was sharply illustrated by one young woman who, when discussing her first experience of condom use, explained that her boyfriend had been certain that the condom should be 'blown up' first. She had strongly doubted this but had allowed her views to be overridden on the assumption that men knew better.

There are other more direct modes of the exercise of male power when women accept men's rights or needs to exert control over their sexual behaviour. Men exercise power when they are considered to be the initiators of sex, when they threaten the loss of the relationship if the young woman will not have sex, when they refuse to use a condom even when asked, and when they destroy a young woman's reputation with the epithets such as 'slag' or 'drag' (Lees, 1986). The English language has a rich vocabulary of sexually abusive terms for women (Mahoney, 1985), and it is these behaviours and expectations which constitute a framework of male power within which young women negotiate sexual encounters and relationships. Their sexual understanding and behaviour within this context can demonstrate acceptance of male power, ambivalence towards it or resistance. Variation in these stances means that negotiations around condom use are worked out in a number of different ways.

Where men did agree to use a condom, there was still the problem of how to make the sexual activity pleasurable. Couples need to be relatively sexually experienced to deal with the woman's need for pace and timing. This young woman compared her experience with two different boyfriends:

> Unless you're quite close it does interrupt things, they [the boyfriends] have got to be quite liberated themselves to use them in a way that's really good. It's frustrating because there isn't an equal amount of knowledge on how you use them. Like with David at the moment. I don't think it would have been a problem with Michael because he's really quite experienced and does it [uses a condom] as a matter of course.

These cases did not necessarily entail much, if any, discussion of condom use, since condoms were either taken to be a precondition for intercourse, or intercourse did not take place. Refusing intercourse without protection was not a trouble-free strategy, however, as women's demands for safe sex illustrate.

Women's Demands for Safe Sex

Despite a very general perception that men dislike condoms, our interviewees did not necessarily see that men's needs must always dominate a sexual encounter. Women are not without agency in protecting themselves when they define sexual safety as a priority.[3] Here again, 'love' can complicate protection:

> Q: If you were having a relationship with someone, and they say they don't like using condoms, you know the line, what would you do?
> A: I got that last night, I got that line.
> Q: So what did you do last night?
> A: I made him wear one — we always do if I miss the pill there's no way ... I find it quite interesting, putting it on, it's good fun.

When we asked young women how they felt personally about using condoms, 20 per cent of the interview sample of 150 young women disliked condoms themselves, and 24 per cent reported that they had partners who disliked them; but 52 per cent of the young women did not mind, liked or preferred condoms, and 41 per cent reported this as being the case for their partners. Condom use for safer sex could be seen either as a problem or a solution, or, in a contradictory way, as both.

Where women did insist on sex being safe, they were often able to get men's cooperation:

> *A*: Whether I liked them or not, we — we used them. I mean, he doesn't like them, but we — we did use them, because you — you've got to take the responsibility for it.

Sometimes they had to assert themselves quite strongly:

> *A*: He really hates using them, so I used to say to him, look, right, look, I have no intention of getting pregnant again and you have no intention to become a father, so you put one of these on. And he starts whingeing. He goes, 'Oh, no, do I have to?' I say look Alan, do it or you know —. He's all right, he knows how to do it now.

Insistence on this strategy could mean being prepared to give up the relationship:

> *A*: Some boys are just stupid, but if they don't want to wear a condom then tough, you know, go and find someone else. That's it. But most of them don't mind.

A very small number of young women in our sample seemed to be prepared to attempt to negotiate either non-penetrative sex or condom use in a range of different situations. These young women have some characteristics in common. They all seem to have a fairly strong sense of themselves, rather than being highly dependent on having a relationship with a man, and they also talk about sex in terms of pleasure and their own needs. These women gave more considered responses to the question, 'what do you understand by safe sex?' based on personal experience:

> *A*: Safe sex is as pleasurable an experience as actual penetration. Oral sex, things like touching somebody else's body in a very gentle way, kissing, appreciating one another's bodies.

A more common way for young women to counter young men's rejection of condoms is to assert their fear of pregnancy. There could be considerable embarrassment about telling a new partner that a condom was wanted for protection against possible infection, but it is allowable for women to be concerned with pregnancy (Cossey, 1979; Spencer, 1984). In one case even a rapist used a condom:

A: I was 16, we just went for a drive. He locked the door and wouldn't let me out. But he used something though. But I wasn't willing.

Q: So you did not want to do it?

A: No he was forcing me.

Q: But he used a condom?

A: Yes, I thought it was weird as it goes — but I bet he was afraid that if he got me pregnant you know — because I knew where he works and so he was scared I would go down.

Fear of pregnancy might well lead young women to feel able to *ask* for condoms to be used, but this does not necessarily mean that condoms will be used. Fear of HIV could also be presented as a fear of pregnancy. One young woman had discussed this strategy with a girl friend:

A: Rather than saying, 'Will you wear something, because I don't want to get AIDS?' which sounds really bad, doesn't it, we would say, 'you'll have to wear something because I'm not on the pill.'

A way of using fear of pregnancy to resist unwanted intercourse was to refuse to have sex without a condom, assuming that a young man would rather forego sex than use a condom. This could be a short-term strategy if the young man finally decided to buy a packet, leaving the young woman without an argument.

Women's Opposition to Condoms

While some young women were refusing or resisting unprotected intercourse, other young women (or the same young women on other occasions) had picked on a range of reasons for not using condoms. This could be interpreted as a form of self-assertion, but equally could indicate an accommodation to their own relative powerlessness in sexual encounters. Their reasons for having unprotected intercourse could be a diversion from, or perhaps a deflection of, women's understanding of this relative powerlessness.

A: Well, it would be nice if it was easier for girls to actually initiate things with men without feeling difficult about it. But I don't really know how it happens.

The reasons given varied, but seemed often to be a means of incorporating aspects of the ideology of male sexual dominance into women's definitions of sexual encounters.

When it is expected and accepted that what men want from sex is pleasure and penetration, avoidance of practices which limit male pleasure is understandable. Where women had accepted this legitimation, they entered into sexual encounters with a general acceptance of the idea that men do not like nor want to use condoms:

Q: What about using a condom?
A: No he wouldn't.
Q: He wouldn't?
A: No, a lot of guy don't really like them'.

A: I really don't know that many blokes who I think would use a condom or are even concerned about it. I mean they've never been concerned about getting women pregnant have they?

The young women also reported a wide range of negative descriptions of condom use which seemed to reflect male perceptions, for example: 'like picking your nose with a rubber glove', 'going to bed with your wellingtons on', 'washing your feet with your socks on', although these perceptions were not necessarily presented as male:

A: I mean, they're terrible. I mean, the thing is as well, people just won't use them because they hate them. It spoils the whole effect of it. It's like — I mean, as most people say, you know, it's like chewing toffee with the wrapper on.
Q: Does it — I mean, do you feel that, that that's the effect, that it is like...?
A: I can't — honestly can't abide the things. I really don't like them at all. I mean we got — we got ones which were sort of special, you know, with the bobbly bits on; but I mean, even them, it just — it just come off, it didn't do a lot for me.

A very different approach to accepting that men would not want to use condoms was for the woman to assume that she would be all right without protection (see also Abrams *et al.*, 1990). Some young women felt that they were invulnerable and certainly would not get pregnant:

A: I had this feeling, when I didn't use anything, I had this feeling I'm not going to get pregnant, you know, I was really sure.

Or they did not think about it at all:

> *A:*   I can't imagine myself getting pregnant.

At least one reported pregnancy was the result of this attitude. Others employed a method based on 'condoms or cross your fingers', using condoms when they were available or agreed upon, but going ahead anyway when they were not. In this way women justified relinquishing the control they desired.

A further group of reasons for reluctance to use condoms came from the women's fear of upsetting men by asserting their own needs. These reasons were partly to do with the fear of losing a boyfriend and the hope of a more committed or steady relationship, and partly a general unwillingness to hurt the man's feelings:

> *A:*   The climax to intercourse is all passion and kissing and I think to actually just stop and he puts a condom on, or me to turn around and say I want you to put this on, it just ruins the whole thing then.

Another said that, 'if you want the relationship, I didn't want to, like, fuck around with questions', and another, 'I just thought it's all right, I just decided he had to be safe.' Another had been having unprotected sex for eighteen months because she did not want to upset her boyfriend: 'Yeah, I think that's what it is, you don't want to hurt his feelings.'

A clear way of avoiding control was to enter into a sexual relationship with no specific expectation that there would be sexual intercourse on this occasion:

> *A:*   You meet a lad, and you start kissing, and before you know it, it's happening — and then it's too late [to use a condom].

One young woman described a situation where she had asked a man to use a condom because she was worried about HIV and AIDS, although she could not tell him that. He had no condom, and she did not want to offend him, nor cause an embarrassing social situation by refusing sex. She convinced herself that he must be OK, and went ahead, asking him to withdraw, 'whether he did or not I can't remember.' These types of explanations were used by young women who feared both pregnancy and HIV infection and occurred in the context of both steady and more casual relationships.

Going Steady and Trusting to Love

There is a common-sense assumption that negotiations around sex are easier in the context of steady relationships, but this is not necessarily the case. Going steady implies a degree of trust which is lacking in less persistent sexual relationships. Trust then becomes a significant aspect of the context of decision-making about condoms (see also Koller, 1988; Gambetta, 1990). If love is assumed to be the greatest prophylactic, then trust comes a close second:

> A: If you want to have relationships then you've got to trust them [men]. Otherwise it's no good from the start. Yeah, you have to believe what they tell you. You just hope that they tell you the truth. You can't find out if it's lies or not.

Condoms can be seen as a strategy for occasions when it is not clear whether partners can be trusted. Some young women who were on the pill told new partners that they were not, so that condoms were used as well. There was, though, a powerful ideological understanding that 'steady' relationships are based on trust. Trust can even develop into a euphemism for monogamy.

A trusting relationship can provide a social context in which condom use may be relatively unproblematic. Where young couples had been going steady for some time before their first experience of intercourse, their shared inexperience could provide a basis of trust so that they could discuss the problems of using condoms, and their own embarrassment. Reaching the stage of going to Boots together to buy condoms could become a joint commitment to a deepening relationship. Once the relationship was felt to be well established, the young woman was likely to go on the pill.

This transition from condoms with new partners to the pill with steady partners is laden with symbolic meaning and can be used to signify the seriousness of a relationship, a way of showing someone that they are special. As one of our respondents put it, 'I went on the pill for him.' There is, though, a good deal of pressure to define a relationship as 'serious' in order to justify sex. For the current generation of young women, the pill, despite the problems associated with it, is closely associated with grown up status and grown up sex. This makes the prospect of long-term condom use highly problematic, as two of our respondents clearly indicated:

> A: You've got to trust somebody at some time, you can't meet somebody and start, first time say, 'I know let's use condoms I'm not on the pill' (even if you are), and then a week later still be saying 'let's use condoms'....
>
> Q: You don't think you could do that long-term?
>
> A: I'd like to think that I would want to use one [condom] but I mean, you start off using one but are you going to carry on using one every single time?

Further exploration of this neglected area of long-term condom use should clarify the relation between risk and trust in long-term relationships. The circumstances in which condom use can be renegotiated in steady relationships, when one or both partners have intercourse with other people, remains unclear at present.

The question of what counts as a steady relationship is clouded by the meanings associated with particular types of relationship, and fears for loss of reputation, particularly by the younger women. Most young women are reluctant to describe themselves as having casual sex when the culturally approved objective is to be in a steady, preferably monogamous relationship, supported by the ideologies of romance and love. Conversely, they are likely to expect or to express the hope that relationships of short duration, including one-night stands, will in fact last. The positive associations of sex as leisure and pleasure, which have been espoused by the gay movement, tend not to be available to heterosexual young women. The tendency seems to be to expect that relationships ought to last:

> *A:* If I sleep with anyone I intend it to be a long-term relationship — so I don't know, because you don't like to think of the end of a relationship when you start it. So you think it's going to be the right one, but you never know.

Respondents who described themselves as being in steady relationships did not think of themselves as at risk in relation to HIV and focused their attention on avoiding pregnancy. This obviously makes some sense when each was the other's first and only sexual partner, but it assumes that the relationship is, and will continue to be, monogamous. Another young woman illustrates this tension very clearly.

> *Q:* When you decided to sleep with him did you think it was going to last quite a long time?
>
> *A:* Yes, I think that was the only reason I did sleep with him really. I think I wanted to do it, but I didn't in a way, but because it was him I did, and I thought it would last a long time really.

This young woman goes on to explain that she was very scared the first time because they used no contraception, but she subsequently went on to insist that he used a condom:

> *A:* I don't know because I couldn't really go on the pill [because she was under 16 at the time] and I shouldn't have used a cap or something like that, it was easier for him to do it. But before I did it with him I made him put it on. I didn't watch him but I stood there as if to say, 'make sure you put it on', and he did put it on.

She saw condoms as her only option, and her fear of pregnancy gave her the strength to insist on their use. It seems clear, though, that she saw protection as something she would have to fight for, and men as untrustworthy in this respect. She felt it necessary, literally, to stand over her partner while he did what she wanted.

Often the young women's experience of sexual pressure and physically unpleasant sexual encounters conflicted with their desire for love, romance, caring, closeness and trust. The contradictions of female subordination in loving relationships were expressed in this desire for close, loving relationships without a very positive sexual identity for young women. There was a widespread negative perception of male sexuality, typical comments being that, 'lads don't care', and 'women want love and men want sex.' One young woman commented: 'I don't trust boys today — I don't trust them at all.' Others insisted that they would not have sex, or they would not be in a relationship with a man, if they did not trust him. The very fact of being in a steady relationship implied the existence of trust. Where there are social pressures on young women to police sexual encounters and be alert for problems, particularly the risk of pregnancy, this militates against developing trust, even when a steady relationship is wanted. Many women took risks with partners they loved but did not wholly trust. (A different perspective on trusting to love is provided by Thomson, 1988.)

A small number of the young women clearly stated that they had casual sex or one-night stands. Some of these had taken on the idea that it is legitimate for women to be sexually active, to have their own sexual identity, but they were not necessarily any more in control of their encounters. One young woman who was very clear that she wanted to be in control of her life, which included 'choosing' to be sexually active and child-free, was in fact having unprotected sex, including intercourse with partners who were potential health risks. She said that she had come to be interviewed to make her think about what she was doing.

Condom use tends to be associated with one-night stands rather than 'steady relationships' (see also Day *et al.*, 1988; Nix *et al.*, 1988), but if young women's relationships are conceived as 'steady' until proved otherwise, this makes condom use rather unpredictable. Where men see sex as a process of attrition, as wearing a girl down until she says yes, there are problems in producing a condom at the right moment:

> A: About two weeks ago I ended up not asking him and had to go and get the morning-after pill. I wouldn't say anything, and kept thinking I'll say something in a minute, it's just so difficult. I thought I'd say something in a minute and then it was too late, and I thought, 'Oh no! I didn't even know this person anyway.'

There are problems not only in asking about partners' sexual histories, but also deciding whether to believe the answers (see also Cochrance and Mays, 1990). The most confident young women in this respect were those from a small inner city area where they claimed that they knew the sexual histories of all the local lads who constituted their pool of sexual partners.

Abandoning condoms for the pill in a steady relationship is not necessarily empowering for women. It depends on the strength of their sense of self and of individual agency.[4] Research shows that both inexperience and experience can lead to changing conceptions of male versus female responsibility for safety, and so to shifting patterns of risk and safety in condom use (Pleck *et al.*, 1988).

Asking Him to Use a Condom: Contradictory Discourse and Practices

The mixture of positive and negative ways in which the young women we have interviewed react to sexual safety makes it clear that young women cannot be treated as a unified category. A number of couples used condoms with few apparent problems in negotiation, particularly where couples were young and inexperienced, where women were assertive, or where men habitually used condoms with new partners for their own protection. Public education campaigns need to be sensitive to the different ways in which young women are positioned in relation to safer sex. Our sample indicates not only a range of sexual experiences, but also variations in levels of power and autonomy in the negotiation of these sexual relationships. While most of the young women do not use condoms most of the time, they are coping with considerable and conflicting social pressures in organizing their sexual behaviour. When they do not use condoms, most of them perceive themselves as employing some strategy of risk reduction, such as 'not going with dodgy guys' or trying to check sexual histories.

We found embarrassment about every stage of condom use. When young women put their reputations first, then buying condoms, carrying them and, of course, asking for their use are all embarrassing. Having a condom on one's person indicates a lack of sexual innocence, an unfeminine identity, that of a woman actively seeking sex. The sexual woman is, then, easy, fair game, a slag and generally at men's disposal. Advertizing has had to counter this level of meaning by associating condoms with personal responsibility (see also Winn, 1986). But the contradictions of sexual safety mean that when the risk of pregnancy or a sexually transmitted disease is a possibility which women feel strongly about, they may be willing to ignore the risk to their reputation:

Q: Do you think that you'd feel OK asking somebody to use a condom?
A: Definitely, because it would be my embarrassment, or being in danger, and there's no contest if you ask me.

Young men may well be just as embarrassed in sexual encounters as young women, especially when they are inexperienced, but the meanings carried by condoms allow them to hide embarrassment by recourse to a public discourse which legitimates the rejection of condoms. Young men can be fearful of sexual inadequacy and apprehensive about sexual encounters, but as these emotions are not defined as natural aspects of male sexuality, there is no discourse around this issue to which women have access. Condoms are seen to limit male sexual pleasure in situations in which male satisfaction is the main point of the encounter. Dworkin (1987:159) argues that male sexual discourse on the subject of sexual intercourse is the only language available to women. The 'rational' discourse of safer sex promoted as official information can be seen as antithetical to an ideology of femininity which constructs sex as the relinquishment of control in the face of love. Thus young women are constantly working through these contradictions in sexual encounters.

In the course of talking about their sexual experiences, many young women who were unable to negotiate condom use, even when they saw condoms as necessary for their own protection, recognized that what they were doing was not in their best interest. This was particularly so for those who were informed and concerned about HIV infection. These contradictions sometimes became apparent to them. One young woman was engaging in what she described as 'short flings' with men of whose sexual history she had no knowledge. She was having sex unprotected against AIDS or pregnancy. It was her concern about this pattern of sexual behaviour which had brought her to the interview. She appeared to be a confident young woman of 19, with a good job, 'A' levels and plans for continuing her education at some stage. She was very well informed about HIV and AIDS, and worried about the spread of HIV in general and about her own likelihood of becoming infected in particular. But she still found it impossible to negotiate the use of condoms that *she* saw as appropriate for her own protection. Her comments indicate the contradictions with which she is struggling:

A: But although I really do think about it a lot, I don't know why, it goes straight out the window if I'm — no not straight out the window it doesn't, no, it's always — there's always this nagging at the back of my mind you know, you don't know what you could catch, you could get AIDS, and it's always immediately afterwards I really start panicking — the last two guys, okay, they're probably bastards — whatever, you know — I said something I think, and one of them said, 'oh you're not going to make me wear one of those are you'. And I could have said — I should have said, 'yes', you know; but I wanted sex as much as they did and I didn't want any aggro. I thought straight after, 'you stupid, stupid girl' — and immediately resolved that next time I would, you know.

But this resolution, often expressed by these young women, particularly after frightening or risky sexual experiences, is not so easily realized. One young woman had experienced pregnancy, abortion and a scare about cervical cancer in the most unpleasant circumstances. Together with her current boyfriend she had had an HIV test because she thought that she might have the virus. She felt that she had changed, become more responsible and could and would take control of her own life and sexuality, — or at least this was what she wanted to think she would do. She described her inability to take control of the situation in the past, and inability to voice her wishes:

> *A:*   I know I have been in situations where I haven't [used a condom]. I have simply thought to myself, well look, well. When I got pregnant, I thought to myself, 'I'm not using a condom here, I'm not using anything', but I just couldn't say, just couldn't force myself to say, 'look, you know —' and then the consequences were disastrous. But at the time I knew what I was doing, and I knew that I just couldn't say it and I knew that it was wrong.

When she was asked if she felt confident that she could be more assertive (her term) in a future relationship, her ambivalence persisted. She said:

> *A:*   I don't know how I would be, because I was telling myself, if this relationship comes to an end, I'm never falling in the same trap as before, that I won't, I'll make sure that I'm sort of thinking that — Oh, God, I bet I will. I don't want to but I don't know whether I am really trying to say look, if all these things happen, you should learn from it. I'm more than fifty per cent confident that it won't, but not a full hundred per cent.

Another young woman, who very successfully negotiated condom use in her current steady relationship, had doubts about her ability to do so if she was in another in which she was really keen on the man:

> *A:*   But, you know — some men ... you can get some men which refuse to use them, which makes it really difficult. You think 'Oh, God!', say you really like them a lot.

For another, her own doubts about her capacity to insist on protection on a one-night stand brought the dramatic plea, 'I would like to think that I would, I hope to death I would.'

It is these varied patterns of condom use which can alert us to the unpredictable outcomes of situations in which women have to respond to conflicting pressures.

To unravel the variability in women's experience of using and not using condoms, we need to develop a theoretical framework which can account for the gendered power relations and the contradictory pressures which constitute the context of sexual risk and safety. The AIDS epidemic has provided a spur for attempts both to examine what actually takes place in sexual encounters and to understand the complex social processes, pressures and power relations which permeate and construct such encounters. The data emerging from our study provide an illustration of the major elements in sexual relationships and encounters which remain to be explored, explained and restructured if young heterosexuals are to be able to protect themselves against the spread of HIV and AIDS. One key facilitating factor would be to develop a challenge to the language of heterosexuality which privileges male over female sexual experience and desire. A transformation and expansion of this discourse to encompass the heterogeneity of male and female desire and experience would enable women and men to recognize and express the contradictions of their own experiences, their own responsibilities and their own agency (Cameron, 1985). Women themselves can develop a positive language which will make public the continuum of sexual pressure, ambivalence and pleasure in sexuality. When women have self-respecting sexual identities which do not depend primarily on being attached to a man, they will be in a stronger position to promote sexual safety. The embarrassment of negotiating condom use with the one you love highlights and illustrates the current contradictions of female subordination in the close encounters of heterosexual sex.

Notes

1 The Women, Risk and AIDS Project (WRAP), staffed by the authors, working collectively, is currently financed by the ESRC. It is carrying out a three-phase study of the sexual relationships, beliefs and practices of purposive samples of young women in London and Manchester. This paper is based primarily on 150 depth interviews. A subsample of the young women is being reinterviewed after an interval of one year, and some have kept diaries.

2 While safe sex is widely associated with condoms, there is less knowledge of chemical barriers to use with condoms. While there is some confusion about how much is the right amount to 'kill' HIV, it has been argued that condoms provide an effective physical barrier to HIV together with Nonoxynol 9 (Conant *et al.*, 1986; Reitmeijer *et al.*, 1988).

3 Insisting on sexual safety, however, may or may not be a successful strategy. Sexual violence is always a possibility. Of the 500 women who completed questionnaires, 11 per cent said they had intercourse against their will, and we found in the course of the interviews that this was a considerable understatement, since a number of women who had been raped or pressured into unwanted intercourse had not stated this on their questionnaire. This issue will be more fully developed in later publications.

4 If their steady partner is seropositive or otherwise carrying infection, trusting to the pill can put young women at risk. Critics have argued that heterosexuals are not at risk in the

West because sexually transmitted diseases which facilitate the spread of HIV are not widespread. Herpes, cervical cancer and sexually transmitted diseases, however, do constitute risks about which many young women are very ill-informed.

References

ABRAMS, D., ABRAHAM, C., SPEARS, R. and MARKS, D. (1990) 'AIDS Invulnerability: Relationships, Sexual Behaviour and Attitudes among 16–19 Year Olds', in P. AGGLETON, P. DAVIES and G. HART (Eds), *AIDS: Individual, Cultural and Policy Dimensions*, Lewes, Falmer Press.

AZJEN, I. and FISHBEIN, M. (1980) *Understanding Attitudes and Predicting Social Behaviour*, New York, Prentice-Hall.

CAMERON, D. (1985) *Feminism and Linguistic Theory*, London, Macmillan.

CLARK, S., EVANS, B.G., KAUNARATNE, M. and KENNEDY, A.R. (1990) 'Adolescents and Young Adults Infected with HIV-1: The Pattern in England, Wales and Northern Ireland', paper presented to the Sixth International Conference on AIDS, San Francisco.

COCHRANE, S.D. and MAYS, V.M. (1990) 'Report', *New England Journal of Medicine*, 322, 7, 774–775.

COI (Central Office of Information)-DHSS (1987) *Attitudes to Condoms: Report on an Exploratory Study*, London, COI.

CONANT, M., *et al.* (1986) 'Condoms Prevent Transmission of AIDS Associated Retrovirus', *Journal of the American Medical Association*, 255, 1706.

COSSEY, D. (1979) *Teenage Birth Control: The Case for the Condom*, London, Brook Advisory Service.

COWARD, R. (1987) 'Sex after AIDS', *The New Internationalist*. March.

DAY, S. and WARD, H. (1990) 'The Praed Street Project: A Cohort of Prostitute Women in London', in M. PLANT (Ed.), *AIDS, Drugs and Prostitution*, London, Tavistock/Routledge.

DAY, S., WARD, H. and HARRIS, J.R.W. (1988) 'Prostitute Women and Public Health', *British Medical Journal*, 297, 1585.

DWORKIN, A. (1987) *Intercourse*, London, Arrow Books.

FITZPATRICK, M. and MILLIGAN, D. (1990) 'Reflections on the AIDS Panic (interviewed by LINDA RYAN)', *Living Marxism*, 15, 14–19.

FREEMAN, R. (1990) 'The Condom in Manchester', *Working Papers in Applied Social Research*, University of Manchester.

FUMENTO, M. (1990) *The Myth of Heterosexual AIDS: How a Tragedy Has Been Distorted by the Media and Partisan Politics*', extracts in *The Sunday Times*, 18 and 25 March.

GAMBETTA, D. (1990) (Ed.) *Trust: Making and Breaking Cooperative Relations*, Oxford, Blackwell.

GATHERER, A., *et al.* (1979) *Is Health Education Effective?* London, Health Education Council.

GROSS, A.E. and BELLEW-SMITH, M. (1983) 'A Social Psychological Approach to Reducing Pregnancy Risk in Adolescence', in D. BYRNE and W.A. FISHER (Eds), *Adolescence, Sex and Contraception*, New Jersey, Lawrence Erlbaum Associates.

GROSS, J. (1987) 'Bleak Lives: Women Carrying AIDS', *New York Times*, 17 August.

HANSON, S.L., MYERS, D.E. and GINSBURG, A.L. (1987) 'The Role of Responsibility and Knowledge in Reducing out of Wedlock Childbearing', *Journal of Marriage and the Family*, 49, 241–256.

HEYWARD, W.L. and CURRAN, J.W. (1988) 'The Epidemiology of AIDS in the US', *Scientific American*, 259, 4, 52–59.

HITE, S. (1989a) *The Hite Report Women and Love: A Cultural Revolution in Progress*, Harmondsworth, Penguin.

HITE, S. (1989b) *The Hite Report on Female Sexuality*, London, Pandora.

HOLLAND, J., RAMAZANOGLU, C. and SCOTT, S. (1990a) 'Managing Risk and Experiencing Danger: Tensions between Government AIDS Education Policy and Young Women's Sexuality', *Gender and Education*, 2, 2, 125–146.

HOLLAND, J., RAMAZANOGLU, C. and SCOTT, S. (1990b) 'AIDS: From Panic Stations to Power Relations', *Sociology*, 24, 3, 499–518.

JOHNSON, A. (1988) 'Heterosexual Transmission of Human Immunodeficiency Virus', *British Medical Journal*, 296, 1017–1020.

KELLY, L. (1988) *Surviving Sexual Violence*, Cambridge, Polity Press.

KOLLER, M. (1988) 'Risk as a Determinant of Trust', *Basic and Applied Psychology*, 9, 4, 265–276.

LEES, S. (1986) *Losing Out: Sexuality and Adolescent Girls*, London, Hutchinson.

MCROBBIE, A. (1978) 'Working Class Girls and the Culture of Femininity', in Birmingham University CCCS, Women's Studies Group, *Women Take Issue*, London, Hutchinson.

MAHONEY, P. (1985) *Schools for the Boys? Co-education Reassessed*, London, Hutchinson/ Explorations in Feminism Collective.

MILLETT, K. (1977) *Sexual Politics*, London, Virago.

MORGAN, D. (1987) 'Masculinity and violence', in J. HANMER and M. MAYNARD (Eds), *Women, Violence and Social Control*, London, Macmillan.

NIX, L.M., PASTEUR, A.B. and SERVANCE, M.A. (1988) 'A Focus Group Study of Sexually Active Black Male Teenagers', *Adolescence*, 23, 91, 741–743.

PADIAN, N.S. (1987) 'Heterosexual Transmission of Acquired Immunodeficiency Syndrome: International Perspectives and National Projections', *Reviews of Infectious Diseases*, 9, 5, 947–960.

PANOS INSTITUTE (1988) *AIDS and the Third World*, London, Panos Publications.

PLECK, J.H., SONENSTEIN, F.L. and SWAIN, S.O. (1988) 'Adolescent Males' Sexual Behaviour and Contraceptive Use: Implications for Male Responsibility', *Journal of Adolescent Research*, 3, 3/4, 275–284.

PYE, M., KAPILA, M., BUCKLEY, G. and CUNNINGHAM, D. (1989) (Eds) *Responding to the AIDS Challenge: A Comparative Study of Local AIDS Programmes in the UK*, London, HEA/ Longman.

REITMEIJER, C.A.M., et al. (1988) 'The Physical and Chemical Effectiveness of the Condom as a Barrier against AIDS', *Journal of the American Medical Association*, 259, 1851–1853.

RICH, A. (1983) 'Compulsory Heterosexuality and Lesbian Existence', in E. ABEL and E. K. ABEL (Eds), *Women, Gender and Scholarship: The Signs Reader*, Chicago, Ill., University of Chicago Press.

RIEDER, I. and RUPPELT, P. (1989) (Eds) *Matters of Life and Death: Women Speak about AIDS*, London, Virago.

SCOTT, S., ALDRIDGE, J. and TEMPLE, B. (1990) Data presented at Methodology Conference, University of Manchester, March.

SHULMAN, A. (1971) 'Organs and Orgasms', in V. GORNICK and B.K. MORAN (Eds), *Women in Sexist Society: Studies in Power and Powerlessness*, New York, Mentor Books.

SPENCER, B. (1984) 'Young Men: Their Attitudes towards Sexuality and Birth Control', *British Journal of Family Planning*, 10, 13–19.

SPENCER, L., FAULKNER, A. and KEEGAN, J. (1988) *Talking about Sex: Asking the Public about Sexual Behaviour and Attitudes*, London, Social and Community Planning Research.

THOMSON, R. (1988) 'Women, AIDS and the Social Construction of a Disease', undergraduate dissertation, University of Manchester.

VANCE, C.S. (1984) 'Pleasure and Danger: Towards a Politics of Sexuality', in C.S. VANCE (Ed.), *Pleasure and Danger: Exploring Female Sexuality*, London, Routledge and Kegan Paul.

WATNEY, S. (1987) *Policing Desire: Pornography, AIDS and the Media*, London, Methuen.

WEEKS, J. (1989) 'AIDS: The Intellectual Agenda', in P. AGGLETON, G. HART and P. DAVIES (Eds), *AIDS: Social Representations, Social Practices*, Lewes, Falmer Press.

WINN, D. (1986) 'Smart Girls Carry Condoms', *Cosmopolitan*. November.

Chapter 10

Condoms, Coercion and Control: Heterosexuality and the Limits to HIV/AIDS Education

Tamsin Wilton and Peter Aggleton

It is generally accepted that, in the continued and continuing absence of a vaccine or cure for HIV disease, education to bring about the widespread adoption of those sexual and drug injecting practices which do not transmit the virus is the only realistic option open to us by which to halt the global epidemic. Given the current state of medical knowledge about sexual transmission, coupled with the range of technologies which enable information to be disseminated around the world, it might be expected that the rate at which HIV is transmitted by sexual contact would by now have slowed almost to a standstill. At one level the information needed to prevent sexual transmission is so simple and straightforward that it should theoretically be possible for each and every individual to avoid infection and, if infected, to protect their sexual partners. Yet this is clearly not happening. Indeed, recent figures show that in Britain, where vast sums of money have been spent on public education campaigns, the rate of sexual transmission among heterosexuals is on the increase (Adler, 1990).

As research into the effectiveness of different models of health education has long indicated, information giving is simply insufficient to bring about clearcut and lasting behaviour change (Gatherer *et al.*, 1979). Individuals do not simply absorb information and respond logically by modifying their health-related behaviour. Rather, people actively 'make sense' of new ideas they encounter by assessing them in the light of pre-existing beliefs, interpreting them accordingly, and fitting them in with what they already know (Warwick, Aggleton and Homans, 1988). Thus new health-related information is responded to, often unconsciously, in the light of pre-existing biomedical understanding, as well as culturally and generationally specific lay beliefs about health. Many of us, for example, believe that an apple a day keeps the doctor away, despite more modern concerns about horticultural pesticides. In the same way thousands of people ritualistically swallow a daily dose of vitamins of contested prophylactic value. In the case of AIDS the conceptual matrix into which safer sex information must be fitted includes not only lay beliefs about the origins, aetiology and effects of the syndrome but also socially, culturally, ethnically, religiously and politically specific significations of sexual desire and practice.

It is also important to recognize that safer sex guidelines are not themselves free from ideological contamination. Information is produced, reproduced, distributed and transformed by and within social groups, each of which may have its own ideological motivation for promoting certain ideas at the expense of others. Paradigmatic of this are some of the attitudes espoused by the present government, informed as they are by a narrow, putatively Christian, moralism which privileges above all other forms of sexuality a reproductive, familial heterosexuality organized around rigid gender divisions. Allied to this is an increasingly punitive social ostracism of all groups defined as 'deviant' by reference to that narrow norm. Thus politicians, religious leaders and key decision-makers in Britain, unable to resist the opportunity offered by early constructions of AIDS as a 'gay plague', the supposedly natural consequence of promiscuity and deviant object-choice, have perverted simple messages about safer sex into a set of justifications whereby a reactionary set of ideologies can be promulgated. As a result, the fundamental safer sex message, which Patton (1989a) has, somewhat simplistically, reduced to 'Don't get semen in your anus or vagina', has been transformed into an ever more urgent insistence on the prophylactic properties of chastity, fidelity and marriage (Wilton and Aggleton, 1990a).

Safer sex work, although predicated upon simple and straightforward changes in sexual practice, is made more problematic by the fact that sex in our culture has become, as Weeks (1985) puts it, 'a contested zone...a moral and political battlefield'. This chapter offers an attempt to identify some of the ways in which work around safer sex engages with one profoundly contested aspect of sexuality, sexual identity. It also aims to demonstrate how the gendered relations of power within heterosexuality differentially influence the capacity of women and men to initiate and/or maintain the practice of safer sex in their close and loving relationships.

Practice and Identity: Safer Sex in the Gay Community

It remains vitally important to recognize that safe sex was not something dreamed up in recent years by medical professionals. Instead it was an intrinsic component of the USA gay community response to AIDS long before HIV was identified, and well before a medical consensus was established concerning the viral aetiology of AIDS (Watney, 1989; Patton, 1989b). Its significance was twofold. Faced with a mounting death toll, safer sex was above all a community practice with which to counter grief and fear. But the epidemic of disease was accompanied by an equally deadly epidemic of discrimination, ostracism and attacks on civil rights (Frankenberg, 1989). In the face of government negligence and the widespread social legitimation of AIDS-related homophobia and queer-bashing, safer sex practices became for many gay men the core of an oppositional discourse which reinforced a sense of community identity and provided the collective strength essential for survival (Weeks, 1985; Patton, 1990).

The notion of the 'gay community' is, of course, not unproblematic, and a crucial issue for HIV/AIDS education is that many men who have sex with men do not self-identify as gay, and there are many lesbians and gay men who live their lives entirely untouched by any notion of community. Even among those who do see themselves as part of the lesbian and gay movement it is clear that homosexuality encompasses heterogeneity and diversity no less than does heterosexuality. Yet it is important to recognize that issues to do with sex and sexuality have a resonance in lesbian and gay culture which simply does not exist for the majority of heterosexuals. Lesbians and gay men are obliged, in our intensely erotophobic and homophobic culture, to construct their social and political identities around sexual object choice. Inherent in this process is the creation of discourses of sexuality and sexual practice into which it is relatively straightforward to fit notions of safer sex and sexual responsibility. Notions of safer sexual practices simply become one more item on a pre-existing agenda.

Discourses of Desire: 'Coming to Power' vs 'The Joy of Sex'

While it would be overly simplistic to suggest that all lesbians and gay men are accustomed to participation in free and frank debate about sexual matters, it is true that many have access to rich and wide-ranging discourses of sexuality. Questions of sado-masochism, of monogamy, of erotics and of desire have been well theorized, often through a close engagement with allied feminist discourses around relations of power and sexual politics. In contrast, the discursive structuration of heterosexual practice and desire is most usually encoded within a more limited set of options, varying from the more repressive forms of mass market pornography to technique manuals such as 'The Joy of Sex'.

Oppositional discourses on sex and sexuality offered by radical feminists (and some gay writers) have no counterpart among heterosexual men, though a few are taking up the challenge of tentatively deconstructing masculinity (Reynaud, 1981). It is precisely this lack of any sustained critique of heterosexual practice outside feminism which makes feminists' personal experience of heterosexuality so painful, and which leads to the radical feminist assertion that a precondition for the overthrow of patriarchy is that all women identify as lesbian (Jeffreys, 1990).

The paucity of heterosexual discourses of desire and sexual practice has two sets of implications for HIV/AIDS health promotion. First, as Rule (1985) points out, the dominant heterosexual culture is predicated not only on homophobia, but on erotophobia. The Judaeo–Christian legacy of guilt and shame pervades much of Western culture, and heterosexuality offers no oppositional discourse within which to challenge this. As Rule says, 'If straight people have the decency to be modestly ashamed of their own sexual natures, what right have we to be proud of ours?' p. 118.

It is clear, therefore, that the challenge to homophobia that is so central a part of HIV/AIDS health promotion can only be effective in the context of a broad challenge to the erotophobia that pervades heterosexual culture. In the absence of a pre-existing heterosexual critique of the erotic, such a challenge has little with which to engage systematically.

The second issue for HIV/AIDS education follows from this awareness. To be effective, safer sex work must be explicit, and specific sexual practices must be discussed in relation to HIV transmission. We know that vague generalizations about 'body fluids', and even terms like 'sexual intercourse', are open to conflicting interpretations, and need careful deconstruction. The problem is that heterosexual women and men lack a context in which to engage with issues of sexual practice in ways which are distinct from notions of morality or 'good' and 'bad' behaviour. Indeed, the present government has made the provision of safer sex information in schools *conditional* upon the overt promotion of familial ideology. For example, the teachers' booklet accompanying the HIV/AIDS education video sent to all British secondary schools insists that:

> It is not sufficient for schools to remain neutral: pupils should understand that the best way for them to avoid AIDS is to refrain from sexual activity until, as adults, they establish a stable, loving and mutually faithful relationship. . . . The central role of marriage in sexual relationships must be emphasised.

Disengaging sexual desire and sexual practice from such notions is a strategy which very many lesbians and gay men are obliged to engage in both individually and collectively. It is not one that is familiar within mainstream heterosexual culture, and the negotiation of safer sex is consequentially problematic.

Normal and Hence Invisible: The Problem of Being Heterosexual

The hegemonic status of the institution of heterosexuality is predicated upon presumptions of naturalness and normality (Rich, 1980). This has specific consequences for heterosexual practice, as well as for notions of heterosexual identity.

The central icon of heterosexual desire is spontaneity (Weeks, 1985; Wilton and Aggleton, 1990a). This is partly contingent upon the idea of naturalness. To be capable of construction as 'natural', with all the concomitant associations with that which is instinctual, visceral and even animal, sexual behaviour must be spontaneous and unpremeditated. Indeed, the idea of premeditation is anathema to ideologically sound *heterosex*. Many complaints about various methods of contraception revolve around the aspect of premeditation which they unavoidably bring to a sexual encounter (Phillips and Rakusen, 1978), and this is a familiar problem for those who would promote condoms as a form of protection against HIV.

The construction of heterosexual desire as instinctual, spontaneous and irresistible is in addition one way in which moral imperatives against sexual pleasure may be overcome. Passion, it is widely accepted, must be expected to override ethical considerations. It is also, crucially, a profoundly gendered construct, which operates to reinforce the sexual oppression, abuse and objectification of women by allowing men to justify their abusive and irresponsible sexual behaviour. It is largely *male* desire which is constructed in this way, through what several writers have characterized as the hydraulic model of male sexuality, whereby the male sexual 'drive' is presumed to be powerful, beyond conscious control and liable at any moment to be set in motion by erotic stimuli in a primitive, neo-Pavlovian way (Jeffreys, 1990). This construction of male desire is not, of course, exclusively heterosexual — some gay men live out such scripted identities — but it maps onto the social relations of power in heterosexual relationships in such a way as to produce specific problems for women in negotiating safer sex. Questions of safer sex, whether involving non-penetrative activities or the use of condoms, are thus inevitably problematic within heterosexuality, predicated as it is upon gendered inequality, and privileging as it does an ideal of spontaneity.

Recognizing that the practice of safer sex engages in an important way with gay identity leads us to ask whether there is anything within the experience of heterosexual identity which could engage in a similarly positive way with safer sex in response to the threat to HIV. The concept of 'heterosexual identity', unfortunately, is far from unproblematic. The hegemonic status of the institution of heterosexuality, radically embedded as it is in Western culture, the dominance of its ideology manifest across wide-ranging religious, social, cultural and political discourses, constructs a monolithic norm whose unproblematic status becomes an ideological tenet. Heterosexuality, we would argue, is best understood as a *relative* identity, predicated upon a collusion with its givenness, which is, in fact, negotiated in continual struggle by negative reference to those who are identifiably 'other'. To be heterosexual is above all to be *not-homosexual*. Moreover, under the relations of power which inhere in patriarchy, it is male heterosexual identity which is the fundamental defended principle.

Some writers have suggested that, in a culture defined and organized by men, the social identity of femininity is ascribed, while masculinity 'has to be achieved in a permanent process of struggle and confirmation' (Mapp, 1982). This is not to deny that femininity has always been a site of struggle for women in opposition to the defining power of men, but rather to assert that masculinity, having no definition imposed upon it by a more powerful other (as is the case with femininity), achieves its own identity by a continual process of negative reference to *less* powerful others, specifically to women and to gay men. As the monolithic norm around which patriarchal culture is constructed, masculinity is unself-conscious, unquestioned and undefined. Its nature is that of the hole in the mint — an organizing absence. Male power, organized around such evanescence, is consequently displaced onto that visible and given symbol of innate maleness, the penis, and onto practices which label and disempower those who are *other*, practices which range from queer-bashing and rape to the construction of the rigid gender demarcations which structure all our social relations. Sexual penetration by the penis thereby becomes the symbolic assertion of male power over disempowered other, an ideological totem which explains why anal intercourse between two men is regarded by many with such abhorrence, representing as it does the pre-eminent betrayal of masculinity. It also reveals the ideological mechanism whereby lesbian sexuality, where a penis is by definition not involved, is so absolutely devalued and denigrated.

Male Power and Sexual Practice

A culture predicated upon the allocation of power to a class whose status inheres in its identity as the supposed norm against which all else is measured, cannot afford to problematize that norm. Feminism offers a powerful critique of the normalizing and normative status of masculinity, but has not, so far, brought that critique to bear on either establishment or radical discourses around AIDS. Without such a critique, the practice of safer sex, the only prophylactic we have against the sexual transmission of HIV, remains a minority concern.

As long as heterosexual masculinity persists in defining itself by negative reference to those who are 'other' than itself, the adoption of safer sexual practices, specifically those which dispense with penetration, will remain ideologically intolerable. Disempowering the act of penetration creates profound anxieties around masculine identity against which heterosexuality, lacking a critique of its own nature, has no language with which to defend itself. Feminists have pointed to the sustained silence about the clitoris which has pervaded safer sex discourse, precisely that discourse within which the significance of clitoral sexuality should be foregrounded (Jackson, 1988). This is unsurprising: the very existence of the clitoris is intolerable within the discourses of a dominant ideology dependent upon the social and cultural construction of sex as that which involves bodily penetration. Within such an ideological context, exhortations to practise non-penetrative sex are merely incomprehensible.

As long as straight men continue to define their heterosexuality as non-homosexuality, gay men will continue to be oppressed, and straight men will in turn be obliged to deny that HIV, historically constructed in the West as a *consequence of homosexuality* (Weeks, 1985; Watney, 1989), has any relevance to them. Similarly, as long as masculinity is defined in opposition to femininity, a social construction, crucially, in which inhere notions of responsibility about health, personal relationships and sex (Chapman, 1988), non-penetrative sex, or even the wearing of condoms, will be seen as emasculating. Heterosexual women who attempt to ensure their own and their partner's safety by suggesting the use of a condom, therefore, not only challenge their partner's inalienable right to the full sensations of penetration, but also introduce an element of premeditation into an act justified largely by its spontaneity. They impugn the heterosexuality of their partner by association with a virus stubbornly elided with homosexuality, and they ask their partner to behave with a responsibility which is simply dissonant with the construction of the male sex 'drive'. Furthermore, to purchase and carry condoms is, for a woman, to challenge the patriarchal definition of her sexuality as innately responsive to male initiative — as reactive rather than proactive. Such a challenge demands more than mere assertiveness training for women. It demands a paradigmatic shift around the nexus of gender identity and sexual identity.

Conclusions

Throughout this chapter we have argued that ideologies of heterosexual masculinity represent a powerful counterforce to the promotion of safer sex. If safer sex practices are to become established among more than a minority, initiatives to challenge this counterforce must be established at the level of theory and practice, ideology and policy. A systematic deconstruction of masculinity is central, not merely tangential, to radical HIV/AIDS discourse. In relation to policy even a sustained survey of the literature reveals heterosexual man as the great undiscussed, a ghostly presence made manifest by his absence. Admittedly, in health promotion policies constructed to target discrete population groups, heterosexual men may well be addressed incidentally, inasmuch as they may inject drugs, or partake of other identified risk behaviours, but with the exception of a tiny handful of locally produced leaflets, they remain unengaged with *as* heterosexual men.

For heterosexual women the need to respond to the HIV epidemic has made sex still more dangerous, and violence against women is central to the concerns of those who struggle to construct around HIV and AIDS oppositional discourses of gender and sexual identity, desire and sexual practice, within which to promote safer sex. Women who attempt to negotiate safer sex with male partners risk abuse, physical violence or the loss of that partner, often with profound social and economic consequences. As long as this is true, the widespread adoption of safer sexual practices will remain a pipe-dream. And as long as the hegemony of patriarchal ideology offers men free and full access to womens' bodies (Jeffreys, 1990), women will remain powerless to insist on safer sex.

HIV/AIDS is, of course, of crucial concern to the gay community. It is also, in the face of an incredible and murderous denial, of crucial concern to what would be a heterosexual community if there were such a thing. It is the hegemonic status of masculinity, predicated upon the subordination of women, which represents the greatest challenge in our struggle against the epidemic. Women's oppression, no less than the oppression of lesbians and gay men, is central to those social and cultural structures of a heteropatriarchy which acts to impede the effectiveness of safer sex against the HIV/AIDS epidemic. For those working in HIV/AIDS to ignore this, is to build upon sand. HIV/AIDS is, and must remain, a feminist issue.

References

ADLER, M. (1990) *AIDS Newsletter*, 5, 1, London, Bureau of Hygiene and Tropical Diseases.
CHAPMAN, K. (1988) 'Safer Sex for Some', *Lib Ed,* Summer 1988, Leicester, LIB ED Collective.
DEPARTMENT OF EDUCATION AND SCIENCE (1988) *Your Choice for Life* (teachers' handbook to accompany video of the same name).
FRANKENBURG, R. (1989) 'One Epidemic or Three?' in P. AGGLETON, G. HART and P. DAVIES (Eds), *AIDS: Social Representations, Social Practices*, Lewes, Falmer Press.
GATHERER, A., *et al.* (1979) *Is Health Education Effective?* London, Health Education Council.
JACKSON, G. (1988) 'Promotion of Safer Sex or the Patriarchy, Misogyny and the Condom', unpublished paper.
JEFFREYS, S. (1990) *Anticlimax: A Feminist Perspective on the Sexual Revolution*, London, Women's Press.
MAPP, L. (1982) quoted in *Equal Opportunities — What's in It for Boys*, London, ILEA/Schools Council.
PATTON, C. (1989a) 'Safer Sex, Community and Porn', *Rites*, April, 10.
PATTON, C. (1989b) 'The AIDS Industry', in E. CARTER and S. WATNEY (Eds), *Taking Liberties*, London, Serpents Tail Press/Institute of Contemporary Arts.
PATTON, C. (1990) 'Safer Sex as Resistance to Societal Control and Moralism', paper presented at the First Nordic Conference on Safer Sex, Stockholm, March.
PHILLIPS, A. and RAKUSEN, J. (Eds) (1978) *Our Bodies, Ourselves*, Harmondsworth, Penguin.
REYNAUD, E. (1981) *Holy Virility*, London, Pluto Press.
RICH, A. (1980) 'Compulsory Heterosexuality and Lesbian Existence', in A. RICH, *Blood, Bread and Poetry*, London, Virago.
RULE, J. (1985) 'Straights, Come Out', in *A Hot-eyed Moderate, Talahassee*, Florida, Naiad Press.
WARWICK, I., AGGLETON, P. and HOMANS, H. (1988) 'Young People's Health Beliefs and AIDS', in P. AGGLETON and H. HOMANS (Eds), *Social Aspects of AIDS*, Lewes, Falmer Press.
WATNEY, S. (1989) 'Taking Liberties: An Introduction', in E. CARTER and S. WATNEY (Eds), *Taking Liberties*, London, Serpents Tail.
WEEKS, J. (1985) *Sexuality and Its Discontents*, London, Routledge and Kegan Paul.
WILTON, T. and AGGLETON, P. (1990a) 'AIDS — Don't Die of Misinformation', *Youth Clubs with The Edge*, 56, 19–21, Youth Clubs UK.
WILTON, T. and AGGLETON, P. (1990b) 'Young People and Safer Sex', paper presented at the First Nordic Conference on Safer Sex, Stockholm, March.

Chapter 11

Perceptions of AIDS Vulnerability: The Role of Attributions and Social Context

Amina Memon

In the last three years there has been an increasing amount of research on risk perception and HIV/AIDS. Much of this work has been concerned with attitudes and behaviour change as a result of public education campaigns or local education strategies. More recently, emphasis has been placed upon perceptions of severity and vulnerability to HIV and AIDS and the influence of these variables on the intention to engage in safer sex and drug practices. This work has been guided by a variety of social psychological models (e.g. the Health Belief Model, Rosenstock, 1966, 1974; Protection Motivation Theory, Rogers, 1975). While it is clear that the seriousness of HIV has been communicated through health education campaigns (e.g. Wober, 1988), among some a general feeling of 'invulnerability' to HIV and AIDS still prevails (e.g. Abrams *et al.*, 1990a, 1990b).

The aim of this chapter is to consider the extent to which perceptions of HIV/AIDS risk can be accommodated within the cognitive framework of attribution theory (Heider, 1958; Kelley, 1967). 'Attributions' essentially represent people's ideas about what causes things to occur (causal inferences) and why things happen as they do (Fiske and Taylor, 1984). They also reflect the need to predict and control future events, both behaviour and other people. With reference to recent research on perceptions of HIV/AIDS, this chapter will discuss the ways in which attributional biases influence personal assessments of HIV risk, create 'illusions of invulnerability' (Perloff and Fetzer, 1986) and influence social comparison processes to do with perceived *personal risk* versus the risk to *others*. Attributions of 'responsibility', 'freedom' and 'control' will be examined with reference to qualitative data on young people's lay beliefs about HIV transmission and their social constructions of people with AIDS (PWAs). Finally, following Hewstone and Jaspars (1984), it is proposed that attributions are unlikely to tell us much about behaviour, unless they are considered in a wider social context. This has been neglected in questionnaire research (Memon, 1990) but is being incorporated in more recent work using the 'ethnographic' approach (e.g. Ingham and Woodcock, 1990; Holland *et al.*, 1989). The potential value of such an approach in informing us about the social conditions underlying HIV/AIDS-related risk behaviour will be examined with reference to some recently published research.

Attribution Theory: An Introduction

From a young age children form hypotheses about the causes of events, and this preoccupation with understanding causes persists into adulthood. The attribution theory approach asks, how does the social perceiver (you and I) use information in the social environment to arrive at a causal explanation for an event? (Heider, 1958). Thus it examines what information is gathered and how it is combined to form an attribution. The social perceiver tends to be viewed as a naive scientist who accomplishes many of the same tasks as a formal scientist. In an attempt to infer causes for behaviour the social perceiver can rely either on dispositional qualities or on internal attributes of a person or on situational or external factors. An example of a dispositional attribution for engaging in unsafe sexual behaviour could be 'selfishness' where an attribution to external causes may be 'can't afford to buy a condom' (e.g. the unavailability of a condom).

There appears to be a strong tendency to attribute behaviour to dispositional qualities rather than situational factors. This effect, described as the 'fundamental attribution error', is well documented in social psychology (Fiske and Taylor, 1984). However, attributions are not merely products of cognitive processing; they are, as Hewstone and Jaspars (1984) have argued, social in origin. Deschamps (1978) proposed a theory of social attribution building on work on social representations (e.g. Moscovici, 1981) and social categorization (e.g. Taylor and Jaggi, 1974). According to social attribution theory: 'In a situation of less than complete information...an individual attributes behaviour of another individual not simply to individual characteristics or intentions, but to the characteristics or intentions associated with the group to which the other belongs' (Hewstone and Jaspars, 1984:387).

Thus, according to Deschamps, 'stereotypes' are essentially characteristics attributed to members of one group by members of another group. Group members are expected to show a more favourable pattern of attitudes for an in-group member than an out-group member. Deschamps refers to this as 'ethnocentric attribution bias'. There is evidence to suggest that the tendency to make internal attributions will be enhanced when a member of an out-group performs what is perceived to be a 'negative' act. The negative actions of an in-group member, however, will tend to be attributed to external causes (Taylor and Jaggi, 1974; Pettigrew, 1979).

The impact of social attributions is illustrated by the work of Stockdale *et al.* (1989) in a study of perceptions of AIDS campaign posters. The two target groups were gay men and heterosexuals, and they were asked to comment on media messages. As expected, the responses for the two groups differed. Gay men had a clear perception of personal relevance and recognized some risk of AIDS (a subjective estimate of risk), but only in 'unstable' relationships. Interestingly, gay men perceive other gay men in stable relationships as less at risk than heterosexuals in unstable relationships. In contrast, the heterosexual sample endorsed a stereo-typical view of gay men, bisexuals and injecting drug users (IDUs) as being most at risk from HIV, and the incidence of HIV among heterosexuals was attributed to external factors (e.g. unstable relationships). Stockdale *et al.* (1989) draw the following conclusions, illustrating quite clearly the operation of ethnocentric attributional biases in perceptions of AIDS vulnerability:

> ...There is a clear indication that the heterosexual and homosexual subjects agree about the groups that are more at risk than others. Equally, it is clear that gays, including those in stable relationships recognize their potential susceptibility but feel they have got the message. However, heterosexuals still do not see themselves as at risk. It is still someone else's problem: 'others' are likely to contract HIV not them; 'others' only have themselves to blame if they do contract HIV whereas in the unlikely event that heterosexuals do contract HIV, it's not their fault; and those people who are at risk are *not like me*. (Stockdale *et al.*, 1989:23)

Attributions of 'Responsibility' and 'Control': Media Representations

In addition to individual and group factors influencing judgments, work on causal attribution has generally assumed that motivational factors can be the impetus for causal analysis. The importance of motivational factors is seen in the need to predict the future (in this context AIDS vulnerability) and to control events and other people (Rotter, 1966). Let us consider for a moment attitudes towards PWAs. In terms of attribution theory 'credit' or 'blame' for an action will be assigned on the basis of perceived 'responsibility' for an action. Attributions of responsibility may, in turn, depend on attributions of freedom and control over an action; the greater the perceived freedom or control over an action, the more blame or credit is assigned (Weiner, 1980). There are numerous examples of this in AIDS discourse. Alcorn (1988) shows how AIDS has been identified as a disease of difference, and how the origins of AIDS, both individual and social, have been likened to 'choice' and 'destiny' (Warwick *et al.*, 1988a, 1988b).

Wellings (1988b), too, has demonstrated how early newspaper reports on AIDS tended to differentiate between the so-called 'innocent' and 'guilty' victims of the syndrome. On the whole, the deaths of those who have contracted the disease through 'morally unacceptable practices' were evaluated far more negatively by the media than those infected as a result of accidental infection (mainly through blood transfusions and use of contaminated blood products).

Biases in media reporting of AIDS issues can produce quite marked biases in information processing and create stereotypes of the kind of person likely to be susceptible to HIV. Kahneman and Tversky (1972) have identified a number of heuristics or biases that may distort our perception and understanding of relevant information about AIDS. One example is the 'availability' heuristic. We assign a higher probability of occurrence to events that are easier to image or recall (recency) and those that have an impact (emotional salience). In terms of assimilating information about prevention of AIDS, this may be to avoid casual sex and reduce number of partners (i.e. avoid promiscuous behaviour). Another heuristic that may bias our perceptions is that of 'representativeness' (a stereotyped image or 'prototype' of the kind of person likely to get HIV), and this is seen clearly in attributions of HIV/AIDS to specific groups such as gay men (Brown and Fritz, 1988).

Kahneman and Tversky's (1972) 'anchoring mechanism' results in people attaching disproportionate importance to their initial assessments of risk. They may adjust upward or downward to create a final estimate, but such judgments are often biased in the direction of the initial 'anchor' value which may hamper their ability to make revisions in the light of new information. Thus in making assessments of vulnerability, people will resist information that is incongruent with their initial perception (Cervone and Peake, 1986). A good example is the early media publicity surrounding AIDS which clearly labelled it as a 'gay disease' and the more recent appeals to the public that the number of heterosexuals infected is increasing.

The association of AIDS with membership of certain 'risk groups' in media reports has clearly influenced social attributions of 'those at most risk'. Indeed Patton (1990) argues that even when the term 'risk behaviours' rather than 'risk groups' is used, 'identity' is collapsed with 'acts' (even when there is no necessary correlation). This is seen in discourse which refers to 'homosexual behaviours' or 'heterosexual behaviours'. Patton argues that by collapsing together HIV and AIDS, both infection and subsequent development of symptoms are seen as random events which may simply be a matter of luck. Media messages in this way may contribute to a perception of AIDS invulnerability.

Attributions of 'Responsibility' and Controllability' in Young People's Accounts of HIV and AIDS

This section discusses the value of an attributional analysis in understanding young people's views on the transmission of HIV and AIDS and their perceptions of their risk status relative to that of 'others' (see Perloff and Fetzer, 1986). Reference is made to data collected through semi-structured interviews (Warwick *et al.*, 1988a, 1988b), a questionnaire (which included a section for comments, Clift *et al.*, 1989, 1990) and focused group discussions (Boyle *et al.*, 1989).

Warwick *et al.* (1988a, 1988b) were interested in lay constructions of health and illness and the ways in which they may influence changes in health status, understanding of health and risk assessments. Data from fifty young people on Youth Training Schemes and in lesbian and gay groups were collected in late 1986 through the use of tape recorded and semi-structured interviews. Both general and specific questions about a wide range of health-related issues including AIDS were asked. Warwick *et al.* report that the young people they talked to were not clear about the medical distinction between HIV and AIDS. Moreover, a common belief was that there is 'something' out there which can be easily caught. Warwick *et al.* suggest that the distinction between 'exogenous' and 'endogenous' theories of disease causation may be usefully applied here. Exogenous theories attribute infection to factors outside the individual (e.g. bad luck) and tend to be employed when discussing personal risk. Warwick *et al.* argue that these beliefs may serve to undermine feelings of control which people would otherwise have. When respondents are asked how 'others' might become infected, endogenous theories or the personal qualities inherent in an individual come into play. The latter bring in notions of 'innocent' and 'guilty' victims of disease and responsibility for infection (cf. Reader *et al.*, 1989).

Clift *et al.* (1989) in a study of knowledge and beliefs about AIDS obtained a great deal of qualitative data by asking their sample of 14-18-year-old young people in school to comment on their views about AIDS (e.g. their feelings about the possibility of infection and their perceptions of PWAs). In relation to young people's responses to PWAs, attribution theory can readily be applied where 'sympathy' or 'blame' for infection are construed in terms of 'responsibility' and 'control'. Thus, for example, Clift *et al.* (1990) found that among their group of young people who were blaming there was little compassion for 'gay men' and 'drug users' (sometimes intravenous drug use was mentioned) or 'promiscuous' heterosexuals. There was, however, sympathy for the 'innocent' babies and haemophiliacs. In the case of the latter category, infection tended to be attributed to external factors (contact with infected blood products), while those in the former category were seen as having themselves to blame (e.g. through 'sleeping around', 'being gay', 'sharing needles'). There are, however, exceptions. For example, many young people in the Clift *et al.* sample expressed sympathy towards PWAs regardless of perceived causality or responsibility for infection ('unconditional sympathy').

Clift *et al.* (1990) suggest that the impact of negative attributions will be mediated by a number of factors such as personal experience (knowing someone who has HIV or AIDS). There also appear to be age and gender differences in attributions of blaming and responsibility. There was a tendency for boys and younger groups (14-year-olds versus 16-18-year-olds) to attribute infection to dispositional factors. Also the fact that the girls in the study perceived themselves as being more vulnerable than the boys suggests that the tendency to attribute blame for infection may be related to the illusion of AIDS invulnerability. Indeed, the 'high blame' group tended to perceive themselves as less vulnerable to infection. This needs to be explored in more depth in future research, possibly through focused group discussions.

Boyle *et al.* (1989) explored AIDS attitudes and knowledge among undergraduates by setting up focused group discussions. The discussions were open-ended, but the interviewer had a set of specific aims; one was to look at perceptions of AIDS relative to other health issues. When asked how concerned they were, there was a tendency to respond 'We're all at risk'. At the same time they 'distanced' themselves from the problem. Attributions of 'blame' were particularly prevalent when making reference to 'gay men' and 'drug users'. Terms such as 'responsibility' and 'innocence' were also employed in discussions about PWAs (cf. Marks *et al.*, 1989; Reader *et al.*, 1989; Clift *et al.*, 1990). Discussion groups in this study were useful in providing insights into the perceptions of health education messages. For example, in relation to attitudes to condom use, while the majority of young people were aware of the use of condoms to avoid infection, they expressed a reluctance to use them. Some young people said that they would prefer to 'vet' their partners and believed that discussions with partners would reduce risk. Others suggested that HIV testing and partner screening would eliminate the need for safer sex. A preference for safer partners over safer sex is consistent with a perception of AIDS invulnerability and optimism about health. Also related to this finding is the argument that reduction in number of partners and careful selection of partners pose less of a threat than losing face, embarrassment and loss of self-esteem through inept handling of condoms (Klee, 1990). As Richardson (1990 also points out: 'For the first time men have had to think about sex as a possible danger to themselves whereas women have always had to be in fear of unwanted pregnancy, rape and of health risks associated with use or loss of contraception or loss of reputation' (Richardson, 1990: 173).

Biased Perceptions of AIDS Risk:
The Role of Social Attributions

The saying 'it won't happen to me' generally implies 'it will happen to others' instead. (Perloff and Fetzer, 1986)

Research on the perceived risks associated with a variety of diseases concludes that people have judged themselves as less likely than others to be susceptible to diabetes, cancer, heart attack, strokes, pneumonia, leukaemia, alcoholism and sexually transmitted disease (Weinstein, 1980, 1984). Weinstein (1980) maintains that it may be as a result of attributional processes that individuals tend to underestimate their own risk (i.e. be 'unrealistically optimistic') relative to that of other people, and there is evidence to suggest that people are consistently biased about risk factors perceived to be 'controllable' (Weinstein, 1984). In a recent study of female college students' AIDS-related attitudes and beliefs (Memon, in preparation), I noted half a dozen comments which took the form: 'I am faithful to one partner' (and therefore) 'I am not at risk' (and therefore) 'I don't have to change my behaviour.'

There is also evidence of unrealistic optimism in young people's ratings when asked, for example, to estimate the prevalence of HIV among people of their own age (Abrams *et al.*, 1990a; Clift *et al.*, 1989). Abrams *et al.* (1990b) suggest that 'social identity' (the positive association with a group that is not at risk) and false consensus beliefs (e.g. that others are more irresponsible than themselves) may result in individuals underestimating and discounting factors that put them at risk of HIV. A similar discrepancy between perceptions of risk for self and others was reported in a survey of general public attitudes (British Market Research Bureau). Seventy-nine per cent of the sample did not think they would ever get the virus, and 70 per cent did not think they had to change their lifestyle because of AIDS. However, 92 per cent believed that people who have sex with a lot of different people are likely to get it, and 80 per cent thought there was a bigger risk of getting the virus through sex in some other country (Wellings, 1988b).

Perloff and Fetzer (1986) have addressed some important questions with respect to optimism about health. They argue that we need to look closely at the role of social comparison processes. These may, for example, serve an ego-defensive function reducing anxiety and make one feel 'good' about one's situation relative to that of the 'other' (see Taylor *et al.*, 1983). This is especially true in situations where an individual is being asked to make comparisons with a 'typical' or 'average' person, as in the Abrams *et al.* study. Indeed, Perloff and Fetzer (1986) report that when people are asked to rate the risks of a close friend or family member in relation to a series of illnesses (such as cancer, heart attacks, venereal diseases), they are perceived as equally 'invulnerable'. This suggests that biased perceptions of risk may be extended to include one's close friends and loved ones. The motivational explanation here would be that 'the closer one is emotionally to the comparison target, the more motivated one is to see the target as invulnerable' (see Burger, 1981).

One question that has not been addressed so far is: to what extent are subjective ratings of risk related to behaviour? One of the major limitations of much research on perception of AIDS risk in questionnaire studies is that the subjects are responding individually, in a hypothetical situation and not in the wider social context (see Farquhar, 1900). There is also evidence to suggest the predicted relationship between perceived risk and behaviour may be due to confounders. Baseline perception affects both risk perception and subsequent behaviour (Joseph *et al.*, 1987). The final section addresses this problem in reviewing some research on HIV/AIDS risk and behaviour change in gay men.

HIV/AIDS Risk and Behaviour Change in Gay Men

Exploratory studies have attempted to describe the prevalence and context of risk behaviour and the associated prevalence of HIV by looking at the perceptions of individuals in specific groups. In the United States and in Europe there has been a shift towards monitoring and evaluating changes in the content or stability of behaviour, in order to construct profiles of risk behaviour in gay men and the sexually active populations in general (see Coxon and Carballo, 1989, for a review).

Bauman and Siegel (1987) report data from a study of gay men in New York which was concerned with subjective perceptions of risk in current sexual practices and the relative accuracy of these perceptions in the light of epidemiological data. Data were obtained through structured interviews which asked, for example, for information about frequency of protected and unprotected intercourse, numbers of partners and details of sexual practice. A majority of men who engaged in sex with anonymous partners accurately appraised their practices, whereas men with only one partner or several partners were more likely to underestimate their risk. Bauman and Siegal argue that although safer sex guidelines almost universally recommend reducing the number of sexual partners, these practices do not eliminate risk when sexual practices including exchange of blood and semen occur. They argue that gay men must realistically appraise the riskiness of their sexual behaviour if they are to experience a sense of vulnerability. Some of the gay men in this study had weighed the risk associated with their behaviour based on misconceptions (e.g. showering and inspecting one's partners or lesions would reduce the risk) and were misled by advice such as 'reduce your partners' and 'get to know your partners'. Such health belief schemas can have an influence on the kind of behaviours adopted with the expectation of reducing risk. This work also suggests that we need to look at lay beliefs about risky and safe practices in order to get an insight into decision processes underlying behaviour change.

Fitzpatrick *et al.* (1990), in a recent review of evidence of behaviour change in gay men, stress that the emphasis on the health belief model has resulted in a focus on individual perceptions, when sex is clearly a social action involving two people in some sort of relationship. There is a move in the right direction in recent research. For example, Gold *et al.* (1990) report a detailed study of the thought processes and situational factors underlying decisions to engage in safe/unsafe sex in a study of 279 gay men in Australia. Respondents were asked to recall specific encounters in which they had engaged in high risk situations and encounters where they decided to engage in safe sex. Data were gathered by means of a questionnaire which divided each encounter into a number of sequences and stages from the start to the end of the encounter. This included such information as mood, sexual attractiveness, location, alcohol and so on. Gold *et al.* report that unsafe sex occurs more often with lovers than with casual partners (cf. Fitzpatrick *et al.*, 1990). The majority of respondents were aware that they were engaging in risky practices, but despite this they claimed to have had a desire for this at the start of the evening. If there was a desire for safe sex, communication failed to occur in the majority of cases. Among the self-justifications offered for engaging in unsafe sex was a desire to engage in exciting sex, greater attraction to the partner sexually, inferring from the physical characteristics of the partner that he was not infected, and the intention to have sex without ejaculation.

Conclusions

Self-report questionnaires have been particularly valuable in collecting baseline data on knowledge and beliefs about AIDS and in documenting the general myths and prejudices surrounding HIV and AIDS (see Memon, in press, for a review). Young people's descriptive accounts obtained by using open-ended response formats have enabled us to speculate on the attributions people make about causality and how this may determine attitudes to PWAs. One of the major problems with this research, however, is that subjects are responding in a hypothetical situation (e.g. if someone is expressing worry about infection, it may be limited to worry about a particular sexual encounter). In the absence of information about social context, we have no idea how the response will be shaped by the attitudes of the partner, parents, peers or other 'significant' persons. A related point is that questionnaires are making generalizations about individual decision-making which does not take into account the attitudes and opinions of a partner (see Fitzpatrick *et al.*, 1990). Self-efficacy (one's belief about how one can perform in situations where one is not sure of the skill required) and subjective norms (the influence of others) are important predictors of decisions to engage in safer sex practices (see Phillips *et al.*, 1990; Klee, 1990; Ingham and Woodcock, 1990).

Future Research

It is clear that ethnographic data will be necessary to gain insight into the social and motivational factors influencing choice and judgments about risk. A promising approach is suggested by the work of Gold *et al.* (1990) in which self-justifications for engaging in safe or unsafe practices shed light on the social and cultural barriers to behaviour change. Currie (1990) illustrates the value of a lifestyle approach which looks at the social and environmental contexts in which health behaviour is performed and involves looking at the impact of family, parents and school in relation to other health behaviours such as smoking and drinking.

The attributional approach may be a useful one in understanding the cognitive and social processes that influence our perceptions of HIV risk, and in drawing our attention to the biases in interpretation of AIDS information. However, we need to bring a more social approach to the study of attribution processes (Hewstone and Jaspars, 1984). For example, the social conditions under which different attributional judgments about one's susceptibility to HIV infection occur merit further study. Moreover, we need to look closely at the processes of social categorization if we are to counter HIV/AIDS-related prejudice. Many of the behaviours which place an individual at risk of HIV infection are social. Future research may benefit from an approach that includes a study of social representations, group norms, historical and cultural influences. This approach is, for example, illustrated by current British research such as the Women Risk and AIDS Project (Holland *et al.*, 1989) and by the Social Aspects of Risk Reduction Project at Southampton University.

References

ABRAMS, D., ABRAHAM, C., SPEARS, R. and MARKS, D. (1990a) 'AIDS Invulnerability: Relationships, Sexual Behaviour and Attitudes among 16–19 Year Olds', in P. AGGLETON, P. DAVIES and G. HART (Eds), *AIDS: Individual, Cultural and Policy Dimensions*, Lewes, Falmer Press.

ABRAMS, D., SHEERAN, P. and ABRAHAM, C. (1990b) 'Social Identity, Normative Context and Vulnerability to HIV', paper presented at the British Psychological Society Annual Conference, Swansea, April.

ALCORN, K. (1988) 'Illness, Metaphor and AIDS', in H. HOMANS and P. AGGLETON (Eds), *Social Aspects of AIDS*, Lewes, Falmer Press.

BAUMAN, L.J. and SEIGEL, K. (1987) 'Misconception among Gay Men of the Risk of AIDS Associated with Their Sexual Behaviour', *Journal of Applied Social Psychology*, 17, 329–350.

BOYLE, M.E., PITTS M.K., PHILLIPS, K.C., WHITE, D.G., CLIFFORD, B. and WOOLET, E.A. (1989) 'Exploring Young People's Attitudes to and Knowledge of AIDS: The Value of Focused Group Discussions', *Health Education Journal*, 48, 21–23.

BROWN, L.K. and FRITZ, G.K. (1988) 'Children's Knowledge and Attitudes about AIDS', *Journal of American Academy of Child and Adolescent Psychiatry*, 27, 504–508.

BURGER, J.M. (1981) 'Motivational Biases in the Attribution of Responsibility for an Accident', *Psychological Bulletin*, 90, 496–512.

CERVONE, D. and PEAKE, P.K. (1986) 'Anchoring Efficacy and Action: The Influence of Judgemental Heuristics on Self Efficacy Judgements and Behaviour', *Journal of Personality and Social Psychology*, 50, 49–501.

CLIFT, S.M. and STEARS, D.F. (1988) 'Beliefs and Attitudes Regarding AIDS among British College Students: A Preliminary Study of Change between November 1986 and May 1987', *Health Education Research: Theory and Practice*, 3, 75–88.

CLIFT, S.M., STEARS, D.F., LEGG, S., MEMON, A. and RYAN, L. (1989) *The HIV and AIDS Education and Young People Project: Report on Phase One*, HIV/AIDS Education Unit, Christ Church College, Canterbury.

CLIFT, S.M., STEARS, D.F., LEGG, S., MEMON, A. and RYAN, L. (1990) 'Blame and Young People's Moral Judgments about AIDS', in P. AGGLETON, P. DAVIES and G.HART (Eds) *AIDS: Individual, Cultural and Policy Dimensions*, Lewes, Falmer Press.

COXON, A.P. and CARBALLO, M. (1989) 'Editorial Review: Research on AIDS: Behavioural Perspectives', *AIDS*, 3, 191–197.

CURRIE, C. (1990) 'Young People in Independent Schools, Sexual Behaviour and AIDS', in P. AGGLETON, P. DAVIES and G. HART (Eds), *AIDS: Individual, Cultural and Policy Dimensions*, Lewes, Falmer Press.

DESCHAMPS, J.C. (1978) 'La Perception des Causes du Compartement', in W. DOISE, J.C. DESCHAMPS and G. MUGNY (Eds), Psychologie Sociale Experimentale, Paris, Colin.

FARQUHAR, C. (1990) 'Understanding Young Children's Thinking in Relation to HIV and AIDS', paper presented at the British Psychological Society Annual Conference, Swansea, April.

FISKE, S.T. and TAYLOR, S.E. (1984) *Social Cognition*, New York, Random House.

FITZPATRICK, R., McLEAN, J., BOULTON, M., HART, G. and DAWSON, G. (1990) 'Variation in Sexual Behaviour in Gay Men', in P. AGGLETON, P. DAVIES and G. HART (Eds), *AIDS: Individual, Cultural and Policy Dimensions*, Lewes, Falmer Press.

GOLD, R.S., SKINNER, M.J., GRANT, P. and PLUMMER, D.C. (1990) ' Situation Factors and Thought Processes Associated with Unprotected Intercourse in Gay Men', in submission, Deakin University, Victoria, Australia.

HEIDER, F. (1944) 'Social Perception and Phenomenal Causality', *Psychological Review*, 51, 358–374.

HEIDER, F. (1958) *The Psychology of Interpersonal Relations*, New York, Wiley.

HEWSTONE, M. and JASPARS, J.M.F. (1984) 'Social Dimensions of Attribution', in H. TAJFEL (Ed.). *The Social Dimension*, Vol. 2, Cambridge, Cambridge University Press.

HOLLAND, J. RAMAZANOGLU, C. and SCOTT, S. (1989) 'Managing Risk and Experiencing Danger', paper presented at the British Sociological Association Conference: Sociology in Action, Plymouth.

HOLLAND, J., RAMAZANOGLU, C. and SCOTT, S. (1990) 'Managing Risk and Experiencing Danger: Tensions Between Government AIDS Education Policy and Young Women's Sexuality', *Gender and Education*, 2, 125–146.

INGHAM, R. and WOODCOCK, A. (1990) 'Ten Questions about Sexual Behaviour', paper presented at the British Psychological Society Annual Conference, Swansea, April.

JOSEPH, J., MONTGOMERY, S., EMMONS, C. (1987) 'Magnitude and Determinants of Behavioural Risk Reduction: Longitudinal Analysis of a Cohort at Risk for AIDS', *Psychology and Health*, 1, 73–95.

KAHNEMAN, D. and TVERSKY, A. (1972) 'Subjective Probability: A Judgement of Representativeness', *Cognitive Psychology*, 3, 430–454.

KELLEY, H.H. (1967) 'Attribution in Social Interaction', in D. LEVINE (Ed.) Nebraska Symposium on Motivation, Vol., 15, Lincoln, University of Nebraska Press.

KLEE, H. (1990) 'Some Observations of the Sexual Behaviour of Injecting Drug Users: Some Implications for the Spread of HIV Infection', in P. AGGLETON, P. DAVIES and G. HART (Eds), *AIDS: Individual, Cultural and Policy Dimensions*, Lewes, Falmer Press.

MARKS, D., ABRAMS, W.D., SPEARS, R. and ABRAHAM, S.C.S. (1989) 'Exploring AIDS Relevant Behaviours and Cognitions in 16–19 year olds', paper presented at the Annual Conference of the British Psychological Society, April.

MEMON, A. (1990) 'Young People's Knowledge, Beliefs and Attitudes about AIDS', *Health Education Research: Theory and Practice*, 5, 327–335.

MEMON, A. (in preparation) *Perceptions of HIV Risk: Attitudes, Intentions and Behaviour.*

MOSCOVICI, S. (1981) 'On Social Representations', in J.F. FORGAS (Ed.) *Social Cognition*, London, Academic Press.

PATTON, C. (1990) 'What Science Knows: Formation of AIDS Knowledge', in: P. AGGLETON, P. DAVIES and G. HART (Eds), *AIDS: Individual, Cultural and Policy Dimensions*, Lewes, Falmer Press.

PERLOFF, L.S. and FETZER, B. (1986) 'Self-Other Judgements and Perceived Vulnerability to Victimisation', *Journal of Personality and Social Psychology*, 50, 502–510.

PETTIGREW, F. (1979) 'The Ultimate Attribution Error: Extending Allport's Cognitive Analysis of Prejudice', *Personality and Social Psychology Bulletin*, 5, 461–476.

PHILLIPS, K., WHITE, D., ELLIOT, J. and WILSON, P. (1990) 'Planning for Sex? The Role of Sexual Diaries to Monitor Sexual Intentions and Behaviour', paper presented at the Annual Conference of the British Psychological Society, Swansea, April.

READER, E.G., CARTER, R.P. and CRAWFORD, A. (1989) 'AIDS Knowledge, Attitudes and Behaviour: A Study with University Students', *Health Education Journal*, 47, 4, 125–127.

RICHARDSON, D. (1990) 'AIDS Education and Women: Sexual and Reproductive Issues', in P. AGGLETON, P. DAVIES and G. HART (Eds), *AIDS: Individual, Cultural and Policy Dimensions*, Lewes, Falmer Press.

ROGERS, R. (1975) 'A Protection Motivation Theory of Fear Appeals and Attitude Change', *Journal of Psychology*, 91, 93–114.

ROSENSTOCK, K. (1966) 'Why People Use Health Services', *Millbank Fund Quarterly*, 44, 94–124.

ROSENSTOCK, K. (1974) 'The Health Belief Model and Preventative Behaviour', *Health Education Monographs*, 2, 354–365.

ROTTER, J.B. (1966) 'Generalised Expectancies for Internal versus External Control of Reinforcement', *Psychological Monographs*, 80, 1 (whole number), 609.

SIEGEL, K. CHEN, J.Y., MESANGO, F. and CHRIST, G. (1987) 'Persistence and Change in Sexual Behaviour and Perceptions of Risk for AIDS among Homosexual Men', paper presented at the Third International Conference on AIDS, Washington, D.C.

STOCKDALE, J.E., DOCKRELL, J.E. and WELLS, A.J. (1989) 'The Self in Relation to Media Representations: Match or Mismatch?' paper presented at the British Psychological Society Annual Conference, St Andrews, Scotland.

TAYLOR, D.M. and JAGGI, V. (1974) 'Ethnocentrism and Causal Attributions in a South Indian Context', *Journal of Cross Cultural Psychology*, 5, 162–171.

TAYLOR, S.E., WOOD, J.V. and LICHTMAN, R.R. (1983) 'It Could Be Worse: Selective Evaluation as a Response to Victimisation', *Journal of Social Issues*, 39, 19–40.

TVERSKY and KAHNEMAN, D. (1974) 'Judgements under Uncertainty: Heuristics and Biases', *Cognitive Psychology*, 5, 207–232.

WARWICK, I., AGGLETON, P.J. and HOMANS, H. (1988a) 'Young People's Beliefs about AIDS', in P. AGGLETON and H. HOMANS (Eds), *Social Aspects of AIDS*, Lewes, Falmer Press.

WARWICK, I., AGGLETON, P.J. and HOMANS, H. (1988b) 'Constructing Commonsense in Young People's Beliefs about AIDS', *Sociology of Health and Illness*, 10, 213–233.

WATNEY, S. (1987) 'Visual AIDS and Advertising Ignorance', in P. AGGLETON and H. HOMANS (Eds), *Social Aspects of AIDS*, Lewes, Falmer Press.

WEINER, B. (1980) *Human Motivation*, New York, Rinehart and Winston.

WEINSTEIN, N.D. (1980) 'Unrealistic Optimism about Future Life Events', *Journal of Personality and Social Psychology*, 89, 808–820.

WEINSTEIN, N.D. (1984) 'Why It Won't Happen to Me: Perception of Risk Factors and Susceptibility', *Health Psychology*, 3, 431–457.

WELLINGS, K. (1988a) 'Perceptions of Risk: Media Treatment of AIDS', in P. AGGLETON and H. HOMANS (Eds), *Social Aspects of AIDS*, Lewes, Falmer Press.

WELLINGS, K. (1988b) 'Tracking Public Views on AIDS', *Health Education Journal*, 47, 1, 34–36.

WOBER, J.M. (1988) 'Informing the British Public about AIDS', *Health Education Research: Theory and Practice*, 3, 19–24.

Chapter 12

Moral Perspectives and Safer Sex Practice: Two Themes in Teaching about HIV and AIDS in Secondary Schools

Stephen Clift and David Stears

Within schools the impact of HIV/AIDS on what is talked about in the area of sex has been significant. Teachers and their pupils have begun to discuss issues and practices which only five years ago would not have been acceptable topics of pedagogic discourse. Inevitably, such increased openness has provoked concern in some quarters, and debate continues regarding such issues as the proper aims of HIV/AIDS education for young people; the range of issues which should be examined; the language which should be used to discuss sexual activities; the age at which issues to do with HIV/AIDS should be introduced into the secondary curriculum; whether and how the topic should be addressed within junior schools (see Farquhar, Ch. 13, this volume); the best teaching methods to use and so on.

The seriousness of AIDS as a medical and social problem and the consequent concern of the government to intervene in the processes regulating individual desire and sexual practice have been reflected not only in the sponsoring of public information campaigns, but more significantly in the production of two substantial teaching resources. These have been developed to help teachers provide education on HIV and AIDS and have been directly distributed, or made available, free of charge to secondary schools. The first of these, the DES video resource package *Your Choice for Life*, consists of a five-part video about AIDS and a booklet which gives advice on how the video should be used and the proper value/ideological framework within which information on AIDS and HIV infection should be contextualized. The guide states, for instance, that:

> For school-age youngsters...teaching must focus on the positive benefits of responsible sexual behaviour and the virtues of abstinence and restraint. Care must be taken to ensure that, in discussing aspects of sexual behaviour with this age group, there is no assumption that the pupils themselves are already sexually active. Responsible sex education should

encourage pupils to appreciate the physical, emotional and moral risks of casual and promiscuous sexual behaviour and should help them to resist societal and peer group pressures for early sexual experimentation. (DES Guide to *Your Choice for Life*: 9)

The second major resource available to schools is the Health Education Authority (HEA) pack, *Teaching about HIV and AIDS*, developed by Doreen Massey of the Family Planning Association. This consists of three units, each of which contains plans and notes for five lessons on HIV/AIDS. The resource is structured on a spiral curriculum model, with Unit 1 intended for use with 12–14-year-olds, Unit 2 with 14–16-year-olds and the third unit with young people 16 and older. It is clearly recommended that the materials be used in a flexible way to assist teaching on AIDS, which ideally would be given within a course of sex education, set within the broader context of a structured programme of personal, social and health education. Again, the need to place information on AIDS within a particular framework of values is stressed. The major objectives of the pack are said to be:

to provide information and to correct misinformation about AIDS and the transmission and prevention of HIV infection

to encourage responsible behaviour in relation to sexuality through development of personal and interpersonal skills, having regard to moral and legal considerations

to provide information and encourage responsible behaviour in relation to drugs, through the development of personal and interpersonal skills

to help young people develop supportive networks which encourage informed and responsible decision-making.

In addition, the pack includes extracts from relevant Acts of Parliament, DES circulars and HMI documents which have a bearing on the provision of HIV/AIDS education. These include section 19 from DES Circular 11/87, DES/Welsh Office Circular 45/87, which includes the following directives:

Teaching about the physical aspects of sexual behaviour should be set within a clear moral framework in which pupils are encouraged to consider the importance of self restraint, dignity and respect for themselves and others and helped to recognize the physical, emotional and moral risks of casual and promiscuous sexual behaviour. Schools should foster a recognition that both sexes should behave responsibly in sexual matters. Pupils should be helped to appreciate the benefits of stable married and family life and the responsibilities of parenthood.

In addition to government sponsored resources a wide variety of materials has been produced both commercially and by charitable trusts (e.g. the AIDS Education and Research Trust, AVERT) which aim to assist teachers and other professional workers in providing education on HIV/AIDS for young people. These have taken the form of teaching packs (e.g. Strathclyde Regional Council, 1989; Aggleton *et al.*, 1990); booklets (e.g. Clift, 1989), videos (e.g. Wandsworth Health Promotion Services, 1990) and board and card games of various kinds (e.g. British Medical Association, 1989; Riverside Health Education Service, n.d.; Lambert *et al.*, 1990).

Most of these materials aim to help young people understand the nature of HIV/AIDS and to appreciate how the virus is transmitted and how transmission can be avoided. In addition, however, materials aim to help young people appreciate the moral issues associated with HIV/AIDS, understand the personal and social dimensions of HIV/AIDS, and develop the decision-making, assertiveness and negotiating skills needed to avoid behaviours which could lead to infection. Materials devised to assist educational work with young people are of interest, therefore, for the insight they provide into the assumptions and decisions currently made by various producers of resources (e.g. government departments, BMA, HEA, Health Education Units, etc.) regarding the needs of professionals and young people in the area of HIV/AIDS education.

Moralism vs Realism in HIV/AIDS Education

With respect to the central concerns of AIDS education for young people, two American commentators have recently drawn a distinction between 'moralism' and 'ethical realism' in characterizing different approaches to education on AIDS. In discussing 'obstacles to effective AIDS education', for example, Fineberg has highlighted what he describes as a 'fundamental disagreement about the propriety of educational messages to prevent AIDS':

For some, the only socially acceptable change is to have people altogether abandon certain behaviours. In this moralistic view, it is wrong to have sexual relations outside of marriage and it is wrong to use drugs, hence it is wrong to advocate or even discuss anything (such as use of condoms or sterile needles) that would appear to condone these activities. Others take what might be called a rationalist view: behaviours that will occur and are dangerous should be modified so as to make them safer. Such philosophical differences underlie the reticence of many national leaders about AIDS education, controversies over the propriety of specific educational materials, and debates among Catholic prelates over teaching about condoms. (Fineberg, 1988:593)

Similarly, Eisenberg, in considering ethical issues in public health policy in the United States, argues that public debate can be characterized in terms of two opposing viewpoints which are held by 'public health advocates' and 'moralizers'. Those holding strongly moralist views, he suggests, believe that:

Sex education is the primary responsibility of family and church. If it is to be permitted in schools, moral context must take precedence over physiology. Those who believe that intercourse is licit only when it permits procreation regard instruction about condoms as unacceptable; condoms are contraceptives, even if they are ostensibly used for disease prevention. (Eisenberg, 1989:759)

Those, on the other hand, who adopt a 'pragmatic, consequentialist position' take a quite different view of sex education:

The consequentialist position on sexuality begins with the recognition that pre-marital experimentation is widespread in contemporary society.... Because ignorance about sex not only fails to delay sexual expression but transmutes it into a high-risk activity, public health advocates focus on what is feasible; namely, the provision of full information about how disease transmission can be minimised, and ready access to condoms to increase their use when intercourse does occur. (Eisenberg, 1989:759–60)

Given the central significance of aims and objectives in the structuring of education on HIV/AIDS, in assessing its outcomes and evaluating its effectiveness, it is clearly an important part of any assessment of current practice to collect information on the aims being pursued. In a school context, where pressures from government via legislation, official guidelines and centrally produced resources promote a particular ideological flavour to provision of education on this subject, it is of interest to assess the extent to which schools and individual teachers have absorbed the official line — in policy and in practice — or have adopted a position which has a different ideological underpinning. In this chapter we report on some of the findings from the second phase of the HIV/AIDS Education and Young People Project which are relevant to these issues.

Table 12.1   Details of Schools (and Teachers) in the Survey

LEA of School
Kent   81 (154)
East Sussex   28 (55)
Bromley   16 (22)
Bexley   7 (10)

ILEA (within SETRHA)   19 (42)

Independent   35 (63)

Selective Type
Selective   54 (101)
Non-selective   412 (76)
All ability   60 (12)

Tameside (selection at 13+)   16 (25)
Special   6 (8)
No information   9 (12)

Sex Composition
Co-education   95 (190)
No information   2 (2)

Boys   40 (66)
Girls   49 (88)

Denominational Status
Non-denominational   164 (306)
Church of England   9 (20)

Catholic   12 (19)
Methodist   1 (1)

Size
Up to 499   56 (96)
500–749   60 (103)
750–999   42 (86)
1000+   24 (56)
No information   4 (5)

Phase 2 of the HIV/AIDS Education and Young People Project

Following Phase 1 of the HIV/AIDS Education and Young People Project (Clift, *et al.*, 1989, 1990), Phase 2 has investigated the provision of education for young people in secondary schools within the South East Thames Regional Health Authority area (this includes all of Kent, East Sussex, the Boroughs of Bromley and Bexley and approximately half the former ILEA area). All state and independent schools within this area were sent copies of a detailed questionnaire regarding provision of HIV/AIDS education half way through the summer term of 1989. All teachers with experience of formal 'timetabled' teaching about HIV/AIDS were asked to complete the questionnaire, giving details of thier teaching during the academic year 1988–1989. By the end of the summer term, following two postal reminders, completed questionnaires had been received from 346 teachers working in 186 schools across the region.

The overall response rate from schools was 50.5 per cent although this varied quite substantially from one part of the region to another (e.g. 80 per cent from Bromley schools, 31.6 per cent from London schools). Table 12.1 provides a brief description of the schools in the sample and the number of teachers from each type of school. Full details of the procedures followed in gaining access to schools, the letters sent, the questionnaire design, etc. can be found in the full report on Phase 2 (Stears and Clift, 1990).

The Questionnaire

The ten-page questionnaire requested information on the respondent and the school (e.g. selective/non-selective type, age range catered for); curriculum context of teaching on HIV/AIDS; whether external support had been used (e.g. health education officers, doctors); what materials/resources were used (e.g. DES video, teaching packs); what objectives had been pursued; what methods were employed; whether any evaluation of teaching had been attempted; and whether teachers felt they needed further information to help them in their teaching. A final section asked teachers to write an account of any issues or problems which had arisen for them in connection with teaching young people about HIV/AIDS.

Teachers' Objectives in Teaching About AIDS

This section focuses on the results from the section of the questionnaire designed to collect information on teachers' objectives in teaching about HIV/AIDS. This section consisted of twenty-four objectives statements, and teachers were asked to indicate whether the statements were true of their teaching on HIV/AIDS. The statements were selected on the basis of results from pilot studies involving secondary schools on the Isle of Wight and in the London Borough of Hillingdon in which a larger number of objectives statements were presented to teachers. The objectives statements included were written to represent five main themes: eight statements were concerned with teaching about risks and safety; four statements based on the guidelines given in the booklet accompanying the DES video were concerned with moral issues; and four objectives each related to pupils' attitudes and feelings, scientific/medical aspects of AIDS and broader social issues (see Table 12.2 for details of the objective statements employed). Teachers were asked to indicate the extent to which each objective was true of their work with young people on HIV/AIDS during 1988–89, using a five-point scale. The instructions given were as follows:

> The purpose of this section is to collect information on the specific content of teaching on HIV and AIDS. Below are 24 statements describing possible objectives which could be pursued in teaching on this subject.

If you have taught 4th formers or above about AIDS, please indicate the extent to which these statements are true of your teaching using the following scale (circle the relevant number):

1   Definitely true — I have given this PARTICULAR emphasis.
2   True — I have covered this.
3   True to some extent — I have touched on this.
4   Not true — but I would do this given more time.
5   Definitely not true — and I would NOT DO THIS even given more time/resources.

Findings

It is of interest to examine the patterns of answers to each set of objectives. Table 12.2 reports the percentage frequency distributions for responses to each set.

Risks and Safety

The results for these objectives are of special interest because they cast light on the extent to which teaching on HIV/AIDS is explicitly oriented towards the prevention of viral transmission. The percentages giving particular emphasis provide the best indication of the extent to which teachers are giving this aspect prominence in their teaching relative to other concerns. It is clear from the findings that over two-thirds of teachers see it as important to dispel any myths or misconceptions young people might have regarding casual social transmission. Almost two-thirds are concerned with making young people aware of the risks involved in being sexually active, and just under 60 per cent place particular emphasis on safer sex. If we take account of both 'definitely true' and 'true' answers it is clear that around 90 per cent of teachers in the sample claim that these issues are at least true of their teaching on HIV/AIDS.

However, responses to the remaining items on risk and safer sex show very clearly that teachers are reluctant to be explicit and precise in their teaching about risks and prevention in relation to sexual activity. Just over a third give particular emphasis to use of condoms, and almost 70 per cent say that this is at least true of their teaching, but the percentage of teachers giving attention to specific safer sex practices or to buying condoms is very low. Only 11 per cent give particular emphasis to the skills involved in negotiating safer sex, while a further 23.7 per cent say this is true of their teaching. Similarly, only 11.1 per cent give particular

Table 12.2 Teachers' Responses to Twenty-four Objectives in Teaching about HIV/AIDS

In my teaching on HIV/AIDS I have tried to ensure that young people	N	Definitely true	True	Response categories True to some extent	Not true	Definitely not true
Risks and safety						
understand that HIV cannot be caught from everyday contact with an infected person	320	68.4	23.4	4.1	0.6	3.4
are aware of the risks they may be running if they are sexually active	324	65.4	26.2	4.0	1.5	2.8
understand what is meant by 'safer sex'	320	57.5	29.7	7.2	1.9	3.8
understand how to use condoms properly	320	34.1	35.6	16.6	9.1	4.7
understand the risks involved in sexual activities such as oral and anal sex	319	22.6	27.9	29.8	11.3	8.5
understand that many sexual activities (e.g. mutual masturbation, massage, etc.) are safe and pleasurable	318	11.9	22.3	29.6	21.4	14.8
understand clearly what to look for if buying condoms	315	11.1	13.0	23.2	37.5	15.2
develop the skills needed to talk about 'safer sex' with a potential sexual partner	317	11.0	23.7	26.2	32.8	6.3

Moral issues						
understand that sexual relationships should involve care and responsibility for one's partner	325	53.2	24.6	9.8	4.0	2.3
appreciate the emotional and moral risks of promiscuous behaviour	320	36.3	34.1	19.1	6.6	4.1
develop the skills needed to resist social pressures for early sexual experimentation	319	25.1	34.2	22.9	15.4	2.5
understand the virtues of sexual abstinence and restraint	312	13.8	27.2	34.0	13.8	11.2
Feelings/attitudes						
feel compassion for all people with HIV/AIDS no matter how they became infected	319	32.3	33.2	23.5	7.8	3.1
feel sympathetic towards gay men and injecting drug users who develop AIDS	312	13.5	31.4	33.0	14.7	10.1
question the view that certain individuals who develop AIDS (e.g. gay men, injecting drug users) only have themselves to blame	316	13.9	23.7	35.8	16.5	7.4
are aware of what it means for a person to live with AIDS	318	12.3	25.8	35.8	23.9	2.2

Table 12.2 (Continued)

In my teaching on HIV/AIDS I have tried to ensure that young people	N	Definitely true	True	True to some extent	Not true	Definitely not true
				Response categories		
Social aspects						
recognize and reject any racist assumptions about AIDS	315	27.6	22.9	19.4	23.8	6.3
are aware of the social and economic issues raised by AIDS	318	7.5	22.3	32.1	34.9	3.1
are aware of different religious and cultural views of AIDS	318	6.9	13.2	24.8	43.4	11.6
know about local sources of support for young lesbian women and gay men	306	2.3	2.9	13.1	48.7	33.0
Scientific aspects						
have an adequate scientific understanding of HIV infection and AIDS	317	29.0	32.2	23.7	11.7	3.5
understand how the immune system works and how it is damaged by HIV	320	28.4	35.0	21.9	12.5	2.2
are aware of the health problems which people with AIDS can develop	318	19.5	38.7	31.8	8.8	1.3
understand what a test for HIV antibodies does and does not reveal	316	11.1	23.7	33.9	27.8	3.5

Table 12.3   Teachers' Responses to the 'Safer Sex' Objectives (percentages)

	Definitely true	True	At least true
Safer sex	57.5	29.7	87.2
Using condoms	34.1	35.6	69.7
Skills to talk	11.0	23.7	34.7
Safe and pleasurable	11.9	22.3	34.3
Buying condoms	11.1	13.0	24.1

emphasis to ensuring that young people know what to look for in buying condoms, and a further 13 per cent describe this as true of their teaching.

The results for objectives regarding specific sexual practices are also illuminating: 22.6 per cent of teachers report giving particular emphasis to discussing the risks attached to oral and anal sex, and just over 50 per cent say it is at least true of their teaching. In contrast, only 11.9 per cent report giving emphasis to what is safe and pleasurable, and only just over a third say this is at least true of their teaching. These results indicate that teachers find it problematic to talk in detail about sexual practice, but if they do, it is easier to talk explicitly about activities which are risky than it is to discuss activities which are safe. In a pedagogic context, therefore, the logic underlying the transmission process is peculiarly inverted: what is safe in practice appears risky to teach, and what is risky in practice appears safe to teach. To underline this point it is interesting to compare the percentages of teachers indicating that the safer sex objectives are at least true of their teaching (see Table 12.3). The gaps here are very striking and point to different interpretations on the part of teachers of the phrase 'safer sex'. Over 50 per cent of teachers claim to be talking about safer sex, for example, without clear reference to what is safe and pleasurable, and 17.5 per cent appear to be talking about safer sex without clear reference to the use of condoms.

Moral Issues

The percentages of teachers giving particular emphasis to the moral objectives vary quite widely depending on the specific wording of the objective. Over half give particular emphasis to issues of responsibility in the context of sexual relationships, and over a third to the moral risks of being promiscuous. But fewer give emphasis to attempting to help young people resist social pressures, perhaps via some form of skills-based work, and even fewer see their role as being to promote the virtues of sexual abstinence and restraint. In other words, the moral issue raised by HIV infection via sexual activity appears to be addressed at the level of being responsible, whereas more active attempts to facilitate skills to resist pressure, or

Table 12.4   Teachers' Responses to Objectives Making Reference to People with AIDS and Specific Groups (percentages)

	Definitely true	True	At least true
Compassion	32.3	33.2	65.5
Sympathy	13.5	31.4	44.9
Blame	13.9	23.7	37.7
Local sources	2.3	2.9	5.2

encourage a positive attitude towards delaying or avoiding sexual activity, are less widely endorsed. This same pattern is apparent when the percentages of teachers who answer that these objectives are at least true of their teaching are examined. Over 80 per cent place stress on being responsible, and over 70 per cent address the issue of moral risks, whereas just under 60 per cent consider ways of resisting social pressures, and less than half emphasize the virtues of abstinence and restraint.

Feelings, Attitudes and Social Aspects

Less than a third of teachers report giving particular emphasis to any of the objectives concerned with feelings and attitudes towards people with HIV/AIDS, or with a variety of associated social issues. The most widely endorsed objectives relate to feelings of compassion and expressions of racism, with 32.3 per cent giving particular emphasis to encouraging compassionate feelings towards all people infected, and 27.6 per cent challenging racist assumptions; 65.5 per cent and 50.5 per cent respectively report that this is at least true of their teaching. There is, however, a sizable gap between the compassion objective and three others which make reference to specific groups particularly affected by HIV so far: gay men and injecting drug users. It is revealing to compare the percentage giving emphasis to compassion for all people and those endorsing the more specific items (Table 12.4). It appears from these figures that while almost two-thirds of teachers report that they attempted to encourage compassion in their teaching, a sizable proportion of these teachers did so without placing equal stress on encouraging sympathy for gay men and drug users with HIV, and without challenging the idea that certain individuals with HIV only have themselves to blame. In the sample as a whole teachers who report attempting to encourage sympathy and challenge blaming attributions are clearly in a minority. Not surprisingly, perhaps, given the sensitivity of the issue of lesbian and gay sexuality and the existence of Section 28 of the 1988 Local Government Act, very few teachers claim to have given their pupils any 'positive' information about local sources of support for lesbian and gay people. In total only just over 5 per cent of teachers report giving such information.

The item 'live with AIDS' was included to assess the extent to which teaching on AIDS addressed the personal significance of HIV infection and AIDS and its psychological and social consequences. Attention to this topic would seem to be needed if teachers are to be effective in addressing young people's feelings towards people affected by HIV and AIDS. The more a person appreciates the seriousness of HIV infection and the severity of AIDS, the more one might expect they would empathize with the plight of someone with HIV or AIDS. In fact, however, 'what it means for a person to live with AIDS' was given particular emphasis by only 12.8 per cent of teachers, and just over a third reported that it was at least true of their teaching. Thus, while 32.3 per cent of teachers claimed to give particular emphasis to encouraging compassion, considerably fewer (12.3 per cent) placed an emphasis on what might appear to be an effective means of encouraging compassion — exploring the consequences of HIV for those individuals affected.

Two further objectives concerned with cultural and social dimensions of AIDS were similarly given a high priority by a small minority of teachers. Only 7.5 per cent reported giving particular emphasis to 'the social and economic dimensions of AIDS', while 29.8 per cent reported that this was least true of their teaching. Similarly, only 6.9 per cent of teachers gave particular emphasis to different religious and cultural perspectives on AIDS, while for 20.1 per cent of teachers this was at least true of their teaching.

Science

If we consider the percentage of teachers giving particular emphasis to science objectives, it appears that less than a third place emphasis on understanding the scientific dimensions of HIV infection and AIDS. This percentage endorsement is even lower when specific issues are presented: less than a fifth give particular attention to health problems, and just over 10 per cent of teachers place emphasis on the test for HIV. Combining the 'definitely true' and 'true' responses reveals that 61.2 per cent are addressing scientific issues, 58.2 per cent 'health' problems, and 63.4 per cent damage to the immune system, while just over a third, (34.8 per cent) give attention to the HIV antibody test.

The 'true to some extent' rating is interpreted as indicating that the objective is seen as having some relevance but is not given priority when compared with other issues. The 'not true' and 'definitely not true' ratings appear to signal an active avoidance or rejection of scientific perspectives on HIV/AIDS. There appears to be, therefore, a roughly three-way split among a definite science emphasis, a recognition of science without giving it particular emphasis, and a perspective in teaching about HIV/AIDS which places little emphasis on science. It may be a cause for concern that 15.2 per cent of teachers indicate that encouraging a scientific understanding was not part of their teaching on HIV/AIDS. This would depend, however, on whether or not a scientific education was provided elsewhere in the curriculum and was effectively coordinated with teaching from a 'non-science' perspective.

Analysis of the Interrelationships Between Objectives

To explore the interrelationships between objectives pursued and to test the validity of the thematic distinctions already presented, responses to objective statements were numerically coded (from zero, 'definitely not true', to four, 'definitely true'), product moment correlations were computed and the resultant matrix subjected to factor analysis. Factoring was performed using principal components analysis followed by varimax rotation. Six factors were identified with eigen values greater than unity. Table 12.5 reports item loadings of + or − 0.4 or higher on the rotated factors.

A number of the items are factorially complex and show loadings on two or even three factors. Nevertheless, simple structure is closely approximated and the factors are clearly identifiable from their strongest loadings as concerned with the following issues:

1 moral issues
2 scientific aspects
3 attitudes and feelings
4 explicit teaching about safer sex
5 risks and safety
6 social aspects.

It is interesting to consider the factorially complex items as these provide some insight into the different ways in which particular items may have been interpreted differently by different teachers depending upon their approach to education on HIV/AIDS. The most complex item is 'skills to talk about safer sex', which loads on both the 'moral' and 'explicit sex teaching' factors. One might hypothesize that for some teachers such skills are necessary for young people to resist or avoid sexual activity altogether, whereas for others the predominant concern is to try and ensure that young people are helped to keep themselves safe, given that they are likely to be sexually active. The 'skills' objective also loads equally strongly on factor 6, social aspects. This suggests that teachers who see the need to address broader social issues in teaching about HIV/AIDS — beyond the facts and an exploration of personal values and attitudes — also have a commitment to skills-based teaching around HIV/AIDS.

The item concerned with the test for HIV loads on both the 'science' and 'social aspects' factors. This again is reasonable as discussion of the HIV antibody

Table 12.5   Six Objectives Factors Identified from Teachers' Responses to Twenty-four Objectives in Teaching about HIV/AIDS
(Listwise Deletion of Cases with Missing Values N = 262)

Objectives	Factors					
	1	2	3	4	5	6
Moral risks	.82					
Social pressures	.74					
Virtues	.68					
Responsibility	.64					
Scientific		.82				
Immune system		.81				
Health problems		.67				
Test for HIV		.55				.48
Sympathetic			.79			
Compassion			.71			
Racist			.63			
Blame			.50			
Buying condoms				.78		
Use condoms				.73		
Safe/pleasurable				.65		
Oral/anal			.41	.56		
Skills to talk	.42			.46		.44
Safer sex					.76	
Sexually active	.40				.70	
Everyday contact					.69	
Religious views	.43				− .49	
Social issues						.63
Live with AIDS		.40				.54
Local sources						.41

test could focus either on the technical issues of what it measures and how it does so, or on the personal and social implications raised by a decision to be tested and the range of possible consequences which follow from a positive test result. The objective 'what it means to live with AIDS' also loads on the 'science' and 'social aspects' factors. The reasons are the same, as this objective might be approached from a biomedical standpoint, with emphasis on the health problems individuals experience, or it could address the many personal and social implications of developing AIDS (the psychological impact on the individual, the consequences for their relationships with others, or broader social issues of discrimination and oppression). The last complex item is concerned with religious and cultural views of HIV/AIDS. This loads on the first factor concerned with moral issues and indicates, not surprisingly, that those teachers who report pursuing a range of moral concerns in teaching about HIV/AIDS tend to be concerned also with religious issues. Interestingly, however, this item also loads negatively on factor 5,

Table 12.6   Five Scales for Assessing Teachers' Priorities in Teaching about
HIV and AIDS

Scale	Number of component items	Range of scores	Cronbach alpha
1 Risks/safety	3	0–12	0.80
2 Morality	4	0–16	0.80
3 Safer sex	4	0–16	0.71
4 Attitudes/feelings	4	0–16	0.74
5 Science	4	0–16	0.79

'risks and safety'. This is the only substantial negative loading to emerge, which suggests that teachers who strongly endorse a concern with 'risks and safety' tend to reject a concern with religious and cultural issues.

Summated Objectives Scales

On the basis of the rotated factor solution, it is reasonable to construct summary indices related to teachers' objectives. Five such indices were constructed corresponding to the first five factors and based on items with loadings equal to or greater than + or − 0.5. The sixth factor, while readily interpretable, involved too many factorially complex items and too few simple structure items to allow for the construction of a meaningful index. Table 12.6 reports the number of items in each index and Cronbach alpha co-efficients. It is clear from this table that each set of items serves to assess five aspects of teachers' objectives in teaching about HIV/AIDS with a substantial degree of reliability. In computing composite scores, responses to individual items were scored such that the higher the total score, the greater the emphasis on each area (e.g. a teacher rejecting the four 'moral' objectives would score 0, and a teacher definitely endorsing each would score 16). Having constructed these summary measures, it is possible to explore relationships between the objectives pursued and a number of personal and educational factors which might be expected to influence the character of HIV/AIDS education produced in a predictable fashion. A brief summary of a preliminary analysis is presented in Table 12.7 by way of illustration.

It is clear, as might be expected, that the denominational status of the school has a strong relationship with the character of teaching on HIV/AIDS; teachers in denominational schools give greater emphasis to moral issues and avoid explicit 'safer sex' education.

It is also possible to examine the relative emphasis placed by teachers on different themes by cross-tabulating the summary scores. Table 12.8 shows the percentages of teachers reporting combinations of low and high emphasis on the

Table 12.7   Associations among Five Themes in Teaching about HIV and AIDS and School/Teacher Characteristics[1]

		Risks	Morality	Science	Attitudes/ feelings	Safer sex
				Themes		
1	LEA	—	—	—	ILEA > Bexley[2]	—
2	Selective type	—	—	select > non-select	all ability > non-select	—
3	State vs independent	—	—	—	—	—
4	Sex composition	coed > girls	—	—	—	—
5	Denominational status	—	C of E > non-denom	—	Catholic > non-denom	non-denom > Catholic
6	Teacher sex	—	—	—	—	—
7	Teacher age	—	older > younger	older > younger	—	—

Notes: 1 Table indicates the most marked differences where statistically significant effects are detected (p ≤ 0.05).

2 The 'greater than' sign indicates that ILEA teachers placed greater emphasis on encouraging compassionate attitudes than did teachers in Bexley. All other entries in the table should be interpreted in the same way.

Table 12.8   The Relative Emphasis on Moral Perspectives and Safer Sex Practice among Teachers in Non-Denominational and Denominational Schools (percentages)

		Non-denominational (N = 266)		Denominational (N = 33)	
		Safer sex emphasis		Safer sex emphasis	
		Low[1]	High[2]	Low[1]	High[2]
Moral perspective emphasis	Low[1]	17.3	5.6	9.1	3.0
	High[2]	23.6	53.0	57.6	30.3

Notes: 1 Low emphasis corresponds to a score of 8 or less on the scale.

2 High emphasis corresponds to a score of 9 or more on the scale.

safer sex and moral issues in non-denominational and denominational schools. From this table it is clear that, in their teaching on HIV/AIDS, a substantial proportion of teachers gave either equally high priority to both a moral perspective and to safer sex practice or higher priority to the former compared with the latter. These teachers, in other words, would appear to be following the DES line, expressed in Circular 11/87 that, 'Teaching about the physical aspects of sexual behaviour should be set within a clear moral framework.' Interestingly, it is also clear that very few teachers reported giving greater emphasis to safer sex issues compared with moral issues — only 5.6 per cent in non-denominational schools and 3.0 in denominational schools.

Discussion

There are limitations associated with the use of questionnaires to collect information from teachers regarding their educational practice, and it is appropriate to acknowledge these before discussing the results obtained and considering their implications. Data collected via questionnaires are subject to biases of both a conscious and unconscious kind. In the present case teachers may have wished to present a particular picture of their teaching which gave emphasis to issues which were not given such emphasis in practice, or they may believe that certain objectives were being pursued when the actual content of lessons may not have effectively addressed the objectives concerned. What teachers say they do and what they actually do may not correspond, and the extent of the correspondence cannot be addressed using the data collected in the survey. Similarly, we have no information which allows us to assess the extent to which teachers were successful in achieving the objectives they report attempting to pursue. Such an assessment would necessitate our having data on changes in pupils' understanding, attitudes and behaviour over time which could, in theory at least, be considered in relation to the stated objectives of teaching and details of the content and process of that teaching. Despite these difficulties, we would argue that certain educationally significant issues have been identified by the study of objectives undertaken, and that the analysis of teachers' responses has supported the idea that a number of distinct themes in education on HIV/AIDS in schools can be assessed simply with an acceptable level of reliability.

Perhaps the most interesting areas addressed concern the nature of objectives pursued in respect of moral issues and sexual practice in the context of teaching on HIV/AIDS. In the two American discussions on HIV/AIDS education referred to earlier, a clear dichotomy is described between a 'realist' approach to HIV/AIDS education on the one hand and a 'moralist' approach on the other. While the extreme positions identified have their vocal advocates, the present study provides evidence that this contrast has only limited usefulness for characterizing the positions adopted by most schools/teachers in this study in providing education on HIV/AIDS. While the fifth factor emerging from the analysis of the objectives data reflects such a polarization (in being positively defined by risks and safety objectives and negatively defined by the objective concerned with religious/cultural perspectives on AIDS), this is only one of six factors identified. More significant is the fact that four objectives concerned with moral issues and four with safer sex practice define two clearly distinct factors, suggesting that teachers may adopt positions which emphasize or de-emphasize both, as well as emphasizing one at the expense of the other. There is a balance to be struck here — as several teachers acknowledged in their written comments. A deputy head wrote, for example:

> The dilemma for the teacher is whether to focus discussion on keeping sexual activity within a stable relationship (i.e. marriage) or preventing AIDS spreading through the use of condoms. It is easier to put the emphasis on the latter — but not in my judgment right to do so.

A second comment from a social education coordinator is also of interest in highlighting the intrastaff conflicts which can arise in relation to the relative emphasis on moral issues and safer sex: 'How do you cope with staff who object to oral, anal sex etc., being mentioned and discussed in the classroom? Too many teachers in my school seem to think I should preach moral values instead of getting to the grass roots.'

It is also important to note that while teaching on both moral issues and safer sex is widely supported by teachers, the levels of endorsement vary widely according to the wording of the objectives. It would appear that as the statements become more explicit and specific with respect to the messages transmitted, so the proportions of teachers who claim to be giving them particular emphasis tends to decline. Thus 53 per cent of teachers agree that they emphasize care and responsibility, whereas only 14 per cent give the same degree of emphasis to the virtues of abstinence and restraint. Similarly, although 57 per cent emphasize safer sex, only 12 per cent give a similar degree of emphasis to safe and pleasurable activities. In some cases teachers expressed reservations about going too far in discussing sexual activities with pupils who were not ready for explicit details. As one teacher in charge of religious education put it:

> I was aware when teaching that whilst the pupils who were fairly streetwise took it OK, some of the more middle class/sheltered types of pupils looked incredibly shocked at the mention of such activities as anal and oral sex, etc. Not really a problem, but I felt some people were being thrust into an area of knowledge that they were not really ready for.

The relative positions adopted with respect to the moral and safer sex objectives are of particular interest because they reflect the operation of personal, institutional and ideological barriers to the provision of explicit and effective safer sex education in schools. The most obvious of the institutional/ideological barriers is presented by a school having a religious foundation. Here it is interesting to compare teachers in Church of England and Catholic schools. Teachers in both types of denominational school are distinct from teachers in non-denominational schools in giving greater emphasis to moral perspectives. On the other hand, teachers in Church of England schools are similar to those in non-denominational schools in the level of emphasis given to safer sex education, whereas Catholic teachers clearly differ in de-emphasizing this area. It was clear from some Catholic teachers' comments that they felt they were placed in a difficult position in teaching about HIV/AIDS by the 'clash' of moral standards around sex. A head of religious education in a Catholic school wrote: 'As a Catholic teacher in a Catholic school I am very aware of the clash that exists between the prevailing moral climate in sexual matters and the high moral ideals as a Christian. One can feel very alone in going against the tide.' A personal and social education coordinator in a Catholic school also pointed to the constraints emanating from the governing body with respect to sex education: 'As a Catholic school we have to tread very warily. There is a history of nervousness in the school because past governors were very critical of anything mentioned of a sexual nature.'

In conclusion, we have explored some of the findings on teachers' objectives in teaching about HIV/AIDS from a survey of schools across the South East Thames Regional Health Authority area. The results show that it is possible to assess the emphasis placed by teachers on a number of distinct thematic areas. The relationship between emphasis on moral perspectives and on safer sex practice was examined, and it appears that most teachers gave either equally high priority to both areas or a higher emphasis to the moral issues than to safer sex. This second pattern was particularly prevalent among teachers working in denominational schools, as might be expected. Very few teachers reported giving a high emphasis to education on safer sex practices together with a low emphasis on moral issues.

While the work reported here has certain limitations, it does provide a starting point for the systematic assessment of teachers' priorities in providing HIV/AIDS education for young people in schools. In future research attempts should be made to explore the relationships among teachers' priorities in HIV/AIDS education, content and process of HIV/AIDS education in schools and the assessment of cognitive, attitudinal and behavioural outcomes among pupils.

Acknowledgments

Thanks are due to AIDS Education and Research Trust (AVERT) and South East Thames Regional Health Authority for their financial support, and to the teachers who participated in this study.

References

AGGLETON, P., HORSLEY, C., WARWICK, I. and WILTON, T. (1990) *AIDS: Working with Young People*, Horsham, AVERT.

BRITISH MEDICAL ASSOCIATION (1988) *AIDS and You Game*, Cambridge, Cambridge Resource Packs.

CLIFT, S. (1989) *AIDS and Young People*, Horsham, AVERT.

CLIFT, S.M., STEARS, D., LEGG, S., MEMON, A. and RYAN, L. (1989) *The HIV/AIDS Education and Young People Project: Report on Phase One*, HIV/AIDS Education Unit, Christ Church College, Canterbury.

CLIFT, S.M., STEARS, D., LEGG, S., MEMON, A. and RYAN, L. (1990) 'Blame and Young People's Moral Judgements about AIDS', in P. AGGLETON, P. DAVIES and G,. HART (Eds) *AIDS: Individual, Cultural and Policy Dimensions*, Lewes, Falmer Press.

DES/WELSH OFFICE (1987) *Your Choice for Life: AIDS Education for 14–16 year olds*, London, HMSO.

EISENBERG, L. (1989) 'Health Education and the AIDS Epidemic', *British Journal of Psychiatry*, 154, 754–767.

FINEBERG, H.V. (1988) 'Education to Prevent AIDS: Prospects and Obstacles', *Science*, 239, 592–596.

HEALTH EDUCATION AUTHORITY (1988) *Teaching about HIV and AIDS*, London, HEA.

LAMBERT, C., COLEMAN, S. and JOHNSON, M. (1990) *Put Yourself in My Shoes*, North Manchester Health promotion.

RIVERSIDE HEALTH EDUCATION SERVICE AND HAMMERSMITH AND FULHAM YOUTH SERVICE (n.d.) *Opinions: A Game for Young People on Issues around HIV and AIDS*, London.

STEARS, D. and CLIFT, S. (1990) *The HIV/AIDS Education and Young People Project: Report on Phase Two*, The HIV/AIDS Education Research Unit, Christ Church College, Canterbury.

STRATHCLYDE REGIONAL COUNCIL (1989) *Escape-AIDS: Aids Education for Five to Sixteen Year Olds*, Glasgow, Jordan Hill Publications.

WANDSWORTH HEALTH PROMOTION SERVICES (1990) *Whose Problem? A Video Package for AIDS Education*, London, Wandsworth Health Authority.

Chapter 13

Answering Children's Questions about HIV/AIDS in the Primary School: Are Teachers Prepared?

Clare Farquhar

Since 1981 increasing government and media attention has been paid to the implications of HIV/AIDS, and much debate has focused on ways of minimizing the spread and impact of the virus through research and education. Although health education has been widely recognized as having a crucial role to play, little consideration has been given in Britain, either at the research or the policy level, to the implications of HIV/AIDS for primary school education.

Yet HIV/AIDS may be particularly salient for primary school children both now and in the future. Young people are currently growing up in an environment where the numbers of people identified as HIV positive, or as suffering from ARC or AIDS, are on the increase, and where mention of AIDS in the media is becoming more commonplace. The virus affects children as well as adults, and more and more children born with HIV will themselves soon be reaching primary school age. It is also possible that some young people may be at risk through sexual and drug-taking activities. Despite ongoing research, there is no immediate prospect of either a vaccine against HIV or a cure for those affected by it, and today's primary school children are likely to live with the reality of HIV/AIDS throughout their adolescent and probably young adult lives. Given that health-related beliefs, attitudes and values may be laid down at an early age, the content of the messages to which today's primary school children are being exposed, both formally and informally, may well have implications for their attitudes and behaviour in later life.

The Research

In 1987 researchers at Thomas Coram Research Unit (TCRU) in London were concerned with the lack of information about the nature and sources of primary school children's health-related beliefs and knowledge in general, and more specifically, their knowledge and beliefs about HIV/AIDS. As a result, a programme of research was prepared, employing a wide variety of data collection techniques within a range of different contexts (including the home and the school). The aim of this research was to explore the complexity of young children's thinking about health-related issues (including HIV/AIDS). Considerable information was already emerging about young adults' and secondary school children's knowledge, beliefs and attitudes about HIV/AIDS. In Britain this information had been obtained largely through questionnaire studies, and in some cases through group discussions (for a useful review of relevant studies, see Clift *et al.*, 1989). However, only limited research had been undertaken concerning younger children's knowledge, views or questions about health and illness in general (e.g. Bibace and Walsh, 1986; Bush and Ianotti, 1989; Campbell, 1975; Eiser, 1983; Prout, 1986; Wilkinson, 1988; Williams, Wetton and Moon, 1989a), and in 1987 no research data were available which were specifically concerned with young children's understanding of HIV/AIDS. The breadth of data which our study was designed to obtain was viewed as essential, given the profound influence that context is known to play on the expression of particular health-related attitudes and beliefs, as well as on health-related behaviour. It was hoped that the results of the study would provide an invaluable resource to those responsible for drawing up appropriate health education policies at the primary school level.

Discussions with potential funders of this research revealed some concern that a study of primary school children's HIV/AIDS-related knowledge might prove so controversial as to make such research impossible. For this reason, a one-year feasibility study was established in April 1988, funded by the Economic and Social Research Council, to establish whether access for such research could be successfully negotiated, and to explore different methods of collecting reliable and valid data from children.

The feasibility study was small-scale, and was based predominantly in one suburban primary school. Additional discussions and interviews were carried out in two further primary schools (one suburban and one inner city), in order to sample the attitudes and beliefs of those working in different contexts and different areas. It is perhaps important to note that, in comparison with certain other parts of the country (for example, inner London or Edinburgh), the catchment area of the case study school did not contain a large publicly identified population of people with HIV infection, ARC or AIDS. Nor did the fieldwork with children, which was carried out in the autumn of 1988, coincide with any of the national advertizing campaigns related to general AIDS awareness or safer sex.

The feasibility study was designed as a small-scale qualitative study, rather than as a quantitative survey. It is therefore not possible to generalize the findings to other schools or other areas, nor to draw conclusions about the proportion of adults or children who might hold views or beliefs similar to those expressed in the study. The aim of the research was to examine the feasibility of exploring young children's understanding of HIV/AIDS, and the work was designed to highlight some of the educational issues involved in the development of HIV/AIDS policy at the primary school level.

The Educational Context

To set the findings of the study in context, it is necessary first to provide a brief outline of certain aspects of current primary school policy and practice in Britain.

The Primary School Curriculum

In Britain, primary school education differs from secondary school education in the degree to which the curriculum is separated into different subject areas. In most primary schools each group or class of children is taught almost exclusively by one teacher, rather than by a range of subject specialists. Although it is difficult to predict the degree of impact that the new national curriculum will have on primary school practice, current policy allows individual schools and teachers a great deal of control over curriculum content. The extent to which individual primary teachers are therefore already consciously (or even unconsciously) tackling many of the issues raised by HIV/AIDS will be informed and influenced by their own perspective on health and sex education, and on primary school education as a whole, as well as by their personal comfort or discomfort with these issues.

Sex education in schools in England and Wales has recently been subject to important legislative changes (e.g. the Education (No. 2) Act, 1986), and school governors have been given the responsibility for deciding whether or not sex education will take place in any particular school. Meanwhile, the position of health education within the national curriculum has yet to be clarified. Current practice therefore differs considerably from teacher to teacher and from school to school. While some teachers may see health education as an essential element of education as a whole, and something which pervades all their teaching, others undoubtedly perceive health education as a finite area of the primary school curriculum, which can be subdivided into a number of separate topics (drugs, diet, transmission of illness, sex education and so on). Teachers holding a topic-based perspective on health could be expected to view an issue such as HIV/AIDS as a separate topic, which they may or may not choose to cover. On the other hand, teachers who take a broader perspective on health education could be expected to view an issue such as HIV/AIDS as something to be absorbed into their teaching as a whole.

The freedom under which individual teachers operate has implications for curriculum consistency and continuity in health and sex education, and means that certain issues can easily be neglected by some teachers at the primary school level. This is likely to be particularly true for issues that are perceived as high risk, crisis issues, such as HIV/AIDS. Of course, HIV/AIDS raises a wide range of concerns which are relevant not only to sex and health education, but also to other areas of the primary school curriculum. For example, it may raise discussions of morality, of prejudice and discrimination, of social responsibility, of the role of the media and so on. All teachers will have their own feelings about HIV/AIDS and related issues (however broadly or narrowly these are perceived), and, as has been acknowledged by many packages aimed at educating HIV trainers, these feelings may be of paramount importance in determining whether and how teachers are prepared to take on these issue in the classroom.

DES Policy on HIV/AIDS Education and Primary Schools

Any consideration of the role of British primary schools in HIV/AIDS-related education must be set against the stated policy of the Department of Education and Science (DES) in this area. This policy is laid out in DES Circular 11/87, which states: 'The Secretary of State believes that education about AIDS is an important element in the teaching programme offered to pupils in the later years of compulsory schooling. Schools should also be prepared to respond to questions about AIDS from younger pupils' (DES, 1987). Neither the meaning of the word 'prepared', nor the term 'younger pupils' is clearly defined. The phrase 'should ... be prepared to respond to questions' might be taken as placing responsibility on the individual teacher, who would be willing (prepared) to answer questions, or on some other person or persons, who should equip (prepare) teachers to answer such questions.

The implication of this policy for primary school teachers is that they should take a reactive, as opposed to a proactive, stance in relation to HIV/AIDS. That is, teachers should respond to children's questions, rather than engage in any direct teaching or instigation of discussion of the issues. Such an approach could theoretically be described as child-centred, giving control of the curriculum to children, and focusing on children's individual needs as revealed in questions.

The DES has distributed two information booklets to all schools (DES and Welsh Office, 1986; DES, Welsh/Scottish/Northern Ireland Office, 1987). These booklets are an information resource for teachers and do not attempt to examine, either at the primary or the secondary level, any of the educational issues raised by HIV/AIDS.

Findings

In order to examine teachers' views and experiences in relation to HIV/AIDS and primary school teaching, separate group discussions were held with the staff of each of the three participating schools, and these discussions were supplemented by individual interviews with fifteen teachers.[1] Interviews with teachers were designed to explore their experiences and feelings about discussing HIV/AIDS-related issues with young children in the classroom. Teachers were asked to describe their feelings about the DES guidelines, their experience of tackling children's questions about HIV/AIDS, and their experience and feelings about being involved in direct instigation of discussions about HIV/AIDS with children. They were also asked whether and how they believed that HIV/AIDS had relevance for primary school children, and for primary school teaching as a whole, and how they believed that policy and practice could best be developed.

Sex Education in the Schools

It was difficult to obtain a clear picture of health and sex education practice in the schools. As one teacher said, 'It is very much left up to the individual class teacher — so it's a bit, you know ... what is said and what is unsaid, nobody knows really' A number of teachers expressed some dissatisfaction with the lack of any agreed approach, and indicated that attempts were under way to formulate agreed school policies for the future.

> Last year it was a great hotchpotch, really, because we didn't particularly get a good input of sex education, and we are very aware of that — which is why we are trying to sort it out for this year.

> I think the biggest danger with primary teaching is that you actually do want to make sure that in a year you do cover it, because you can get to the end of a year and you think 'oh, I haven't done any health ed.' So that is why we are making a conscious effort at the moment to try and formalize it.

Some teachers mentioned particular factors which they saw as blocking either policy development or the implementation of policy. These included the stance of the head teacher, the availability of appropriate resources, the need for consultation with governors and parents, and the need to balance health and sex education against competing demands. The following quotation summarizes the situation in at least one of the project schools.

It was all a big thing at the end of last term that, well, we hadn't done our sex ed. But it had to be approved by the governors first, and shown to the parents, and to be quite honest by the time we had been away on school journey for two weeks, it was the end of June, we had got sports and everything, and we just couldn't organize parents and governors to actually say, well 'yes, I want the children to see it'. I mean, I felt a bit uncomfortable that we hadn't done much but it was just how it happened.

The apparent lack of a coherent approach to health education in the study schools is important when considering teachers' feelings about tackling HIV/AIDS-related issues in the classroom. As one teacher said,

We don't really discuss health to a great extent.... But you see, if we did, then if we were discussing diseases generally, then perhaps I would feel slightly different about talking about (HIV/AIDS). Because I might think, well, you know, that you can't leave it — that it's a gaping hole to leave, to not discuss AIDS. And they will think, by not discussing it, that there is obviously something a bit dodgy here, because that is the one they hear about all the time ...

There was clearly no agreement among teachers as to whether sex education and education related to HIV/AIDS should be carried out at home or at school. Some teachers clearly felt that it would be 'easier' at home, 'because they know their children'. On the other hand, others anticipated that not all parents would talk to their children about the issues: 'I know you can't leave it completely, that sort of education, because the children that it's not discussed with at home are at a disadvantage, but ...'. Some expressed concern about the way that parents might talk about HIV/AIDS: 'If parents are embarrassed about it, and a lot of them probably would be embarrassed about discussing these things with their children, then it might just be discussed in a very sort of "Oh well, only gays and prostitutes and black people and drug users will get it" ...'. However, whereas some teachers felt that they had to make up for whatever had not been done by parents, others explicitly stated that they did not see this as their role.

Teachers' Experiences of Talking to Young Children about HIV/AIDS and Related Issues in the Classroom

Although most teachers were aware that some young children do mention AIDS at school (for example, in playground games), few had actually heard AIDS mentioned by children in their presence, and quite a number of teachers reported that they had never been asked questions about HIV/AIDS by children. 'It's not just an issue that comes up, you know. I sit with them in the playground sometimes, and sit informally chatting or at lunch times and things, and it's not an issue that I've heard any mention of'. Some teachers saw the lack of questions about HIV/AIDS as a reflection of the difficulty that children experience in articulating questions in general: 'They *might* ask questions, but I think they are most trying to sort of fit it into their knowledge of the world somehow, and it is too difficult to ask questions about, because they don't really know what to ask, they are not certain what to say'. Others saw children's lack of questions as indicative of children's reluctance to ask questions about health and sexual issues in general: 'They don't really ask questions about the whole area, the whole area of health. I mean, they don't really ask you questions about sex or things. If they think it's something a bit naughty, they don't really ask you questions about that whole area'.

In contrast, some teachers who had been asked questions about HIV/AIDS saw children as having lots of questions about sex and health issues.

> A lot of questions — you know, partly just telling you about it in a very sort of trying to be grown up sort of way, but mainly I suppose asking questions, wanting to know things, wanting to know when I started my periods, and what I did about it, and who I told, and what about sex education — what happens in sex education at secondary school? What do you find out about? ...

Some teachers who had been asked questions had chosen to ignore them: 'I just didn't know what to say to that, as I don't know what sort of response I should give. So I end up saying nothing. Or just fobbing them off'. But others had responded, and had discussed issues such as transmission of the virus, the lack of a cure, the suffering involved for those affected, and the importance of medical research. One teacher described the discussion that he had had with children as 'current affairs' discussion, and another reported the fact that 'nobody seemed panicky about it'.

The contrast between different teachers' experiences of children's questions, particularly in relation to potentially sensitive issues, suggests that there are particular teacher characteristics which encourage or discourage questions of this nature. As one teacher said, 'It will come up in a school that allows it to come up, it won't come up in a school that won't'.

Teachers' Attitudes to Answering Children's Questions about HIV/AIDS

Individual teachers in the project schools voiced a range of policies in relation to answering children's questions about HIV/AIDS. Some teachers — including some who had not been asked questions — stated that they saw children's questions as a valuable opportunity, and would try to answer any questions as honestly as they could, as and when they arose, although they would not raise the topic themselves. In many cases this attitude was articulated as part of their general approach to education: 'Any information I've imparted has always started off from the questions they've asked'.

Although they stated that they were willing to answer questions, some of these teachers expressed doubts about their ability to do so well as they would like: 'I am never afraid of talking honestly with the children, and I think if it crops up 'that is a great opportunity — but I think the biggest danger is are my facts correct?' However, some teachers were extremely reluctant to take on discussions of HIV/ AIDS in the classroom. As one teacher said, 'politically it's a minefield' (School X), and another commented 'I would be grateful if they don't ask' (School X). Some teachers who were reluctant to answer questions stated that they would suggest that the children should ask their parents or would write a letter to the parents, informing them that their child had raised a particular question at school.

Teachers' Views on Circular 11/87

When teachers were asked about their views on the DES policy which states that teachers should 'be prepared to respond to questions about AIDS from younger pupils', a number of themes emerged. Teachers were in disagreement over the appropriateness of the policy, and, as has been described above, the policy was not being implemented consistently across all classrooms. Some teachers felt that the policy was appropriate, since, 'If they don't ask, it means they're not worried, and don't need to know'. Others, however, felt that the policy would lead to inconsistency in the education provided in different schools and classes. One teacher commented, 'It really depends on what the children ask you at the time, and it will be different in each class, so that the children have a different experience, depending on who asks what question in what class'. Some teachers expressed fears about implementing the policy: for example, the fear that it would be difficult to balance the needs of the class as a whole against those of the individual questioner; the fear that one question might lead on to lots more questions and they wouldn't know how far to go with the discussion; and the fear of being faced with particular questions, for example, 'How *do* you catch it by sleeping with someone?'. Some teachers were concerned whether children would be able to treat any discussion of HIV/AIDS with the seriousness that they felt it warranted.[2]

When teachers talked about the prospect of implementing Circular 11/87, one of the strongest themes to emerge was concern about the potential risks to children involved in discussions of HIV/AIDS. Some teachers were concerned about increasing children's worries by giving them too much or incorrect information: 'You don't want them getting very anxious, and they may have got anxious because of seeing some of the adverts'. The need to balance the needs of individual children against those of others who 'it would worry to death because they don't want to know', coupled with the need to balance an awareness of children's possible fears against their need for information, were seen as particularly problematic issues.

> You don't want them to think that all sex is going to lead on to disease. That is the problem. You don't want to frighten them, and you don't want to put them off the whole thing. But on the other hand, you want them to realize the dangers involved, don't you.

The concern that children would overgeneralize information so that 'love will become linked with AIDS in children's minds' was voiced by several teachers. The difficulties involved in handling discussions about sex and about death featured strongly in these teachers' comments.

> It worries me, because they have only just got used to the idea of sex anyway. And they might link it with their parents, and think 'Oh, mum and dad must be able to get it — they might have it.' So to eliminate that fear, you would have to say 'well it's not a problem, you know, if you have sex with the same person only.' Then that gets into an area that I would never in a million years have discussed with 2nd year juniors.

And again, 'With 9-year-old children, I think you would have to be very sensitive about death altogether'.

Other issues which were seen as being particularly difficult to address with young children included promiscuity, homosexuality, drug abuse, morality and contraception. Teachers who stated that they would normally attempt to relate their teaching directly to the children's own experiences could see no way of maintaining this approach with topics of this nature. Furthermore, attempting to adopt a neutral, factual approach was also perceived as problematic: 'You can't explain to children about body fluids mingling without it sounding completely repulsive and sordid and horrible'.

Few teachers were clear as to when — that is, at what age — they felt that it was appropriate to introduce some of these issues to children. It was suggested that if information, particularly about sex, was given too soon, children might be worried by it and unable to cope. However, teachers were also aware of the possible dangers of waiting: 'Quite frankly, I think you want to get in there first with information, before there is a lot of misinformation spread. I think that at that age they are very much at the stage where they are going to get a lot of misinformation'. The balance between protecting and informing children was seen by some as extremely delicate: 'There are all these issues which they must know, just before they need to know it, sort of thing. But I often think if you tell children too early, you could worry them'.

In general, teachers seemed to be expressing concern not only about how children could handle or 'cope with' discussions about HIV/AIDS-related issues, but also how they would then go on to interpret and use the information that they had received. For example, there was concern that children would use information about HIV/AIDS to attribute blame: 'I think that children are very sort of tuned in to the idea of having someone to blame. It's the same with anything. "It's his fault." That's just the way they operate'. Some teachers also expressed fears about what children might say to their parents at home. One teacher said she was worried '... about the child going back home and saying, "Miss X told us all about AIDS", and I can quite see parents being horrified'.

The risk of parental disapproval emerged as an important theme in teachers' discussions of Circular 11/87. Teachers anticipated that parents might feel that their children were too young or not ready for information about HIV. They also anticipated particular resistance to school-based discussions of HIV/AIDS from parents from strongly religious backgrounds, or from minority cultures. Teachers differed in the ways in which they felt that schools should approach parents over the issue. Some believed that parents should have the right to withdraw their children from any discussions of which they disapproved; some believed that parents should be *informed* about what was happening at school; some felt that whatever happened should be *negotiated* with parents; while others felt that the parents had to be *manipulated* into agreeing with school policy. Overall, discussions with parents were seen as a highly sensitive area.

> I think that you have got to be very careful about your negotiation with parents about what you are dealing with in school. Because parents are all members of the public, like me. We are all very racist, we are all very sexist. We have been brought up in that model. I think if we are actually going to break that mould, we have got to do it very gently, in a non-threatening way.

Given teachers' comments about the potential risks they felt they might run if they answered children's questions about HIV/AIDS, it is not surprising that some teachers were extremely reluctant to take on a more active role in instigating discussion of HIV/AIDS in the classroom: 'My reaction would be that you would be opening up an unnecessary, unknown can of worms, you know. They haven't thought about it, they haven't expressed any concerns to me about it, so why go stirring them up'. However, it is important to stress that there were a number of teachers who not only expressed positive feelings about answering children's questions in the classroom, but who also indicated that they would welcome being able to take a more proactive approach to facilitating children's understanding of HIV/AIDS.

Teachers' Views on the Relevance of HIV/AIDS for Primary School Children

As has been noted, some of the teachers in the three project schools found it difficult to imagine how they could relate any discussion of the issues raised by HIV/AIDS directly to young children's own experiences. This was due to children's assumed lack of knowledge about sex, sexuality and drugs. Children's perceived innocence in these areas was attributed not only to their age, but also sometimes to their home circumstances. One teacher said, 'It is generally speaking a very middle-class school, and that is not the kind of thing that is going on'. Another commented, 'I think it is easier in this school than it would be in some other schools where you have got a great deal more odd — I shouldn't say odd — but you know, the man at home is changing all the time ...'. Some teachers argued that if children are as yet sexually inexperienced, and do not engage in other potentially risky behaviours such as injecting drugs, then they are not themselves at risk of HIV infection, and therefore have no need of education concerning HIV/AIDS. Others were ambivalent.

> I mean, I think the main reason that they need to know about it is so that you would not put yourself in a situation where you would transmit it or you would catch AIDS. Now that doesn't quite follow, because that would mean you wouldn't have to know about sex until you were in a position where you would have it. I don't know. It's just somehow I feel that it is not relevant to them.

However, while some teachers expressed doubts, others felt that HIV/AIDS education was clearly relevant to young children, both because they perceived some young children as maturing and becoming sexually active at an earlier and earlier age, and also because they believed it was important to enable the next generation to protect itself against the virus. Some mentioned the need for children to be informed about the virus because of the increasing likelihood that they would come into contact with people with HIV infection or AIDS. Finally, some teachers mentioned the importance of tackling the issues of prejudice, misinformation and ignorance at as early an age as possible.

It's important I think in the primary school, because I mean, you have got children who come out with the most ridiculous comments about poofters and all sorts of things, and you feel, well, if they are talking about it like that now, then they have obviously got misinformation.

Despite differing views as to the relevance of HIV/AIDS to young children, and the need to protect or inform children, most teachers agreed that the majority of young children are likely to have some, albeit limited, knowledge about AIDS. As one teacher said, 'They have all heard the word AIDS. I mean, they couldn't fail to have heard it. So they will all know that there is a disease'.

Teachers mentioned the presence (described as 'obligatory') of AIDS in the 'soaps', in media advertizing, on the news and in the tabloid newspapers. They also described comments overheard in the playground: 'You know, "he's got AIDS" as in "he's got nits" or "he's got...." You know, you're not quite sure whether they know all about it, but it just seems that it's the kind of "in" thing to say, a real put down'. The extent of children's knowledge was difficult for many teachers to ascertain: 'I suppose all children know about homosexuals now, don't they? I don't know, do they?'. While acknowledging that some children might have only very limited knowledge and understanding of AIDS, there was a feeling that at least some children might have a far deeper understanding of the issues.

Actually, sometimes you don't always give them enough credit for what they know. They are very on the ball with current affairs issues and that type of thing. So as I say, don't underestimate them. I mean, I would probably be staggered by some of their sexual knowledge and that type of thing....

Teachers' Personal Views on HIV/AIDS

Open questions were used to elicit teachers' personal views about HIV/AIDS, and the extent to which they perceived the virus as having relevance for their own lives. Generally speaking, although some teachers saw HIV/AIDS as an important issue, most of them did not see the virus as having direct personal relevance. Lack of personal relevance was in some cases translated into lack of interest.

This is a big turn-off. It's a big bore for me, because I know I've got nothing to worry about. I've led a monogamous life, I know I'm clear, and I'll always be clear, and I'm not going to come into touch with it. I'm not going to get caught up in drugs, I'm not going to go injecting myself. It's the blood contamination is the only one that could get me.

Some teachers voiced particular personal views and beliefs about some of the issues raised by HIV/AIDS — for example, that homosexuality is wrong, that sex is only for within marriage, and that HIV/AIDS is just a propaganda issue, used as an excuse for 'returning the country to Victorian standards of morality.' Although the range of beliefs expressed cannot be generalized to other groups of teachers, it is important to reflect on the relationship between teachers' attitudes and beliefs and their teaching practice. Indeed, the teachers themselves commented on this relationship. Many appeared to subscribe to the belief that personal feelings should be kept totally separate from teaching activity, and described the primary school as a place where 'we present a neutral sort of attitude to facts ... mostly school for teachers is, at least in the dissemination of knowledge, a neutral kind of thing' Some teachers put this more forcefully:

> It would be very wrong of me to put my personal interpretation, the standards I use for living my life, to tell them 'this is how you should live'.... It is not the place of the school to criticize in that way, or the teacher to criticize or to imply that one way is right and another way is wrong.

Others were less sure that it was possible to hide their personal beliefs in this way.

> The way that you deliver information is of paramount importance. It may be that you give the information in a way which you think is terribly democratic and terribly wonderful, but your body language is saying other things. I think we have got to look at those issues as well.

Teachers' Need for Support and Training

Before adopting any particular approach to HIV/AIDS education, it was clear that many teachers needed to feel that they would have the backing and support of others. As one teacher said, 'I would *only* teach sex education with the blessing of all the powers that be — the staff, parents, governing body after meetings'.

Discussion among the staff, as well as with others, was seen as an essential prerequisite to addressing the issues in the classroom. Those who saw discussion as of paramount importance did so predominantly for two reasons. First, some teachers felt the need for colleagues to discuss and share their own feelings about certain issues: 'I think the only way that you can actually approach HIV and AIDS is through exploring attitudes of adults. I mean, until we have actually addressed ourselves as adults, to see how we feel about these issues, and what kinds of prejudices we have personally ...'. Second, staff discussion (including both teaching and non-teaching staff) was seen as a prerequisite for *developing a common approach*: 'Because learning does not take place in a vacuum of one classroom. The kids talk about something in class, and they are going to share it with other people outside. What are we going to do about the helper, who overhears a child talking about condoms or whatever?'. Many teachers also commented on the need to be well-informed, and stated that they felt ill-prepared to talk about HIV/AIDS, through lack of training and resources.

> Teachers don't know what to do and they want a resource to do it with...they want a tool to be able to help them if it comes up. And it's like sex education...if there were more sex education primary books then you would have more sex education going on in primary schools — but there isn't.

Political and Legal Issues

Some of the risks that teachers believed to be attached to talking to young children about HIV/AIDS were related to issues beyond the immediate context of the school and the individuals within it. These perceived risks revealed the extent to which wider political and legal issues may impinge on practice in the classrooms. For example, some teachers feared the possible long-term career effects of answering certain questions from children without approval at all levels, and they were uncertain as to whether this approval would be forthcoming. In particular, some teachers were concerned about their legal responsibility to comply with whatever policy on sex education might have been decided by the school governors (under the Education (No. 2) Act, 1986). At the time of the research none of the project schools possessed a clear sex education policy. In addition, some teachers were concerned about the implications of Section (previously clause) 28 of the Local Government Act (1986), which states that 'A local authority shall not...promote the teaching in any maintained school of the acceptability of homosexuality as a pretended family relationship.' One teacher said,

> 'I think the head would probably be nervous because of Clause 28, you know, and I don't know what rulings they've had from the borough and things like that.... Our head does sort of toe the borough line on things, so if a ruling came down, she is not terribly flexible about it.'

Some teachers saw the section as a very real block on their teaching practice: 'It's so difficult, because you can't talk about homosexuality and lesbianism.... Nothing has come down from above — you just get the feeling that it could be taken as promoting it'. Sometimes fear of the section was reflected in a belief that talking to children about homosexuality could lay teachers open to disciplinary or even legal action. 'People are terribly nervous of it, nervous that there's risks of parents taking people to court or whatever. I would like to see the borough take a firm stand on it, and test it'. Finally, it is important to remember that many teachers felt bound to adhere to whatever national curriculum guidelines might emerge.

Summary of Teachers' Views

To summarize, the risks that the teachers in the three project schools saw in talking to children about HIV were many and various. They believed that they could be subject to confrontation and anger from a number of parties, including colleagues, parents and governors. They believed that they might be challenged on the relevance of HIV for children of primary school age. They believed that they might be challenged on the appropriateness of such discussions taking place within the school rather than within the home. They believed that they might be accused of destroying children's innocence, of encouraging children to experiment with sex or drugs, of indoctrinating children with their own personal beliefs and of increasing children's anxieties and fears. They believed that children might themselves react negatively, disbelieving or rejecting what they told them, becoming even more confused about the issues, or asking more uncomfortable questions. They believed they might be accused of acting unilaterally, and of ignoring or failing to wait for school policy to be agreed. Perhaps most seriously, they believed they might be open to prosecution under the law.

Of course, teachers were not only reluctant to talk about HIV/AIDS with children because of how others — including governors, colleagues and parents, as well as children — might react. Many teachers were *themselves* uncomfortable about HIV/AIDS. If teachers feel *personally* uneasy about the issues, and about the relevance of these issues for children, then the prospect of raising or dealing with HIV/AIDS-related topics in the classroom may feel extremely risky and uncomfortable. Teachers may risk damaging their own sense of integrity (by acting against their moral, religious or educational principles). They may risk making themselves vulnerable through giving away power (that is, letting children's questions govern the content of discussion rather than keeping control of the curriculum). They may risk revealing their own ignorance of the isssues. They may risk revealing their own personal standpoint or identity and risk being stereotyped and possibly rejected by colleagues and parents. Finally, they may risk confronting their own, possibly deep-seated, attitudes, beliefs and behaviours.

Children's Knowledge about HIV/AIDS

Data from this study on young children's knowledge of HIV/AIDS are available elsewhere (Farquhar, 1990). However, it would be inappropriate to discuss the possible implications of the teachers' views and experiences without brief reference to them.

Methods of exploring children's knowledge and beliefs were piloted in four primary school classes in the case study school (two second year junior classes of 8-year-olds, and two fourth year junior classes of 10-year-olds). Work involved participant and non-participant observation of children, both inside and outside the classroom, health-related surveys, group and paired discussions, and other group activities such as writing and drawing. More than 100 children participated in the research, but as has already been pointed out, the study was not a quantitative survey, and no attempt was made to establish the number of children holding specific beliefs or attitudes. The research was carried out within the constraints set by the DES and the funding body — that no child should be asked direct questions about HIV/AIDS.

The study found that both 8- and 10-year-old children can be encouraged to discuss the issue of HIV/AIDS with relative ease. Many children made spontaneous comments which gave considerable insight into their understanding of the issues surrounding HIV/AIDS, and these comments were most likely to arise in small group discussions. Though most children appeared to be familiar with the term 'AIDS', some showed very limited understanding of its meaning, while others revealed a wealth of knowledge and beliefs about the subject. Children referred to a variety of sources of information, including television news and newspapers, posters, magazines, soap operas and parents. When discussing transmission of the virus, they mentioned blood, sex, drugs and breastmilk. However, they also mentioned a variety of other things, including toilet seats, ear-piercing, razors, pins and ordinary needles. Children's emergent understanding of HIV/AIDS appeared to be closely linked with, and embedded in, their knowledge of related topics, such as sexual behaviour or drug use. This complex interdependence of knowledge was well illustrated by some of their comments. For example, the statement by a second year child (aged 8) that you could 'catch AIDS ... when you go to bed in the same bed' was not surprising given that this child described 'sex' as going to bed with somebody. Similarly, the statement that 'smoking causes AIDS' made by another second year child is best understood in the context of her knowledge that cigarettes contain nicotine, that nicotine is a drug, and that drugs are somehow implicated in HIV transmission.

Although some children's beliefs about HIV/AIDS appeared to be dependent upon related knowledge, their age or state of maturity, others did not. Indeed, many of the children's beliefs reflected myths and stereotypes reported among the adult population (e.g. that you can 'catch' AIDS from toilet seats). Overall, young children both mirrored the beliefs and attitudes of the adults on whom they were dependent for information, and also constructed beliefs of their own, as they struggled to incorporate what they had heard about HIV/AIDS into a complex network of related concepts and ideas.

Implications for Policy and Practice

Perhaps the most striking finding to emerge from this study was the contrast between the children's and the teachers' views. While a number of teachers were reluctant to contemplate children's possible need for education on HIV/AIDS, and consciously discouraged or avoided their questions, a number of children were building up complex beliefs and attitudes on the basis of information derived from a variety of sources.

The fact that some teachers in the study were not only reluctant to answer children's questions but also unwilling to engage in *any* form of discussion with young children about HIV, AIDS and related issues could have serious implications for the implementation of the DES guidelines issued in Circular 11/87. Of course, it is impossible to say whether the attitudes expressed by teachers in three individual primary schools are indicative of any *widespread* reluctance on the part of primary teachers to implement these guidelines. However, their comments do raise questions about the policy and illustrate some of the possible barriers to its successful implementation. If teachers are not 'prepared' (in both senses of the word) to carry out a broadly responsive policy of this kind, such a policy is in danger of being not only impractical but also tokenistic. While some children may feel encouraged by their teachers to ask questions, and may feel supported in their search for understanding, others may be left to make whatever sense they can of the information that they receive from the media and other sources. The result may be an uncritical acceptance of media myths, the transmission of prejudice to the next generation and continued widespread vulnerability to the virus through lack of understanding of transmission and of risky behaviour. Indeed, prejudice may well be passed on more easily than the virus itself.

Even under the national curriculum, it is likely that individual primary schools will have a certain degree of control over the content of cross-curricular areas such as health education or personal and social education. It could be argued, therefore, that a great deal of responsibility for policy in relation to HIV/AIDS education lies with schools rather than with the government. However, given that any school-based policy must conform first to policies laid down by the DES, it is essential that the DES takes a lead in ensuring that national policies are both appropriate and workable. Current policy advocated by the DES may well result in some children reaching secondary school with little or no understanding of the issues.

Individual teachers in the study described a range of risks or possible repercussions which might result from answering young children's questions about HIV/AIDS. These risks had acted in many cases to block them from tackling the issues in the classroom. Given that the decision to provide or withhold information about HIV/AIDS has implications beyond the individual teacher or child, it seems essential to explore the factors which impinge on decision-making in this area. If the DES wishes to maintain a reactive policy, it is important to look seriously at the apparent barriers to its implementation, and to take steps to remove them.

The risks that teachers perceived in answering children's questions were both intrapersonal (i.e. how *they* would feel if they did so) and interpersonal (i.e. how *others* would feel and react if they did so). Interpersonal risks included risks within the context of the school (e.g. how children, colleagues, parents and governors might react) and within the broader context of the community (e.g. how the LEA as their employer or the legal system might react). If primary education is to play a role in furthering children's understanding of HIV/AIDS, then steps need to be taken to change the balance of risk in favour of answering, rather than avoiding, children's questions.

Teachers have a right to clear *information*, to *training* which enables them to explore the issues for themselves, to *consultation* with parents, governors and non-teaching staff, to *participation* in decision-making and to *resources*. Without these, they will continue to feel unsupported in the classrooms. For them to obtain these things, the DES and the LEAs have to recognize their importance. If policies are to be developed *within* schools, from the bottom up (that is, involving all parties within the school), then a lead has to come from the top. The development of school policies takes time, and will not happen unless it is encouraged and supported.

The DES has already gone some way towards supplying teachers with basic information about HIV/AIDS. However, teachers also need to know whether talking to young children about HIV/AIDS is 'allowed', not only by law (particularly the Education (No. 2) Act 1986 and Section 28 of the Local Government Act 1986), but also by the local authority, by parents, by the head teacher and so on. The DES and LEAs have responsibilities in this respect.

As so many health education programmes have already demonstrated, information giving alone is not sufficient, and teachers need a forum in which they can discuss the issues raised by HIV/AIDS. Primary schools have an advantage compared with secondary schools in that their staff numbers are generally small and in-service training for the whole staff group is a realistic possibility. In theory, given time for discussion, policy decisions can involve all parties concerned, thus reducing the isolation of individual class teachers. HIV/AIDS is a difficult issue for many schools to tackle because they do not have a well developed personal, social and health education curriculum. Staff of individual primary schools should be enabled to plan their personal, social and health education curriculum and policy together, in cooperation with both parents and governors. In this way collective responsibility could be taken for an agreed curriculum, however limited, thus relieving teachers of individual responsibility for decisions in the classroom.

However, teachers will be unable to reach policy decisions about HIV/AIDS until they are encouraged to explore and clarify their own feelings about the virus, and their own reactions to talking to young children about HIV-related issues. Exploring values, attitudes and feelings is a difficult and often threatening task, and one which many people, including teachers, would prefer to avoid. We cannot expect teachers to do it without support. But any agreed curriculum will not be truly accessible to all children unless a classroom climate can be created which enables children to ask the questions that they need to have answered; and teachers will only feel able to answer these questions if they have had a chance to explore the feelings which currently block them. Similarly, governors and parents may feel unable to support the teachers' responses until they have had a chance to express *their* own doubts and fears. There is a clear need for in-service teacher (and governor) training in this area.

This study has highlighted a number of issues which in-service training and discussion would enable primary teachers to clarify. First, they need to clarify with each other *why* children need to know about HIV. They need to identify whether and how HIV/AIDS may have implications for children's current and future lives and for their learning across the curriculum. They need to consider whether and how particular groups of children may be particularly vulnerable, both now and in the future. This is an enormous challenge, bringing into question many different models of childhood and education (for example, concepts of childhood innocence, and of childhood as preparation for adulthood), and raising issues concerning the structure of our society and in particular the importance of power relationships based on gender, race and sexuality.

Second, both teachers and parents need to clarify *who* has responsibility for the education of young children about HIV/AIDS, and whose rights must take priority. The division of responsibility between, for example, parents and teachers, is less clear for health education than it is for more traditional areas of the curriculum such as reading or maths. The relative rights of children and parents in relation to HIV/AIDS education may on occasion seem to conflict.

Third, teachers need to clarify together *how* they believe it is most appropriate to approach HIV/AIDS in primary schools. They need to explore, for example, the appropriateness of models which give greater emphasis to the content of learning (such as the national curriculum) or to the learning process (for example, concepts such as the spiral curriculum and participatory learning).

Fourth, teachers need to clarify *what* children should know about HIV/AIDS and issues such as sex, sexuality, racism, drugs and death that the virus raises. Decisions of this nature may bring into play teachers' own moral, educational and religious beliefs, as well as their own personal experiences.

Fifth, teachers need to clarify *when*, or at what age, it is appropriate to talk to children about HIV and related issues. Again, different decisions may seem appropriate, depending on different models of learning and of childhood. For example, teachers who believe that children must be 'ready' before they can learn certain things might wait longer before talking about HIV than teachers who believe that children can cope with appropriate information at a very young age.

Only by discussing and clarifying all of the above areas will primary teachers be able to make a realistic assessment of the possible advantages and disadvantages of answering children's questions about HIV/AIDS. Unless they are given the opportunity to explore their assumptions, and the reasons why they make them, they are most likely to assume the worst case — that is, that particular strategies will lead to particular negative consequences. If the barriers to talking about HIV/AIDS in the primary schools are to be overcome, it is important that teachers themselves are enabled to explore these issues fully.

Finally, it is important to recognize that policy building in school is a lengthy process, particularly when teachers are struggling to cope with widespread changes, including the implementation of a new national curriculum. As one teacher in the study commented, 'If you acknowledge that it is a long-term process, in the meantime, where does the issue of HIV and AIDS come in? Does one wait until one has built the approach and the climate up?'

Whether we like it or not, one of the realities of classroom practice is that it is often determined not only by policy, but also by resources. Few, if any, HIV/AIDS resources are currently available in Britain for either teachers or children. Although this research was unsuccessful in obtaining further funding for a large-scale study of young children's knowledge of HIV/AIDS, it has provided the basis for two practical resources for primary schools. A simple book about HIV/AIDS has now been written for 10-year-olds (Sanders and Farquhar, 1989), and materials to be available in late 1990/early 1991 are currently being produced for primary school teachers, funded by AIDS Education and Research Trust.

Acknowledgments

This research was funded by the Economic and Social Research Council (ESRC), reference number: XA44250005. The author would like to express her thanks to the governors, staff, parents and children of the study schools.

Notes

1 Group and individual discussions were also held with parents and with non-teaching staff, but these are not reported here.
2 This latter view was in contrast to the actual experience of teachers who had engaged in discussions about HIV/AIDS in the classroom.

References

BIBACE, R. and WALSH, M.E. (1986) 'Development of Children's Conceptions of Illness', *Pediatrics*, 66, 912–917.

BUSH, P.J. and IANOTTI, R.J. (1989) 'A Children's Health Belief Model', paper presented at the Social Science and Medicine Conference, Leeuwenhorst, The Netherlands.

CAMPBELL, J. (1975) 'Illness Is a Point of View: The Development of Children's Concepts of Illness', *Child Development*, 46, 96–100.

CLIFT, S., STEARS, D., LEGG, S., MEMON, A. and RYAN, L. (1989) *The HIV/AIDS Education and Young People Project: Report on Phase One*, HIV/AIDS Research Unit, Department of Educational Studies, Christchurch College, Canterbury.

DES (1987) *Sex Education at School*, Circular No. 11/87, London, HMSO.

DES AND WELSH OFFICE (1986) *Children at School and Problems Related to AIDS*, London, HMSO.

DES, WELSH/SCOTTISH/NORTHERN IRELAND OFFICE (1987) *AIDS: Some Questions and Answers. Facts for Teachers, Lecturers and Youth Workers*, London, HMSO.

EISER. C. (1983) 'Children's Knowledge of Health and Illness: Implications for Health Education', *Child: Care, Health and Development*, 9, 285–292.

FARQUHAR, C. (1990) *What Do Primary School Children Know about AIDS?* Working Paper No. 1, London, Thomas Coram Research Unit.

PROUT, A. (1986) 'Wet Children' and 'Little Actresses': Going Sick in Primary School', *Sociology of Health and Illness*, 8, 2, 111–136.

SANDERS, P. and FARQUHAR, C. (1989) *AIDS*, London, Franklin Watts.

WILKINSON, S.R. (1988) *The Child's World of Illness: The Development of Health and Illness Behaviour*, Cambridge, Cambridge University Press.

WILLIAMS, T., WETTON, N. and MOON, A. (1989a) *A Picture of Health: What Do You Do That Makes You Healthy and Keeps You Healthy?* London, Health Education Authority.

WILLIAMS, T., WETTON, N. and MOON, A. (1989b) *A Way In: Five Key Areas of Health Education*, London, Health Education Authority.

Chapter 14

Prison, HIV Infection and Drug Use

Graham Hart

Despite concern regarding the spread of HIV infection among prisoners, and the possibility of ex-offenders transmitting the infection to their sexual and drug using partners after release, no large-scale study of the risk behaviours for HIV in the prison population has been undertaken in the UK. Politically this is understandable: from a civil liberties perspective prisoners constitute all too literally a captive population and any large-scale research would be subject to extremely critical scrutiny from the outset. It is also suggested that such a study would be unpopular at government and prison management levels; if it *were* to identify a large number of offenders with HIV, then actions might have to be taken to do something about it. This could be an increase in the use of the viral infectivity restrictions, used to segregate prisoners with HIV disease, or a massively increased level of provision of health education, counselling and care services for prisoners and staff; either strategy would require substantial additional resources. In this chapter some of the issues relating to the problem of HIV infection in prison are discussed. Although the chapter focuses on the situation of drug users and describes a small study of ex-offenders who are also drug users, some of the broader implications of identifying risk behaviours and individuals within the prison context are also addressed.

Risk Behaviours

Although the risk behaviours for HIV infection are the same in prison as outside (with the exception, in the UK at least, of heterosexual intercourse), the *context* of these behaviours is quite specific. Thus it is not possible to use condoms during penetrative sex, unless these have been smuggled in; it is virtually impossible to use clean needles and syringes on each occasion of injecting illicit drugs as, unlike small bags of heroin, it is difficult to secrete injecting equipment into prison.

In men's prisons the primary risk behaviours for contracting the infection are unprotected anal sex, the use of needles and syringes used by someone else and, probably to a lesser extent, the shared use of needles or other sharpened instruments for tattooing. In women's prisons sexual contact poses a theoretical risk, but sharing injecting and tattooing equipment are the primary risks; the unborn child of an infected mother runs the same risk of viral infection as a child whose mother is not in prison.

Determining the risk behaviours for HIV infection in prison is unproblematic; determining the prevalence of these behaviours is impossible. Not only are there no published studies of risk behaviours within prison in the UK, there are no nationwide studies of ex-offenders and their reports of behaviours while in custody. Indeed, with the exception of one study which aims to recruit 400 ex-offenders soon after their release (Dolan, personal communication), it will be some time before we can expect to see any reports of research on this population.

Concern about the situation comes from the medical press because of transmission possibilities both within prison and to the community outside (McMillan, 1988), and in relation to care issues such as counselling (Curran *et al.*, 1989), but disquiet has also been expressed by representatives of non-statutory organizations dedicated to the care of prisoners and ex-offenders (Padel, 1988; Trace, 1990), as well as from a variety of other sources (Vernon, 1987). Yet in the absence of data, individual instances of coerced antibody testing and isolation will continue to serve as currency in discussions of HIV in prisons, and present policies of providing limited health education to staff and prisoners, and the use of viral infectivity restrictions, will remain unchallenged — at least at the level of fully informed debate.

Prevalence of HIV Infection

It has been reported that 0.1 per cent of the 50,000 people held in prison in 1988 in the UK were known to be seropositive for antibodies to HIV infection (Trace, 1990). However, as screening for HIV is not routinely carried out on entry to prison, and there have been no anonymous studies of prevalence, this tells us nothing of the real level of infection. In other circumstances one might be tempted to look elsewhere, such as the USA or Europe, for information which might fill the gap in our understanding of the UK situation. For example, in 1988 in the New York state prison system alone there were 838 cases of AIDS — not asymptomatic HIV infection — and this constituted 1 per cent of *all* US AIDS cases in that year (Morse *et al.*, 1989). In Europe studies report levels of the infection in prison ranging from 0.4 per cent in Portugal (Melico-Sylvestre *et al.*, 1989) and 6 per cent in France (Espinoza *et al.*, 1989) to 59 per cent in one adolescent prison in Spain (Colomo-Gomez *et al.*, 1989). Yet the temptation to seek comparative data elsewhere should be firmly resisted. The epidemiology of HIV infection and AIDS is sufficiently varied within and between countries to make the wholesale transfer of this information to the UK context inadvisable.

Drug Use: A Particular Problem

Discussion so far has been at a general level regarding the possible problem of HIV in prison. In those countries reporting high levels of the disease in prison populations there are also concomitantly high levels of injecting drug use, imprisonment for drug offences, and HIV disease and AIDS in drug using populations. In most of these countries gay men are no more, or less, likely to find themselves in prison than heterosexual men, but drug users — regardless of gender or sexual orientation — are generally at increased risk of the attentions of the criminal justice system. Indeed, studies invariably identify injecting drug use as the primary risk behaviour distinguishing those with HIV infection from the seronegative prison population.

In the UK there are large regional differences in the prevalence of HIV infection among injecting drug users (IDUs). In London rates as low as 2 per cent have recently been reported (Hart *et al.*, 1990), whereas in Edinburgh the most recent report gave a prevalence of 52 per cent (Brettle, *et al.*, 1989). We can, therefore, assume that there are likely to be regional and custodial variations in prevalence, and that prisons in the south of England will have fewer seropositive inmates than those in Scotland; this also implicitly assumes that drug users in different parts of the country are equally likely to be indicted and convicted of drug-related offences. Once again, in the absence of empirical data, this remains conjecture.

In an attempt to investigate the extent to which prisons do provide opportunities for the further spread of HIV we undertook a small study of IDUs who had spent some time in prison since 1982, when the first case of AIDS was identified in the UK. This has been reported fully elsewhere (Carvell and Hart, 1990), but the key findings are presented here to illustrate the circumstances in which risk behaviours take place; certain policy questions also arise from this work and these will be discussed.

The Study

It was known from previous studies that one risk behaviour for HIV infection — the sharing of needles and syringes — does occur in prisons. The national evaluation of needle exchange schemes found that 7 per cent of clients had shared injecting equipment, in the year prior to interview, while in custody; however, it was not known what proportion of the total number of clients interviewed had been in prison (Stimson *et al.*, 1988). In a study of risk behaviours for HIV among IDUs attending a Drug Dependency Unit in central London it was found that eight (25 per cent) of thirty-two clients who had been in prison within the previous five years had shared needles and syringes in custody, but no questions were asked regarding sexual risk behaviours in prison (Hart *et al.*, 1989). The Parole Release Scheme reports that around 5000 people are imprisoned for drug offences each year, but many more drug users are imprisoned for drug-related offences such as theft and fraud in order to fund illicit drug use; they estimate that up to 20,000 regular drug users may be in prison at any one time (Trace, 1990). It seemed appropriate to find out more about drug users' experiences in prison, and in particular to ask about HIV-related risks; to this end we conducted a survey of IDUs attending two drug agencies in central London, recruiting only those people who had been imprisoned since 1982. The study was undertaken between February and July 1989.

Method and Sample

Fifty injecting drug users, forty-two from a needle exchange scheme and a further eight from a Drug Advice and Information Centre, completed an anonymous, self-administered questionnaire regarding custodial sentences, drug use in custody (both illicit and prescribed) and injecting and sexual risk behaviours for HIV infection. The sample was predominantly male (42, 84 per cent) giving a male: female ratio of 5.3:1. The mean age of the sample was 31.2 years (range 21–42), and they had begun injecting on a regular basis (that is, weekly) at the age of 18.2 years on average; they were therefore long-term injectors, having used drugs in this way for a mean of thirteen years. We found no statistically significant differences between clients recruited from the needle exchange and those from the drug advice agency.

The study population had substantial experience of prison life. The average number of prison sentences received in the period since 1982 was 2.4 (range 1–7), and these custodial sentences averaged 8.6 months each. Successful prosecutions were of drug offences such as the possession, supply and importing of restricted drugs, but others included drug-related crimes such as shop-lifting, burglary and cheque fraud.

Findings

Drug Use in Custody

Levels of illicit drug use while in custody were high, with 47 (94 per cent) reporting the use of at least one illicit substance in prison. The substances used, and whether they were injected, are given in Table 14.1; it is clear that heroin was used most frequently, with 84 per cent reporting this. Two-thirds (33, 66 per cent) had injected drugs in prison, and 26 (52 per cent of the total sample) said that they had

Table 14.1   Illicit Drugs Used by a Sample of Drug Users While in Custody
(percentages in brackets)

(*N* = 50)

Substance	Used		Injected	
Heroin	41	(82)	27	(54)
Methadone	28	(56)	6	(12)
Other opiates	36	(72)	20	(40)
Amphetamines	27	(54)	13	(26)
Cocaine	19	(38)	8	(16)
Barbiturates	20	(40)	2	(4)
Tranquilisers	34	(68)	2	(4)
Cannabis	29	(58)	0	(0)

shared injecting equipment. The drug-related risk behaviour for the transmission of HIV infection is lending used equipment, and 21 (42 per cent) reported doing this; borrowing used equipment is the risk behaviour associated with contracting the infection, and 19 (38 per cent) reported that they had borrowed needles and syringes used by others.

Sexual Behaviour

In terms of sexual risk behaviours we found that four men and one woman (5, 10 per cent) reported that they had had sex in custody. Three men reported both oral and anal sex, and one indicated that he had sex other than oral and anal sex; the female respondent reported oral and other sex. The four men had a mean of seven male partners in custody (range 2–16), but the one woman reporting sexual activity did not put a figure to the number of partners she had had in prison. Questions on condom use during sex were not asked.

Part of the interest in the risk behaviours of people in prison relates to the possibility of infection contracted in custody being transmitted to sexual or drug using partners outside prison; similarly, if ex-offenders are reconvicted subsequent to their release, risk behaviours in the community could result in further infections in the prison population. Our questions in this area were limited, however, by the need to keep the questionnaire acceptably short for our respondents. We therefore asked only for the number of sexual partners respondents had had between periods in custody and subsequent to their last sentence. The men reported a mean of eight female partners (range 0–90), and three men reported a mean of six male partners (range 2–11) between custodial sentences. Women reported a mean of one male partner (range 0–3) and no female partners between sentences. Since their last period in prison men reported a mean of two female partners (range 0–18), and of five men reporting that they had had male partners, four had had a mean of twelve partners (range 1–40), and one, a male prostitute, reported over 1000 partners. The women in the study reported a mean of two male partners since their last time in prison (range 1–3) and no female partners.

Drug Treatment in Custody

Finally, respondents were asked whether they had been prescribed drugs while in custody. Thirty had received prescribed drugs during at least one sentence, most frequently oral methadone (10, 20 per cent) as part of a three-day detoxification. Nine (18 per cent) had been prescribed benzodiazepines, on a short-term basis, to combat withdrawal related insomnia. Three (6 per cent) had been prescribed the major phenothiazine chlorpromazine ('Largactyl'). Two (4 per cent) had been given other oral opiates, and one (2 per cent) barbiturates. We found that women were more likely than men to receive such drug treatment in custody; all the women, but only 55 per cent of the men, had been given these drugs ($p < 0.05$, with yates correction). Respondents had been prescribed drugs on an average of 1.4 sentences, half the mean numbers of sentences served by the study group since 1982.

Implications

It should be noted from the outset that the study reported here is extremely limited in its scope. The study population was self-selected — only those people volunteering to participate did so — and no attempt was made to randomize the sample; the exigencies of undertaking such research mean that we are unable to report a response rate. Questions were kept to a minimum, and restricted to issues pertaining directly to HIV transmission, with the exception of those related to drug treatment in custody which have implications for illicit substance use and which we therefore felt that respondents would be happy to answer. Our numbers were also small, partly a reflection of our desire to generate data quickly, and partly from a wish to limit the inconvenience to staff and clients in the drug agencies surveyed. Nevertheless, despite its limitations the study did raise some important issues which are worth discussing, and its findings should be noted by those who are concerned with the health of prison inmates and ex-offenders.

The first point to note is that the use of illicit drugs in prison, widely reported but rarely substantiated by systematically collected data, does occur; that virtually the same range of drugs is used by those in custody as those outside; and that the majority of those who report injecting drug use outside prison are able to use this route of administration while in custody. However, what is also demonstrated is that while drugs of various kinds do seem to be readily available, injecting equipment is scarce. Just over half of all respondents (52 per cent), and the majority of those who had injected (26 of 33, 79 per cent) had shared injecting equipment in prison. We found in an earlier study of drug users in London that the primary reason people gave for sharing equipment is its unavailability (Hart *et al.*, 1989), and it seems likely that this is the explanation for the activity in this context.

This is also the first published study to investigate sexual risk behaviours for HIV infection of offenders in prison and, to a limited extent, after release. A small group of male prisoners may be compounding their drug using risk behaviours for HIV infection with sexual risks, having sex with multiple partners. We have no idea, of course, of the extent of same-sex sexual activity in prisons, and this report is limited to drug users. However, if our finding that 9 per cent of male prisoners engage in some homosexual behaviour is representative, then the possibility of HIV transmission by sexual means is evident. As the number of women in the study was small, it was not possible to determine fully the extent of sexual risks for women in custody. These data should in any case be treated with caution; we were unable to question respondents about condom use, and so do not know whether, when sex involved penetration, this was protected or unprotected.

Our finding that *between* periods in custody our study population were sexually active is significant for two reasons. First, it indicates that, if people have been at risk of HIV infection while in prison, then their sexual and possible sharing partners outside prison are also at risk if they have unprotected penetrative sex and/or do not sterilize shared injecting equipment. This is one of the major concerns of those writing about HIV in prison — that ex-offenders might prove to be a conduit of HIV to what is described as those 'in the community'. However, what tends to be ignored are the risks that ex-offenders themselves might run of contracting the infection in the community. With 47.2 per cent of all male offenders being reconvicted within two years of their release, it may be that to focus on prison risk behaviours in isolation is to ignore the real dynamics of transmission in relation to the prison population. Our findings regarding sexual risk behaviours therefore have consequences not only for ex-offenders and their sexual partners outside prison, but also — in the event that they reoffend and are once more given prison sentences — for any further drug using or sexual partners in prison.

It might appear that, with the majority (60 per cent) of our sample receiving some drug treatment, their drug-related needs were being met while in custody. The importance of appropriate drug treatment in prison — and this includes non-pharmacological aspects of treatment, such as counselling and support — relates primarily to the opportunity that prison offers in theory to re-evaluate one's situation and possible dependency, and to use the period in custody to begin the process of making more positive choices in the direction of becoming permanently drug-free. Sadly, this is probably rarely the case, although we have no information on the number of drug-related offenders who, after release, are able to remain abstinent. A second function of such treatment, and one of more immediate concern in this context, would be its possible contribution to the prevention of HIV infection. If drug use were successfully managed in custody, even if this were to be a temporary respite in terms of the person's drugs career, then this could contribute to reduced need to inject and, by implication, share drug using equipment in prison. However, our data do not provide evidence that either of these aspects of 'treatment' is seriously considered in the management of prisoners who are drug users.

For example, these ex-offenders have received treatment in only half the number of sentences they had served since 1982. Anecdotal evidence from re-spondents suggests that three major factors militate against therapy for drug users in prison. The first is the variability of its provision. Prisons vary widely on a number of dimensions, and one of these is the extent to which the prison medical officer has any interest in working with drug users; even where that interest may exist, inexperience or uncertainty about treatment means that even rapid detoxification in the form of a three-day methadone programme may not be available. In other prisons the 'policy' may be not to do anything at all — what could be called an aggressively abstinence-oriented programme. A second area of concern relates to the nature of the intervention offered. Although the majority of the sample were opiate-dependent, only twelve (24 per cent) had received prescribed opiates, usually over three days. Many of the users felt that such a rapid detoxification was of little help in reducing the effects of withdrawal, and the total absence in most situations of any counselling or support meant that the psychological sequelae of dependency received no attention. For the majority, of course, the only treatment available was non-opiate drug therapy of limited duration.

The third factor militating against treatment for drug use in prison relates not to its availability or appropriateness but to the advisability of its uptake. In those institutions where it was offered some people were unwilling to opt for therapy because of the possibly negative consequences of disclosing previous drug use to prison staff. Those who have not been recognized as IDUs prior to sentencing are loathe to inform medical officers because they are not persuaded that confidentiality will be maintained, and are concerned that the medical officer or other staff will demand HIV antibody testing, isolation if found to be seropositive, or extra security or other restrictive and stigmatizing measures.

Again, in the absence of supporting data it is impossible to be certain as to the extent of justification for such fears. There is evidence that the viral infectivity restrictions are employed — with as much, if not more, demand that they should be used by other inmates as by staff — but information regarding coerced anti-HIV testing or other measures taken against drug users is less easily obtained. Never-theless, drug users clearly have heard or know of the negative consequences of disclosure and avoid this where possible.

Although the focus of this chapter has been the particular situation of drug users, and the context of risk provided by prison for HIV infection, certain policy questions arise which, if addressed, could also have consequences for other non-drug using prisoners and indeed staff.

Policy Questions

It might be assumed that the first policy question to arise relates to the advisability of providing sterile needles and syringes to prisoners, on the assumption that as illicit drugs appear to be available then the same 'right' accorded to IDUs outside — to purchase or be provided with clean injecting equipment — should accrue to those users inside. However, I would suggest that before this question is addressed, or any others related to risk for HIV infection raised, a prior condition should be fulfilled. That is, information regarding the extent of HIV infection in prisons, of risk behaviours and of the efficacy of present health education initiatives should be available so that any subsequent interventions can be properly monitored. Not to collect such information is as much a firm policy decision as any apparently more proactive initiative, and it is one which should be challenged. In this circumstance the plea for more research is not the delaying tactic so frequently adopted as an excuse to do nothing; it is central to the whole enterprise of properly facing up to the problem of HIV infection in prison.

Given the points made in the introduction to this chapter regarding the quite appropriate level of critical scrutiny that any such research would attract, no studies should take place without fully involving organizations representing the interests of prisoners, ex-offenders and prison staff, and that representation should be sought from prisoners themselves in those institutions where any research is conducted. This may not be the usual policy of the Home Office Prison Research Unit, but the particular sensitivity of such work demands that approval and participation should be sought at every level. Previous research in the epidemiology of and risk behaviours for HIV infection has successfully been undertaken in a non-invasive, voluntary and fully informed and consenting manner, and there is no good reason why this should not occur in a penal context.

To come, then, to the question of HIV prevention, and in particular to the provision of sterile injecting equipment and, in male prisons, condoms. Mike Trace of the Parole Release Scheme 'grudgingly accept(s) WHO's line that sterile syringes should be made available' in prisons (Trace, 1990:14). However, he also identifies the problems associated with such provision, including the inevitable disclosure to staff that illicit drugs were being used, and the possibility that injecting equipment could be used as weapons against staff and other inmates. His suggestion, and one which seems to have the support of Home Office minister Douglas Hogg, is that more prominence should be given to methadone treatment

— beyond present three-day detoxifications — and more fully integrated treatment programmes, including counselling and support. This would have staffing implications, such as training and extra personnel, but the use of locally available health professionals and drug workers should also be considered; the culture of prisons is such that they are, not surprisingly, inward-looking and loathe to turn to outside help. In this circumstance a reappraisal of this culture is needed; this also applies to the research mentioned above.

By providing improved drug treatment programmes, and dealing with the consequences of this in prisons where drug users are unpopular and subject to verbal and physical abuse from other inmates, the need to introduce sterile injecting equipment might be obviated. Again, however, thorough monitoring of the efficacy of such interventions is an absolute priority, and the policy option of increased needle availability should remain a possibility.

The policy of not providing prisoners with condoms is one which is perhaps more easily addressed. Even without research on the extent and nature of same-sex sexual activity within prisons there seems to be no good reason for withholding condoms. Home Office arguments that male homosexual activity in prisons is illegal because it does not take place in private are spurious in that they ignore the reality that, at some level, they do take place; it is a matter of determining to what extent these are allowed to be safe. The more important issue relates to the circumstances in which condoms are made available. The very public nature of most aspects of prison life means that this is something that requires some thought; it would be inappropriate for these to be on sale or otherwise collected from a public place, as it is unlikely that most of those engaging in same-sex activity would care for this to be known by others. Improved health education and the open discussion of issues of sexuality and drug use are very distant possibilities, and it is utopian to believe that even if instituted they would end homophobia and the stigmatization of drug users in prison.

Conclusions

The present policy within prisons in relation to HIV is to provide health education to staff and inmates in the form of videos, leaflets and, variably, a short discussion on some of the points relating to the transmission of the virus. Those found to have the infection can be subject to the viral infectivity restrictions which limit contact with other inmates and staff; these are not always imposed by medical staff — antibody positive inmates have requested that they be invoked in order to seek protection from other inmates, while avoiding the hated Rule 43 separation of sex offenders, police informers and others stigmatized and physically abused by prisoners. However, this is not always the case, and the consequence can be even worse living conditions, with fewer opportunities for social integration within the prison.

From an epidemiological viewpoint the viral infectivity restrictions are not necessary in relation to HIV infection. HIV is not contagious, and has recognized and discrete transmission routes; therefore, no health benefits accrue to seropositive inmates, other inmates or staff from the implementation of these restrictions. Merely asserting this, however, does not address the underlying reasons for their use, which include misapprehension of the infectivity of HIV, distrust of those who have contracted the infection, the protection of known seropositive inmates, as well as more specific attributes of prison culture relating to authority, homophobia, 'acceptable' and 'unacceptable' crimes and control. Few, if any, of these issues are going to be dealt with by a few health education discussion groups. In the end it is absolute medical confidentiality and dissuading inmates from the temptation to disclose their HIV antibody status which are most likely to contribute to reduced use of such regulations (Curran *et al.*, 1989).

Finally, what happens once prisoners are released into the community has to be addressed. Regardless of the level of risk run by people while in prison, the desire to enjoy the sexual pleasures and substances — alcohol and/or drugs — denied, for the most part, in custody may be strong; HIV preventive efforts in prison are meaningless if they are not then carried to the outside. Preparation for release, if it occurs at all, should include frank recognition of the reality of people's needs and expectations in terms of sexual and drug using behaviours, and incorporate risk reduction strategies which allow the enjoyment of pleasures long denied, while at the same time avoiding harm to ex-offenders and their sexual and drug using partners.

This chapter has been primarily concerned with the relationship between drug use and HIV infection in prison. It is all too easy to be overwhelmed by the potential problems that these issues raise and to try to seek solutions within the penal system, allowing its restrictions to determine one's response. However, the final policy implications of this, and much other research regarding the penal system, are that prison is an inappropriate place for people whose drug dependency disposes them to property-related crime, and the need to find other means of dealing with this and other small-scale criminal activity is paramount. There have been calls for some time to reduce the size of the prison population in the UK. One contribution could be the realization of alternatives to custody for drug users not implicated in the importing and trafficking of restricted drugs. Although demand reduction strategies in the drugs field are dismissed by many of the representatives of the criminal justice system as ineffectual, the major alternative — supply reduction — has proved to be unachievable in the absence of a global drugs strategy. Alternatives to custody, including varied treatment packages and options, should be properly instituted, monitored and evaluated. It may be that the penal system in the UK has so far escaped the worst ravages of HIV infection and AIDS, but the continued incarceration of drug users, and the failure to face up to the realities of risk behaviours for HIV in prison, could alter this situation dramatically.

References

BRETTLE, R.P., JONES, G., DAVIDSON, J., BISSET, C., BURNS, S.M. and INGLIS, J.M. (1989) 'Transmission of HIV by Mobility in Injecting Drug Users (IDU)', paper given at the Fifth International Conference on AIDS, Montreal, Canada.

CARVELL, A.L.M. and HART, G.J. (1990) 'Risk Behaviours for HIV Infection among Drug Users in Prison', *British Medical Journal*, 300, 1383–1384.

COLOMO-GOMEZ, C., ZUNZUNEGUI, M.V., ESTEBANEZ, P., SASTRE, J., RUA, M. and BABIN, F. (1989) 'Prevalence and Risk Factors for HIV Infection among Adolescent Inmates in Madrid', paper given at the Fifth International Conference on AIDS, Montreal, Canada.

CURRAN, L., McHUGH, M. and MOONEY, K. (1989) 'HIV Counselling in Prisons', *AIDS Care*, 1, 11–25.

ESPINOZA, P., BALIAN, P. and BOUCHARD, I. (1989) 'Etude des Risques de Contamination par les Virus de l'Hepatite B, du VIH1 en Milieu carceral', paper given at the Fifth International Conference on AIDS, Montreal, Canada.

HART, G.J., SONNEX, C., PETHERICK, A., JOHNSON, A.M., FEINMANN, C. and ADLER, M.W. (1989) 'Risk Behaviours for HIV Infection among Injecting Drug Users Attending a Drug Dependency Clinic', *British Medical Journal*, 298, 1081–1083.

HART, G.J., WOODWARD, N.J., JOHNSON, A.M., QURUBIN, G., CONNELL, J. and ADLER, M.W. (1990) 'Risk Behaviour and HIV Infection in Clients of Needle-exchange in Central London', paper given at the Sixth International Conference on AIDS, San Francisco, USA.

McMILLAN, A. (1988) 'HIV in Prisons', *British Medical Journal*, 297, 873–874.

MELICO-SYLVESTRE A., POMBO, V., PEREIRA, A., LOPSES, R. and CORTE-REAL, R. (1989) 'Seroepidemiological Survey of AIDS, Hepatitis and Syphilis in Portuguese Prisoners', paper given at the Fifth International Conference on AIDS, Montreal, Canada.

MORSE, D.L., TRUMAN, B., MIKL, J., SMITH, P., BROADDUS, R. and MAGUIRE, B. (1989) 'The Epidemiology of AIDS among New York State Prison Inmates', paper given at the Fifth International Conference on AIDS, Montreal, Canada.

PADEL, U. (1988) *HIV, AIDS and Prisons*, London, Prison Reform Trust.

STIMSON, G.V., ALLDRITT, L., DOLAN, K. and DONOGHOE, M. (1988) *Injecting Equipment Exchange Schemes: A Final Report*, London, Goldsmiths College.

TRACE, M. (1990) 'HIV and Drugs in British Prisons', *Druglink*, 5, 1, 12–15.

VERNON, G. (1987) (Ed.) *Drug Users and the Prison System*, London, Health Information Trust.

Chapter 15

The Future of Syringe Exchange in the Public Health Prevention of HIV Infection

Gerry Stimson, Rachel Lart,
Kate Dolan and Martin Donoghoe

❧

'Syringe exchange' has been a cornerstone of HIV prevention strategies for people who inject drugs. It has been one of the most rapidly expanding and developing areas of work, and has had major significance as a symbol of new aims, working practices and working ideologies for those seeking to help drug users reduce their risk of HIV infection or of transmitting it to others. Programmes in Britain, Australia and the Netherlands have received international attention and have been held up as models for HIV prevention elsewhere.

The first syringe exchange schemes in Britain were established in 1986, with a major take-off with the government sponsored pilot experiment which ran from 1987 to 1988 (Stimson, 1989). There has been swift expansion since then; we estimate that there were about 120 schemes in England by the end of 1989 (Lart and Stimson, 1990) with additional exchanges in Scotland and a programme starting in Wales.

Much of the publicity about syringe-exchanges focused initially on the large schemes which were set up specifically to offer this service, as in Liverpool, and The Exchange at Cleveland Street and the Caravan at St Mary's Hospital — both in London. However, our recent survey of schemes shows that the special purpose 'stand-alone' schemes are rare (Lart and Stimson, 1990). Most operate from pre-existing drugs agencies. The dominance of drugs agencies in HIV prevention is a theme we elaborate later. There are also a few schemes running in collaboration with high street pharmacies, and from a variety of other health facilities such as genito-urinary medicine (GUM) clinics.

The idea and practice of distributing syringes on an exchange basis is now an accepted part of the UK response to the prevention of HIV transmission among people who inject drugs. It has received ministerial and departmental support, and is supported by many drugs workers. One remarkable feature is how readily the strategy was adopted and how it received so little political, community or

225

professional opposition. The situation has not been the same in some other countries, notably the United States of America. The contrast is extraordinary: in the USA there are guerrilla programmes in San Francisco and New England, and the only ones to run with official sanction or acquiescence are in Portland, Boulder, Tacoma and New York. The New York scheme has now been closed by the Mayor.

Syringe Exchange: The Second Stage

In Britain 'syringe exchange' has now entered a second stage, marked by a shift from an early 'frontier spirit' when many staff thought that they had discovered new ways of working with drug users, to the hard slog of 'getting on with business'. Agencies have moved from an evangelical urgency to sell the message about a new service, to a need for fine-tuning the delivery of the service. Britain is now in the position to discuss this fine-tuning, whereas many countries have not reached the first take-off stage.

'Syringe exchange' has major potential to help reduce the spread of HIV. But the promise of the strategy hides its limitations: moving into the second stage provides the opportunity to analyze critically its contribution and future potential. The question raised in this chapter is whether the shortcomings can be remedied by fine-tuning, or whether a rethinking of the strategy is required.

Achievements

A remarkable feature of the syringe exchange experiment is that it has been extensively documented, monitored and evaluated, and that workers have willingly agreed to have their work scrutinized. Other areas of drug work have not received such critical attention, and few of us would allow our work to come under such examination.

Syringe exchanges are successful on a number of measures. They are good at reaching people who are not reached by conventional drugs services. They attract people who are motivated to make changes in their behaviour. They are able to deliver the basic service — getting syringes out and getting them back (Donoghoe *et al.*, 1989a; Stimson, 1989). Many also offer advice and counselling, practical help with housing, finances and the law, very basic health care, and referral to other helping and treatment agencies (Carvell and Hart, 1990). As a worker in one of the agencies put it, 'we are not just a syringe exchange.'

There is considerable evidence that those who attend exchanges are helped to achieve and maintain lower risk behaviour. The Monitoring Research Group has surveyed clients of syringe exchanges and comparison groups of injectors not using them, with HIV risk behaviour data on over 4000 people since 1987. The various studies show a consistent decline in self-reported syringe sharing, which has been triangulated by interviews in different settings in a number of locations in England, Wales and Scotland, using a variety of interviewers (both professionals and ex-drug users) and a range of questions.

In 1987 the percentage who reported sharing syringes in the last four weeks was around 28 per cent for new syringe exchange clients, and 60 per cent for others. In 1989 the rate for clients had dropped to around 21 per cent, and for others to 32 per cent. All reports from interviews suggest that lack of syringes is now a less common reason for sharing syringes. These changes are of major importance (Donoghoe *et al.*, 1990).

Limitations

Syringe exchanges have a clear role to play in HIV prevention, but as they move into their second stage of development several limitations can be identified. The Monitoring Research Group has continued to monitor exchanges, and has looked at how they have developed since the first evaluation that was conducted between 1987 and 1988.

First, data from 1989 and 1990 show that syringe exchanges continue to attract clients, but that the number of clients coming to individual exchanges is, on average, disappointingly low. Of fifty-five exchanges surveyed in 1989, the average number of clients per week ranged from 1 to 150, with an average of only 21. In 1987–88 exchanges tended to attract older, longer-term injectors, and pro-portionately few were women. Many exchanges were well aware of these shortcomings, and have made creative attempts to recruit such people. But in 1990 the client profile remained substantially unchanged: there had been no improve-ment in reaching younger injectors, newer recruits to injecting, and women (Donoghoe *et al.*, 1990).

Second, syringe sharing rates are reducing, and self-reported sharing is lower than previously, but there remain substantial numbers who continue to share. For example, lower sharing rates were reported in 1989 and 1990, but it is still the case that 21 per cent of syringe exchange clients had shared syringes in the past four weeks, sharing with an average of 1.7 different partners.

Two things underlie these problems facing syringe exchanges. The *first* is a question of resources available to agencies, their capacity and the potential demand for the service; and the *second* is the relationship of syringe distribution, changes in risk behaviour and remaining obstacles to risk reduction.

Reaching Drug Injectors: Resources for Syringe Exchange

In any examination of the potential demand for the syringe exchange service, assumptions must be made about the prevalence of drug injecting. Using data from 'drug indicator projects', and from informed expert assessments from different parts of the country, the consensus of the Advisory Council on the Misuse of Drugs (1988) working group on AIDS Drug Misuse was that there were between 35,000 and 75,000 drug injectors in the UK in 1986. To keep calculations simple, it will be assumed here that there are currently 50,000 regular injectors in England. This is probably a conservative estimate.

How adequate is the current distribution of syringes? Extrapolation from the Monitoring Research Group survey of syringe exchanges indicates that about 2 million syringes were distributed from syringe exchanges in 1989/1990. Alan Glanz's survey of retail pharmacists suggests an additional 2 million syringes from those outlets (Glanz et al., 1990). If there are 50,000 injectors in the UK, and each requires a sterile syringe each day, then 18 million syringes would need to be distributed annually. At 4 million, current distribution falls far short of this.

How adequate is the capacity of the agencies? If 50,000 injectors visited a syringe exchange every two weeks, there would be 24,000 visits per week, and the 120 syringe exchanges would each have a weekly client load of 200. But our survey found that each saw an average of twenty-one people a week (Lart and Stimson, 1990). A few large agencies such as Bristol Drugs Project and the Community Drug Project in London see a total of about 100 to 120 clients a week for all services. Current capacity would have to increase tenfold to meet the potential caseload.

Assuming that *every* drugs agency in England ran an exchange, and there are estimated to be 300 currently funded agencies in England (McGregor et al., 1990), then the client load would be eighty clients each, just for syringe exchange. Another way to look at this is to consider the number of staff required. Drug agencies in England see an average of one client per staff member per day: without any change in current working practices, nearly 5000 staff would be needed to cope with the potential client visits in order to supply syringes on the scale required.

The conclusion must be that the current model for distributing syringes is insufficient to meet potential demand. The scale of the shortfall is such that demand cannot easily be met by increasing resources or by introducing more efficient working practices.

Obstacles to Changes in Risk Behaviour

The *second* relevant area is the relationship between syringe distribution and changes in risk behaviour. In the first stage a simple message was promoted —

'don't share syringes' — along with provision of the means to avoid sharing — supplies of sterile syringes. The evidence is now quite considerable that this strategy is working to help injectors change their behaviour.

On the positive side our qualitative studies show that sharing syringes is no longer viewed as the norm and that most people who inject drugs try to avoid sharing syringes. In 1988 and 1989 we conducted an in-depth study of drug injecting in London and Brighton (Burt and Stimson, 1989) and found that people had adopted a variety of *protective strategies* to avoid the risk of HIV infection. These included obtaining supplies of sterile syringes, cleaning syringes, avoiding risky situations and being selective about sharing partners. They talked about sharing as no longer part of the etiquette of everyday drug use. Occasions when syringes were shared were exceptional events, and they promoted justificatory explanations.

But the changes in behaviour recorded in this and other studies may be insufficient to stop the spread of HIV infection. Indeed, given the percentage who still report sharing syringes, which is around 20 per cent or more, it is questionable what impact there will be on the spread of HIV. We found that sharing still occurred despite attempts to adopt a variety of protective strategies. It happened for a number of situational and personal reasons, such as running out of syringes, being away from home without a syringe, because a syringe broke, or as a consequence of being intoxicated. We concluded that increasing the supply of syringes does not, on its own, ensure that sharing will cease.

The other area for HIV prevention is sexual behaviour. Most people who inject drugs are sexually active. Half of those who are active have partners who themselves do not inject drugs (Donoghoe *et al.*, 1989b). Condom use is uncommon. Both staff and clients at syringe exchanges find it difficult to talk about sex. Because syringe exchanges are located in drugs agencies, the dominant 'frame' is drug use, and this discourages talk of sexual behaviour. We first noted this in 1987 and have little evidence that the situation has changed.

Responding to the Limitations

Drug agencies have responded to these problems of resource limitations and obstacles to behaviour change in two ways. The first is to try to reach out to drug injectors through, for example, mobile schemes and outreach work, and by involving local pharmacists. The second is to use contacts with clients to engage them in counselling in safer drug use and safer sex. The drawback is that both outreach and counselling are extremely labour intensive.

In summary, there remain many obstacles to risk reduction that are poorly tackled by the current strategy. Just as agencies cannot be expanded to reach sufficient injectors, nor can agencies reach people at the point where risky behaviour occurs.

Facilitating and Constraining Factors

We suggest that there are basic philosophical, structural and organizational reasons for the limitations to the current 'syringe exchange' strategy. Before describing these, it is necessary to understand what facilitated the original development of syringe exchanges. It is our thesis that the factors that helped syringe exchanges develop so swiftly now constrain their development.

There are three factors that helped syringe exchanges develop so rapidly and relatively easily in England, and which explain why drugs agencies are prominent in this task. The first was the *debate on harm minimization* that developed in many drugs agencies in the 1980s, and which can be traced as an important theme of the British approach to drug problems in earlier periods. Throughout the last seventy years of British drugs policy, medical advocates have promoted harm minimization (although they may not have employed this term). The practice of prescribing drugs to addicts, dating from the 1920s, was based on the idea that it enabled addicted people to lead relatively normal lives. The notion that harm can be limited was present in the 1960s in both professional and drug user circles; it has been part of the workplace rhetoric in many statutory and non-statutory agencies from the early 1980s.

The second factor that facilitated syringe exchanges was a matter of *institutional sites*. By the time HIV became an important issue, a wide range of agencies, mainly outside the medical arena, was involved in the provision of help and advice to drug users. Most were established from 1984–85 under the Department of Health and Social Security Central Funding Initiative which pump-primed almost one-third of drug services and contributed funds to almost a half. Three-quarters of currently existing drug services in England began operation between 1984 and 1989. This initiative increased accessibility of services and attracted new client groups. When HIV and AIDS became of concern, these agencies were able to adopt HIV prevention work and adapt their work to cope with the new tasks. As MacGregor and colleagues have described it, 'One clear benefit of the CFI [Central Funding Initiative] promotion of the new services was that it provided a base from which AIDS work could be developed and allowed a smoother and more rapid response to this major public health issue than might otherwise have been the case' (MacGregor *et al.*, 1990).

The third factor that influenced their development was the *social policy framework*. English drugs policy in the 1980s was characterized by centralized policy and funding initiatives, accompanied by high levels of local autonomy. This absence of central direction and coordination resulted in a proliferation of different agencies which were responsive to local needs.

It is unlikely that syringe exchanges would have been so swiftly adopted in this country without this combination of an existing debate on harm minimization, a wide variety of existing institutional sites, and a social policy framework that allowed for a central 'nudge' but which left high levels of local autonomy. This also explains why HIV prevention for injecting drug users has developed primarily as a client-oriented service operating from drug agencies: it has been added on to pre-existing drug services with a pre-existing idea of harm minimization through individual client contact.

Public Health and Community Change

What is the way forward? One of the needed practical developments is to increase the supply of syringes and the opportunities for safe disposal. This cannot be achieved through individual client-based services alone, for drug services can never reach sufficient people. It must be done through a proliferation of different outlets: this includes agency-based syringe exchanges, but also pharmacies, outreach, secondary distribution via other health workers and via indigenous workers (current and ex-drug injectors), and impersonal means of delivery (such as vending machines). It requires some separation of syringe supply from disposal. There is also an urgent need to develop a broader conception of safer drug use which recognizes a range of protective strategies in addition to use of sterile syringes. For example, syringe distribution can be supplemented by instruction in a variety of other protective strategies, including syringe decontamination, how to avoid risky situations, and preferred places to use and inject drugs; and it could include promoting social skills in refusing to share, and instruction in safe disposal.

More fundamentally, it is time to rethink the strategy. The factors which enabled syringe exchanges to develop may now hinder their development. The philosophical attachment to targeting individuals for behaviour change, linked with a fixed base agency mode of delivery, make it difficult for syringe exchanges to tackle the twin problems of limited resources and obstacles to behaviour change. A further problem is that the lack of central direction — from the state or from local health or other authorities — makes a redirection of effort difficult to initiate. High levels of local autonomy can encourage creativity, yet discourage progress when a coordinated push and change of perspective are required.

HIV prevention is about promoting healthy behaviour; but health behaviours do not occur in a vacuum. Health behaviours — and risky behaviours — are located within social, economic and cultural practices. There are many good reasons why people engage in harmful behaviour, even when they intend the opposite. All these behaviours take place well away from the territory of the drugs agency. While attempts can be made to tackle these behaviours on an individual client-centred basis, what has changed is the broader culture within which drug use — and syringe-sharing and sexual behaviour — takes place.

Promoting healthy behaviour is thus a massive task of encouraging social change. The task is not so much how an individual will be helped to change his or her behaviour, but how that person can help others to change. The target group is all those drug injectors whom the drugs worker will never meet. This task can only be achieved in collaboration with drug injectors, who will be the main agents of change.

This is a public and community health task: it requires a major reconceptualization of working philosophies to focus on communities and not just individuals; it requires the development of new working practices away from the cosiness of the office; and it requires the development of preventive strategies on a coordinated community-wide level.

Acknowledgments

We are grateful to our colleagues at the Centre for Research on Drugs and Health Behaviour whose work has contributed to this paper, and in particular to Betsy Ettorre and Robert Power for comments on earlier drafts.

References

ADVISORY COUNCIL ON THE MISUSE OF DRUGS (1988) *Report: AIDS and Drug Misuse, Part 1*, London, HMSO.

BURT, J. and STIMSON, G.V. (1989) 'Strategies for Protection: Drug Injecting and the Prevention of HIV Infection', report to the Health Education Authority.

CARVELL, A. and HART, G. (1990) 'Help Seeking and Referrals in a Needle-Exchange: A Comprehensive Service to Injecting Drug Users', *British Journal of Addiction*, 85, 235–240.

DONOGHOE, M.C., STIMSON, G.V., DOLAN, K. and ALLDRITT, L. (1989a), 'Changes in Risk Behaviour in Clients of Syringe-Exchange Schemes in England and Scotland', unpublished paper, London, Centre for Research on Drugs and Health Behaviour.

DONOGHOE, M.C., STIMSON, G.V. and DOLAN K. (1989b) 'Sexual Behaviour of Injecting Drug Users and Associated Risks of HIV Infection for Non-Injecting Sexual Partners', *AIDS Care* 1, 1, 51–58.

DONOGHOE, M., DOLAN, K., JONES, S. and STIMSON, G.V. (1990) *National Syringe Exchange Monitoring Study: An Interim Report*, report to the Department of Health, London, Charing Cross and Westminster Medical School, Centre for Research on Drugs and Health Behaviour.

GLANZ, A., BYRNE, C. and JACKSON, P. (1990) *Prevention of AIDS among Drug Misusers: The Role of the High Street Pharmacy. Findings of a Survey of Community Pharmacies in England and Wales*, London, Institute of Psychiatry, Addiction Research Unit.

LART, R. and STIMSON, G.V. (1990) 'National Survey of Syringe-Exchanges Schemes in England', forthcoming, *British Journal of Addiction*, 85, 1433–1443.

MACGREGOR, S., ETTORRE, B., COOMBER, R., CROSIER, A. and LODGE, H. (1990) 'Central Funding Initiative and the Development of Drug Services in England', London, Birkbeck College, University of London.

STIMSON, G.V. (1989) 'Syringe Exchange Programmes for Injecting Drug Users', Editorial Review, *AIDS* 3, 5, 253–260.

Chapter 16

Reaching the Hard to Reach:
Models of HIV Outreach Health Education

Tim Rhodes and Richard Hartnoll

In recent years outreach health education has come to be viewed as both a central and essential component of wider HIV prevention strategies. But despite this, there is a dearth of published material about the nature and comparative efficacy of national or international interventions. This chapter aims to redress this imbalance by developing a descriptive typology of models of HIV outreach health education in Europe and the United States. This provides a context within which preliminary judgments about the efficacy of differing outreach models and strategies can be made.

Outreach Health Education and HIV Prevention

There are certain populations who are unlikely to be reached by conventional HIV prevention strategies. These include those traditionally more difficult to access, such as injecting drug users, women and men working in the sex industry, and their sexual partners. Although a relatively small proportion of the total population, they are likely to be of increasing HIV epidemiological importance (Des Jarlais and Friedman, 1987; Padian, 1988). This arises both from the prevalence and frequency of HIV transmission behaviours which occur among hard to reach populations (Power *et al.*, 1988; Stimson *et al.*, 1988a; Coleman and Curtis, 1988), and from their high level of mobility and interchange occurring across different social networks and geographical areas (Kinnell, 1989; McDermott, 1988).

The broad objective of HIV outreach health education is to make face to face contact with hard to reach drug injectors and sex industry workers to provide idiosyncratic interventions, such that risk reduction behaviour can be both effected and maintained. Thus 'outreach' may be defined as 'any community oriented activity which is undertaken in order to make contact with individuals or groups from particular populations, who are out of contact or who are not regularly in contact, with existing services' (Hartnoll *et al.*, 1990).

There are two subdivisions of outreach work within this definition: detached and peripatetic. Detached interventions operate in the specific and restricted sense of working outside any agency contact, for example, work undertaken on the streets, in pubs, cafes, squats and at shooting galleries. Their aim is to facilitate change either *directly* in the community, or *indirectly* by attracting individuals into existing treatment and helping services. Peripatetic interventions are organizationally rather than individually focused, such as work undertaken in community institutions, for example, prisons, syringe exchanges and hostels.

Outreach has traditionally been the focus of 'bottom-up' rather than 'top-down' approaches to health (Beattie, 1986), and has more in common with 'self-empowerment' and 'community-oriented' paradigms of health education than those concerned with 'information-giving' (Homans and Aggleton, 1987; French and Adams, 1986). While models of HIV outreach health education have evolved from a diversity of health service perspectives, such as youth and community work, self-help provision, ethnographic research and public health interventions (Des Jarlais, 1989; Hartnoll *et al.*, 1989), in even their most conventional forms (models of self-empowerment) they accept the need for context-related health education and active participation on the part of the client. This is in sharp contrast to the behaviour change and information giving models of health education about HIV infection which remain the dominant paradigms (Homans and Aggleton, 1987).

Models of HIV Outreach Health Education

Outreach health education about HIV infection, safer sex and safer drug use has developed most extensively in the United States (US) and the Netherlands (Rhodes *et al.*, 1990, Friedman *et al.*, 1990; Des Jarlais, 1989; Buning *et al.*, 1988a). Similar interventions in the United Kingdom (UK), although fast expanding, remain in relative infancy (Hartnoll *et al.*, 1990). The models and strategies described here, along with available evaluation findings, come mainly from the US and the Netherlands, and are organized into several types. These include outreach ethnography, indirect change, self-help, bleach and teach, syringe exchange, combined bleach and syringe exchange, and mobile outreach.

Outreach Ethnography

The value of ethnography as a research methodology in the study of illicit drug use has been well documented (Plant and Reeves, 1976; Power, 1989; Weppner, 1977; Feldman, 1974). The combined ethnography–epidemiology outreach model, where ethnographic research informs the nature and parameters of outreach health education, is popular in relation to HIV prevention (Connors, 1988; Feldman and Biernacki, 1988).

The Chicago AIDS Community Outreach Intervention Project is an established example of such a model (Wiebel, 1988; Wiebel and Altman, 1988). Originally developed to intervene and contain community outbreaks of heroin use (Hughes and Crawford, 1972), it combines the principles of medical epidemiology (de Alarcon, 1969) and community ethnography (Becker, 1953). Indigenous outreach workers (current or former drug users/sex industry workers) are used as participant observers and as 'AIDS Prevention Advocates' at sites where drug injectors and those working as street prostitutes congregate.

Rather than addressing atomized individuals within a specified target population, the model aims to achieve subcultural change among target constituencies (Wiebel, 1988). The intervention thus falls within a community-oriented model of health education, as opposed to individualistic behaviour change and self-empowerment models which remain prevalent in the US and UK. A number of specific outreach strategies facilitate this process of subcultural or community change. First, the use of indigenous outreach workers enables immediate identification with target populations. Second, a repetition of outreach contacts, using a series of complementary risk reduction messages at different locations, maximizes health recommendation exposure and reinforces its content. Third, and most significantly, the targeting of 'key people' and the suggestion that they become community outreach representatives or streetworkers themselves, encourages feelings of group social responsibility. Together, this provides a cohesive organizational framework for collective HIV prevention and behaviour change (Wiebel, 1988). The extent to which the intervention has reduced the frequency of clients' HIV transmission behaviour or incidence of HIV infection has yet to be determined.

Indirect Change

Models of detached intervention which place more emphasis on encouraging individuals to use existing helping services are based on the knowledge that street health education results in an increased demand for treatment and helping services (Des Jarlais, 1989; Feldman, 1987), and on beliefs that treatment per se is an effective way of modifying HIV transmission behaviour (Ball *et al.*, 1988). Treatment-oriented outreach programmes specifically designed as HIV prevention strategies have been established in New Jersey, New York, San Francisco and Sweden, while others are planned elsewhere in the United States and Europe.

In 1985 the New Jersey Community AIDS Program (NJCAP) was established (Jackson *et al.*, 1987a, 1987b). At this time it was the first outreach project set up in the US. It is also the best known example of an indirect change model of outreach. Initially the project had focused on the communication of safer injection techniques via street detached work among drug injectors (Jackson and Rotkiewicz, 1987), but demand from clients necessitated referral access into drug treatment and helping agencies. The project thus operates an *indirect* self-empowerment model of outreach health education.

A sharp rise in the prevalence of HIV infection in New Jersey coincided with the institution of charges for detoxification. In response, NJCAP's outreach workers began to distribute coupons to injectors which allowed recipients access to free detoxication services at twenty-five drug treatment facilities (Jackson *et al.*, 1987a). The 'Coupon Program' has met with considerable success: of the 3000 coupons initially distributed, 86 per cent were redeemed. The program effectively reached those previously out of contact with existing services: 45 per cent of those who redeemed their coupons had no previous experience of treatment, and almost 39 per cent completed the free twenty-one day detoxification period (AIDSCOM, 1989). To date there is no information available to assess the degree to which redeemed coupons results in a reduction in the incidence of HIV among target populations.

Self-Help

A number of self-help health education initiatives have begun to incorporate outreach strategies specifically as HIV prevention measures. These initiatives characteristically aim to encompass a wider conception of health and illness than those offered by the majority of outreach models, aiming to achieve change in the community collectively rather than individually, but the more politically motivated self-help outreach groups also make steps towards what Homans and Aggleton (1987) have referred to as 'socially transformatory' models of health education.

The Junkiebonden, a federation of Dutch self-help groups, was established in 1981, and consists primarily of current drug users. It aims to initiate community change through campaigning for the modification of local and national drug policy (Friedman *et al.*, 1990). The Junkiebonden have organized most effectively in Rotterdam and in Amsterdam. In both cases the absence of opposition (from police and authorities) and the presence of support (other community groups) were key factors in assuring its survival (Friedman *et al.*, 1988). The Junkiebonden helped establish the first syringe exchange in the Netherlands in 1984 (Kools and Buurman, 1984), and since this date has distributed education and prevention material, including condoms, to drug users and sex industry workers through detached outreach work.

Operating from a similar self-help perspective as the Junkiebonden is

Amsterdam's Red Thread, established in 1984, by people currently or formerly working in the sex industry. Their broad objectives are to ensure that prostitution is seen as a legitimate form of work, and to improve working conditions for sex industry workers. In 1987, as part of Red Thread's wider social and political action about health, HIV infection and the sex industry, they began detached outreach work with women working as street and window prostitutes. The intervention has effectively implemented a sticker system for women prostitutes to indicate to clients that they only operate 'safe houses' (AIDSCOM, 1989).

The New York AIDS Outreach Program operates from a mixed 'indirect' and 'direct' detached perspective, consisting of four strategies: a programme, similar to that in New Jersey, which aims to improve drug injectors' access to treatment; a programme designed to improve drug injectors' access to HIV testing services; a risk reduction programme providing long-term presence of outreach workers in drug prevalent areas; and a risk reduction programme providing short-term high visibility presence in drug prevalent areas (Des Jarlais, 1989). A self-help group, ADAPT (Association of Drug Abuse Prevention and Treatment), undertakes much of the outreach work in the last two components of the programme (Serrano and Goldsmith, 1988; Des Jarlais, 1989).

Unlike the Junkiebonden, where the impetus to organize came from within the drug using community, ADAPT was an attempt to encourage self-help organization from outside the community by non-drug users, ex-drug users and interested health professionals (Friedman and Casriel, 1989). Increasingly, however, ADAPT has recruited current drug users (from treatment agencies rather than from the streets), and recently has formed a collective for drug users working as prostitutes (Friedman *et al.*, 1989). The need for 'external' facilitation of self-help in the case of ADAPT, as opposed to the 'internal' mobilization characteristic of the Junkiebonden, may reflect national and regional differences between the comparatively more 'liberal' legislation and policing policies of Amsterdam and to those in New York.

While ADAPT provides a public voice for drug users on community, legal and policy drug-related issues, it has also effectively gathered considerable support from the public health sector, and remains funded primarily by the City Department of Health (Des Jarlais, 1989). The project is managed by Narcotic and Drug Research Incorporated (NDRI), which provides ongoing formative evaluation of the outreach strategy. The ADAPT model of outreach has developed from a multi-service perspective, combining 'community', 'professional' and 'research' orientations, while remaining closest to community-oriented intervention. This is in contrast to other drug self-help organizations in the United States, such as Narcotics Anonymous, Drugs Anonymous and Cocaine Anonymous, which lack a collective group identity and emphasize individual rather than social change (Friedman and Casriel, 1989).

A similar social research/self-help collaboration operates in San Francisco between the Association for Women's AIDS Research and Education (AWARE) and the self-help and political activist group COYOTE (Call Off Your Tired Old Ethics). Together they have developed the California Prostitutes Education Project (Cal-Pep) to contact women working in the sex industry (Cohen, 1987). As in the case of ADAPT, the collaboration mixes 'internal' responses to HIV outreach with 'external' ones. The intervention was thus established through intensive prior research and consultation with potential clients about the service provision they required. As a consequence, the project incorporates an outreach strategy first developed in Baltimore by the Street Outreach AIDS Prevalence Programme: the 'AIDS Rap' (McAuliffe *et al.*, 1986). On every detached contact, clients are engaged in conversations about risk reduction before more detailed risk assessment and advice are given.

Bleach and Teach

In most Western European countries and most states in America needles and syringes can be purchased legally in pharmacies, supermarkets and in other commercial outlets (Stimson, 1989; Glanz *et al.*, 1989). In many of the states in America with a high prevalence of injectors, however, prescriptions are required before equipment can be purchased, and pharmacists will refuse to sell equipment to people they suspect to be illicit injectors. As a result of political opposition very few, mainly pilot, syringe exchange schemes exist (Hagan *et al.*, 1989; Clark *et al.*, 1989). Owing to restricted needle and syringe availability, outreach harm reduction strategies in the US differ from most of those in Europe, in that 'bleach and teach' campaigns are advocated. Such campaigns have been organized in San Francisco (Watters, 1987), New York (Des Jarlais, 1989), New Jersey (Jackson *et al.*, 1987a), Chicago (Wiebel, 1988), Baltimore (McAuliffe *et al.*, 1986) and Washington D.C. (Connors and Lewis, 1989).

The bleach and teach strategy was initiated in 1986 by the San Francisco Midcity Project (Feldman and Biernacki, 1988). Developed from a mixed public health and ethnographic research perspective, the intervention uses bleach on the basis of speed of action, cost, safety, effectiveness and accessibility (Resnick *et al.*, 1986). The model operates within a self-empowerment health education paradigm, where clients (in this case drug injectors) are provided with the means (a decontamination method) by which rational health choices can be identified and made about transmission behaviour.

The first bleach intervention in the UK began in late 1988 in rural Berkshire (Druglink, 1988). Noting the success of using dealer networks to provide anti-HIV 'wrap pads' in Brighton, the project distributes 'bleach kits' through local dealers as an added extra to drugs bought. The kits are also distributed through pharmacies, and include a coupon which can be redeemed for clean equipment at local syringe exchanges. In central London a number of projects began partaking in the 'Bleach Project' in early 1990 (Druglink, 1990).

Recent research in the United States suggests that bleach use can be incorporated into drug behaviour. After one year of bleach distribution in Worcester City, using a combined epidemiology-anthropology method, Connors and Lewis (1989) found that bleach use had increased: 29 per cent of injectors used bleach in 1987 compared with 70 per cent in 1988. Similarly, in San Francisco the proportion of bleach users increased from 3 per cent in 1986 to 68 per cent 1987 (Watters, 1987). Although there has been a rise in HIV antibody prevalence in San Francisco over the same period (Wetters, 1987; Moss and Chaisson, 1988), Feldman (1987) has found the rate of new infections to have slowed simultaneously with increased bleach use. The intervention has also brought more referrals to the city's drug treatment programmes than any other source, and despite being aimed at street populations, the message has also reached and been acted on by drug injectors on methadone programmes (Feldman, 1987). Elsewhere, however, findings are less encouraging. In New York an evaluation of the outreach programme shows bleach use to be uneven, and concludes that the bleach communication seems not to have been effective (Sufian *et al.*, 1989).

Syringe Exchange

In the Netherlands and United Kingdom outreach intervention has long incorporated syringe exchange. In Amsterdam the first syringe exchange was established in 1984 as a result of increased Hepatitis B infection (Kools and Buurman, 1984). By 1987 there were fourteen exchange locations in Amsterdam, and over 600,000 needles and syringes had been distributed (Buning, 1987). Evaluation of Amsterdam's syringe exchange network is encouraging: exchange users have been shown to be injecting and sharing less often than non-exchange users. Since the exchange was established, the estimated number of injectors in the city has remained constant (at 3000), and the number of persons entering methadone and drug free treatment has increased (Hoek *et al.*, 1989; Buning *et al.*, 1988a, 1988b). Perhaps most importantly, the existence of the exchange has been associated with a decrease in the rate of new infections of HIV (Haastrecht *et al.*, 1989).

Stimson *et al.*, suggest (Ch. 15, this volume) that findings from the evaluation of syringe exchanges are mixed. On the positive side, and in the UK, 2500 injectors were reached by fifteen exchanges in nine months. About a third of these clients had no previous drug treatment, and the average return rate of equipment was approximately 62 per cent (Stimson, 1989; Stimson *et al.*, 1988b). Clients attending the schemes for over three months show lower rates of sharing than have been reported elsewhere in the UK literature (Stimson, 1989). Preliminary findings from the Tacoma exchange in Washington show exchange users practising better needle hygiene, sharing less frequently than non-attenders, and more likely to use bleach when sharing than non-attenders (Hagan *et al.*, 1989). But both these evaluations also show less encouraging findings. In the Tacoma evaluation as many as 35 per cent of attenders reported injecting more frequently than before they attended. In the UK exchange schemes were less likely to reach those engaging in risky behaviour; only a third of attenders made as many as five visits, and although most clients staying in the schemes for as long as three months made risk reduction changes, 21 per cent continued to share at least as much as when they first attended (Stimson *et al.*, 1988a). As yet there is only suggestive research evidence linking the syringe exchange model to a reduced transmission of HIV infection (Stimson, 1989; Hart *et al.*, 1989).

Combined Bleach and Syringe Exchange

In some situations bleach and syringe exchange strategies have been developed concurrently. This combined strategy may be advantageous for two reasons. First, no matter what the availability of equipment, sharing will inevitably occur, such as for first time injectors (Haw, 1985), when intoxicated (Freidman *et al.*, 1986) or in situations where sharing is both socially acceptable and socially desired (Feldmen and Biernacki, 1988). Second, the use of bleach does not require a radical change in normal injecting behaviour. Bleach, as in San Francisco, can be habitually incorporated into existing injecting patterns, whereas continually returning to syringe exchanges for new equipment remains demanding and unrealistic. The available evidence lends support for this mixed strategy: Tacoma's exchange in Washington, with combined exchange and bleach objectives, managed to keep 90 per cent of its clients injecting safely (not sharing; sharing and cleaning; and not sharing but cleaning) (Hagan *et al.*, 1989).

Mobile Outreach

Mobile outreach units have been developed in Amsterdam, New Jersey and in Plymouth in the UK. The best established of these is the mobile methadone bus in Amsterdam. Methadone distribution is seen as an integral feature of Amsterdam's Municipal Health Service harm minimization programme (Buning *et al.*, 1988a). The methadone buses have been in operation since 1979, and provide methadone, a syringe exchange facility, condoms, information and advice and a general health service. The intervention provides low threshold on-site access to general primary health care services for hard to reach populations, rather than being HIV-specific.

Since 1987 the New Jersey Community AIDS Program has operated a mobile outreach service as an addition to the Coupon Program (Jackson *et al.*, 1987b). Three outreach vans aim to reach drug injectors and their partners in inner city neighbourhoods. The intervention also provides a primary health care service, but with a particular HIV emphasis, including on-site HIV antibody testing, but does not provide prescription drugs. Preliminary evaluation data suggest the vans are well utilized, are particularly effective in reaching the female sex partners of injecting drug users, and are reaching people previously out of contact with existing HIV-related information and advice services (Jackson *et al.*, 1989).

The first mobile HIV outreach service in the UK was established in late 1987 by Plymouth Health Authority (Roberts, 1989; Hassard and Parker, 1989). The outreach bus provides condoms, needles and syringes, risk reduction advice and medical referrals to women working as street prostitutes. No general primary care services are provided, although the bus is staffed by both medical doctors and nurses. More recently (1989), the service split to form a separate mobile syringe exchange. Of Plymouth's estimated eighty streetworking women prostitutes, the mobile outreach service has contacted approximately fifty (Roberts, 1989), although the syringe exchange has been less successful (Hassard and Parker, 1989). There are similar mobile outreach units to Plymouth's currently operating in the UK, for example in Mersey (Newcombe, 1989).

Integrating Outreach Service Provision

Outreach work has traditionally been the concern of voluntary and community-based organizations rather than statutory-based or 'professional' ones. Although hard to reach populations are probably more likely to come into contact with voluntary than statutory agencies, voluntary agencies are often without the necessary resources required to cope with their general health care needs. In recognition of this, a model of outreach work was jointly established in central London by both voluntary and statutory health sectors with the explicit aim of bridging existing gaps in service provision between the two sectors (Rhodes *et al.*, 1991). CLASH (Central London Action on Street Health) was set up in 1986 with the dual purpose of providing in situ street health education about HIV infection and AIDS (traditionally the role of outreach work), as well as referral access into appropriate health care and HIV-specific statutory and voluntary services.

Established models of statutory provision are increasingly being called into question in relation to their applicability and relevance for hard to reach populations. This has led to the setting up of lower threshold interventions in the context of HIV infection and AIDS, of which statutory-based outreach work is now a fast expanding field. While this is encouraging, statutory services may have little hope of attracting previously neglected populations without drawing on the

Figure 16.1   CLASH Management and Service Structure

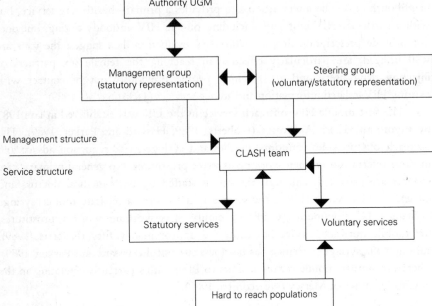

expertise and guidance of organizations which have had a long commitment to and influence in this area. There may be little value in merely providing a 'community mask' for the same 'professional' services. This dominant 'professional–community' model of HIV outreach which is currently emerging in Britain (Hartnoll *et al.*, 1990) runs the risk of merely assuming that given the use of 'community' workers and a 'community' approach, hard to reach populations will be successfully attracted into existing 'professional' services. But the fact that these populations *are* hard to reach indicates that the professional services available may indeed be inappropriate or inadequate. The context within which CLASH was set up attempted to go some way towards acknowledging these conflicts: it was established by both 'community' and 'professional' organizations, and an effort was made to reflect this need in its management structure (Figure 16.1). While being managed on a policy level by the health service, the intention was for the CLASH team to remain as independent as possible within the health authority, and to receive direction through a steering group of both voluntary and statutory representatives.

Reaching the large, often transient, population of young people in central London who are without secure accommodation, involved in drug taking, or exchanging sex for money, drugs or shelter was thus a main objective of CLASH.

Their aims were to provide these populations with HIV-related health education and advice, as well as to facilitate the possibility of their access to health care and other services.

Conclusions

HIV outreach work is fast expanding in the UK. Models of intervention remain innovative and experimental, drawing on the experiences from more established schemes in the US and elsewhere. It is perhaps too early to determine which particular approaches to HIV outreach can or should be generalized and which should be avoided. This is particularly the case when the extent of descriptive and evaluation material available is severely limited. A number of observations can be drawn from this review concerning, first, models of HIV outreach, and second, strategies of HIV outreach.

The objectives of outreach necessitate more innovative approaches to health education and health promotion than conventional HIV prevention measures. In this respect outreach has seen an encouraging departure from 'information giving' paradigms of education. The majority of models lie closest to self-empowerment definitions, although a minority of models aim to achieve community and collective change among target populations. The Chicago model is perhaps the best established example of these. Although evaluation findings determining its efficacy regarding HIV prevention are as yet unavailable, the original model has proved effective in intervening and containing community outbreaks of heroin use (Hughes and Crawford, 1972).

The style of working and ideology of outreach work has most in common with youth and community-based initiatives, although with respect to HIV outreach projects are increasingly being established and managed from 'professional' service perspectives. A number of projects in the US, notably ADAPT and the AWARE-COYOTE collaboration, appear to have effectively combined this professional-community approach. In the UK the CLASH model is a similar collaboration, attempting to provide an interface between community and professional-based services. This type of collaboration, although necessary, may also be a precarious one. First, there may be conflict on an ideological level between the ways in which community workers and their managers define the health needs of target populations. An obvious example would be the extent to which self-help outreach projects such as Red Thread and the Junkiebonden are able to undertake a campaigning role as part of their health education work. Second, there may be conflict on a pragmatic level. There is some preliminary evidence for this with the CLASH project: the statutory sector remains suspicious of the project's relative autonomy within the health service, while the voluntary representatives (and the workers) feel the service is hindered by the unnecessary bureaucratic and authoritarian structures inherent within this managerial setting (Christmas *et al.*, 1988; Rhodes *et al.*, 1991).

The extent to which professional and community outreach collaborations are problematic in terms of realizing clients' needs are as yet unknown. But if the role of outreach is not only to provide an in situ health education service but also to facilitate referral contact of hard to reach populations to existing services, then 'professional' health services will have to be committed not only to innovative ways of accessing clients, but also to innovative developments within the services they plan to offer. The most common criticism of health services by clients, for example, is that they are too judgmental. In this respect it is useful to compare the approach in the Netherlands with those made in the UK and the US. Almost three-quarters of Amsterdam's drug using populations are estimated to be in contact with some form of helping service (Buning *et al.*, 1988a). By comparison, estimates in the UK are in the region of 50 per cent (Hartnoll, 1985). One possible explanation for this difference is that while outreach in the UK and US has attempted to bridge gaps existing between professional services and hard to reach populations, the Netherlands has taken a comprehensive health outreach service out to them, on their own terms and on their home ground. Just one example of this is Amsterdam's mobile outreach unit which offers general health care and methadone prescriptions, as well as specifically HIV-related services. The paucity of general health services provided by outreach in the UK and US, the continued reliance on existing services, and perhaps the reluctance to develop truly accessible, flexible and comprehensive outreach programme may limit the effectiveness and perceived utility of the service for hard to reach populations.

Further observations can be made concerning HIV outreach strategies. First, initial findings suggest outreach appears to be an effective contacting strategy for hard to reach populations. Second, the extent to which outreach has brought about positive risk reduction changes is mixed. There is evidence for the need for complementary strategies to HIV outreach health education. Detached outreach interventions (operating in a 'direct' fashion) should be seen as complementary to treatment-oriented ones (operating in an 'indirect' fashion). Findings in San Francisco (Feldman, 1987) and in New York (Des Jarlais, 1989) both show street detached work to have increased demand for treatment and helping services. Bleach and teach strategies, where possible, should remain complementary to syringe exchange ones. Evidence shows neither strategy alone to be effective, and recent evidence suggests that combined strategies show the potential for greater risk reduction. The communication of safer drug messages must be concomitant with safer sex ones. A review of the literature suggests a greater emphasis, particularly in the US and in the Netherlands, on drug risk reduction programmes. While it is evident that injectors contacted by outreach workers are making some drug risk reduction changes, it is less evident that they are also making appropriate changes in their sexual behaviour.

Lastly, while there is a large and growing literature of evaluation of service delivery and 'output' in the statutory and voluntary sectors for a range of organizations, it is still not the case that monitoring and evaluation are necessarily included in the brief, objectives or practice of any such organizations (Crosier *et al.*, 1988). Few HIV outreach projects systematically monitor and evaluate their service delivery in this way. There is a need for the recognition that models of outreach must remain both experimental and flexible in design while drawing from existing national and international experience, and for the continued and systematic monitoring and evaluation of these approaches.

Ackowledgements

This research was undertaken as part of a wider study relating to HIV-related outreach service provision funded by the Department of Health. We wish to acknowledge further support from our colleagues Janet Holland, Anne Johnson and Janaka Perera, from the CLASH outreach workers, and from Sara Jones at the Centre for Research on Drugs and Health Behaviour.

References

AIDSCOM (1989) *Education and Evaluation: Partners in AIDS Prevention*, Washington, AIDSCOM.

BALL, J., LANGE, W., *et al.* (1988) 'Reducing the Risk of AIDS through Methadone Maintenance Treatment', *Journal of Health and Social Behaviour*, 29, 214–226.

BEATTIE, A. (1986) 'Community Development for Health: From Practice to Theory', *Radical Health Promotion*, 4, 12–18.

BECKER, H. (1953) 'Becoming a Marijuana User', *American Journal of Sociology*, 59, 235–242.

BUNING, E. (1987) *Spuitenomruil in Amsterdam Notitie TBV*, Amsterdam, Beleidsgroep AIDS Amsterdam.

BUNING, E., VAN BRUSSEL, G. and VAN SANTEN, G. (1988a) 'Amsterdam's Drug Policy and Its Implications for Controlling Needle Sharing', in R. BATTJES and R. PICKENS (Eds), *Needle Sharing among Intravenous Drug Abusers: National and International Perspectives*, NIDA Research Monograph 80, Rockville.

BUNING, E., HARTGERS, C., *et al.* (1988b) 'A First Evaluation of the Needle/Syringe Exchange in Amsterdam, Holland', paper given at the Global Impact of AIDS Conference, London.

CHRISTMAS, J., LAZARUS, M., *et al.* (1988) 'Health Outreach Work in the West End of London', *Health Education Journal* 47, 4, 162–163.

CLARK, G., DOWNING, M., *et al.* (1989) 'Street Based Needle Exchange Programs: The Next Step in HIV Prevention', paper given at Fifth International Conference on AIDS, Montreal.

COHEN, J. (1987) 'Three Years Experience Promoting AIDS Prevention among 800 Sexually Active High Risk Women in San Francisco', paper given at NIHA/NIDA Research Conference on Women and AIDS: Promoting Health Behaviours, Bethesda, Md.

COLEMAN, R.M. and CURTIS, D. (1988) 'Distribution of Risk Behaviour for HIV Infection amongst Intravenous Drug Users', *British Journal of Addiction*, 83, 1331–1334.

CONNORS, M. (1988) 'Outreach Ethnography: A Concept Paper', Massachusetts, Spectrum House Inc.

CONNORS, M. and LEWIS B. (1989) 'Anthropological and Epidemiological Observations of Changes in Needle Sharing Practices Following Twelve Months of Bleach Distribution', paper given at the Fifth International Conference on AIDS, Montreal.

CROSIER, A., MacGREGGOR, S., ETTORE, B., *et al.* (1988) *An Assessment of 'The Central Funding Initiative on Services for the Treatment and Rehabilitation of Drug Misusers'*, Fifth Report, London, University of London, Birkbeck College.

DAY, S., WARD, H. and HARRIS, J. (1988) 'Prostitute Women and Public Health', *British Medical Journal*, 297, 1585.

DE ALARCON, R. (1969) 'The Spread of Heroin Abuse in a Community', *Bulletin of Narcotics*, 12, 17–22.

DES JARLAIS (1989) 'AIDS Prevention Programs for Intravenous Drug Users: Diversity and Evolution', *International Review of Psychiatry*, 1, 1, 101–108.

DES JARLAIS D. and FRIEDMAN, S. (1987) 'Editorial Review: HIV Infection and Intravenous Drug Users; Epidemiology and Risk Reduction', *AIDS*, 1, 67–76.

DRUGLINK EDITORIAL (1988) 'US Style 'Bleach and Teach' Tried in Rural Berkshire', *Druglink*, 3, 6, 9.

DRUGLINK EDITORIAL (1990) 'News: The Bleach Project', *Druglink*, 5, 2, 6.

FELDMAN, H. (1974) *Street Status and the Drug Researcher: Issues in Participant-Observation*, Washington, D.C., Drug Abuse Council.

FELDMAN, H. (1987) 'Outreach Education to Intravenous Drug Users', paper given to the Presidential Commission of the HIV Epidemic, Washington.

FELDMAN, H. and BIERNACKI, P. (1988) 'The Ethnography of Needle Sharing among Intravenous Drug Users and Implications of Public Policies and Intervention Strategies', in R. BATTJES and R. PICKENS (Eds), *Needle Sharing among Intravenous Drug Abusers*, NIDA Research Monograph 80, Rockville.

FRENCH, J. and ADAMS, L. (1986) 'From Analysis to Synthesis', *Health Education Journal*, 45, 2, 71–74.

FRIEDMAN, S.R. and CASRIEL, C. (1989) 'Drug Users Organizations and AIDS Policy', *AIDS and Public Policy*, 3, 30–36.

FRIEDMAN, S., DES JARLAIS, D., *et al.* (1986) 'AIDS Health Education for Intravenous Drug Users', *Health Education Ouarterly*, 13, 383–394.

FRIEDMAN, S., DES JARLAIS, D., *et al.* (1987) 'AIDS and Self-Organization among Intravenous Drug Users', *International Journal of the Addictions*, 22, 3, 201–219.

FRIEDMAN, S.R., DE JONG, W.M. and DES JARLAIS, D.C. (1988) 'Problems and Dynamics of Organizing Intravenous Drug Users for AIDS Prevention', *Health Education Research*, 3, 1, 49–57.

FRIEDMAN, S.R., STERK, C., SUFIAN, M., *et al.* (1989) 'Organising Intravenous Drug Users against AIDS', paper given at the Fifth International Conference on AIDS, Montreal.

FRIEDMAN, S.R., STERK, C., *et al.* (1990) 'Reaching out to Injecting Drug Users', in J. STRAND and G. STIMSON (Eds), *AIDS and Drug Misuse: The Challenge for Policy and Practice in the 1990s*, London, Routledge.

GLANZ, A., BYRNE, C. and JACKSON, P. (1989) 'Role of Community Pharmacies in Prevention of AIDS among Injecting Drug Misusers: Findings of a Survey in England and Wales', *British Medical Journal*, 299, 1076–1079.

HAASTRECHT, H., VAN DEN HOEK, J. and COUNTINHO, R.A. (1989) 'No Trend in Yearly HIV-Seroprevalence Rates among IVDUs in Amsterdam: 1986–1988', paper given at the Fifth International Conference on AIDS, Montreal.

HAGAN, H., REID, T., *et al.* (1989) 'Needle Exchange in Tacoma, Washington: Initial Results', paper given at the Fifth International Conference on AIDS, Montreal.

HART, G.J., CARVELL, A., WOODWARD, N., *et al.* (1989) 'Evaluation of Needle Exchange in Central London: Behaviour Change and Anti-HIV Status over One Year', *AIDS*, 3, 5, 261–265.

HARTNOLL, R. (1985) Paper given at Drug Misuse in Camden, Hampstead Regional Health Authority.

HARTNOLL, R., RHODES, T., JOHNSON, A., *et al.* (1989) *A Review of HIV Outreach Intervention in United States, United Kingdom and Netherlands*, Drug Indicators Project, London, University of London, Birkbeck College.

HARTNOLL, R., RHODES, T., JONES, S., *et al.* (1990) 'A Survey of HIV Outreach Intervention in the United Kingdom', Drug Indicators Project, London, University of London, Birkbeck College.

HASSARD, A. and PARKER, K. (1989) *Preliminary Report on Plymouth Syringe Exchange*, Plymouth Health Authority.

HAW, S. (1985) *Drug Problems in Greater Glasgow*, London, Standing Conference on Drug Abuse.

HOEK, A. VAN DEN, HAASTRECHT, H. VAN and COUTINHO, R.A. (1989) 'Evidence for Risk Reduction among IVDU in Amsterdam', paper given at the Fifth International Conference on AIDS, Montreal.

HOMANS, H. and AGGLETON, P. (1987) 'Health Education about HIV Infection and AIDS', in P. AGGLETON and H. HOMANS (Eds), *Social Aspects of AIDS*, Lewes, Falmer Press.

HOPKINS, S., CARLISLE, M., HONEY, J., *et al.* (1989) 'Needle-Sharing and Bleach Use among Intravenous Drug Users (IVDUs) Seeking to Enter an Acute Detoxification Program', paper given at the Fifth International Conference on AIDS, Montreal.

HUGHES, P. and CRAWFORD, G. (1972) 'A Contagious Model for Researching and Intervening in Heroin Epidemics', *Archives of General Psychiatry*, 27, 149–155.

JACKSON, J. and ROTKIEWICZ, L. (1987) 'A Coupon Program: AIDS Education and Drug Treatment', paper given at the Third International Conference on AIDS, Washington.

JACKSON, J., ROTKIEWICZ, L., *et al.* (1987a) *A Coupon Program: Drug Treatment and AIDS Education*, East Orange, New Jersey, New Jersey State Department of Health.

JACKSON, J., ROTKIEWICZ, L., *et al.* (1987b) *AIDS Prevention and Education Programs for Intravenous Drug Users in New Jersey*, East Orange, New Jersey, New Jersey State Department of Health.

JACKSON, J., RODRIGUEZ, G., NELSON, J., *et al.* (1989) *New Jersey Health Van Project*, East Orange, New Jersey, New Jersey State Department of Health, AIDS Community Support Unit.

KINNELL, H. (1989) *Prostitutes, Their Clients and Risks of HIV Infection in Birmingham*, Occasional Paper, Central Birmingham Health Authority.

KOOLS, J. and BUURMAN, J. (1984) Notitie MDHG spuitenomruilsysteem, 5 June.

MCAULIFFE, W. DOERING, *et al.* (1986) *Evaluation of Street Outreach AIDS Prevention Programme (SOAPP)*, Baltimore, Md., Health Education Resource Organization.

MCDERMOTT, P. (1988) *A Survey of Drug Injectors in the Mersey District*, Liverpool, Mersey Regional Health Authority, AIDS Prevention Unit.

MOSS, A. and CHAISSON, R. (1988) 'AIDS and Intravenous Drug Use in San Francisco', *AIDS and Public Policy*, 3, 37–41.

NEWCOMBE, R. (1989) 'Preventing the Spread of HIV Infection among and from Injecting Drug Users in the United Kingdom', *International Journal of Drugs Policy*, 1, 2, 20–27.

PADIAN, N. (1988) 'Editorial Review: Prostitute Women and AIDS; Epidemiology', *AIDS*, 2, 413–419.

PLANT, M. and REEVES, C. (1976) 'Participant Observation as a Method for Collecting Information about Drug Taking: Conclusions from Two English Studies', *British Journal of Addiction*, 71, 155–159.

POWER, R. (1989) 'Participant Observation and Its Place in the Study of Illicit Drug Abuse', *British Journal of Addiction*, 84, 43–52.

POWER R., HARTNOLL, R.L. and DAVIAUD, E. (1988) 'Drug Injecting, AIDS and Risk Behaviour: Potential for Change and Intervention Strategies', *British Journal of Addiction*, 83, 649–654.

PREBLE, E. and CASEY, J. (1969) 'Taking Care of Business: The Heroin Users' Life on the

Street', *International Journal of the Addictions*, 4, 1–24.

RESNICK, L., VEREN, K., *et al.* (1986) 'Stability and Inactivation of HTLV-III/LAV under Clinical and Laboratory Environments', *Journal of the American Medical Association*, 255, 14, 1887–1891.

RHODES, T., HOLLAND, J., HARTNOLL, R. *et al.* (1990) 'Reaching the Hard to Reach', *Druglink*, 5, 6, 12–15.

RHODES, T., HOLLAND, J. and HARTNOLL, R. (1991) 'Hard to Reach or Out of Reach?', Drug Indicator Project, London, University of London, Birkbeck College.

ROBERTS, T. (1989) 'A Street Counselling Service for Prostitutes', paper given at Forum on Communication Issues in HIV Infection and AIDS, Royal Society of Medicine, London.

SERRANO, Y. and GOLDSMITH, D. (1988) 'ADAPT: A Response to HIV Infection in Intravenous Drug Users in New York', paper given at the Fourth International Conference on AIDS, Washington.

STIMSON, G.V. (1989) 'Syringe-Exchange Programmes for Injecting Drug Users', *AIDS*, 5, 3, 253–260.

STIMSON, G.V., ALLDRITT, L., DOLAN, K., *et al.* (1988a) 'HIV Risk Behaviour of Clients Attending Syringe Exchange Schemes in England and Scotland', *British Journal of Addiction*, 83, 1449.

STIMSON, G.V., ALLDRITT, L., DOLAN, K., *et al.* (1988b) 'Syringe Exchange Schemes for Drug Users in England and Scotland', *British Medical Journal*, 296, 1717.

SUFIAN, M., FRIEDMAN, S.R., *et al.* (1989) 'Risk Reduction after Intervention among Intravenous Drug Users', paper given at the Fifth International Conference on AIDS, Montreal.

WATTERS, J.K. (1987) 'A Street Based Outreach Model of AIDS Prevention for Intravenous Drug Users: Preliminary Evaluation', *Contemporary Drug Problems*, Fall, 441–423.

WAPPNER, R. (1977) *Street Ethnography*, London, Sage.

WIEBEL, W. (1988) 'Combining Ethnographic and Epidemiologic Methods in Targeted AIDS Interventions: The Chicago Model', in R. BATTJES and R. PICKENS (Eds), *Needle Sharing among Intravenous Drug Abusers: National and International Perspectives*, NIDA Research Monograph 80, Rockville.

WIEBEL, W. and ALTMAN, N. (1988) 'AIDS Prevention to IDUs in Four US Cities', paper given at the fourth international conference on AIDS, Stockholm.

Chapter 17

Misfortune, Medicine and AIDS Counselling

Anssi Peräkylä

Talking about 'problems' and 'anxieties' is a delicate business. Jefferson, (1980, 1985) and Jefferson and Lee (1981) have described in a series of studies the fine interactional dynamics that people talking about troubles engage in. To depart from a 'business as usual' assumption in favour of talking about worries or anxieties requires skilful manoeuvring on the part of both the 'troubles teller' and the 'troubles recipient'. It is hard to begin suddenly to tell our worries to other people. The teller and the potential recipient first need to give slight hints to each other about their willingness to engage in such talk; and only after proper preparations can the teller reveal his or her concerns. Even then there is the possibility of a mismatch between their expectations and activities. Talking seriously about isssues such as illness and death can be particularly difficult and delicate.

In this chapter the interactional dynamics of HIV counselling will be examined. Particular attention will be given to analyzing talk about fears for the future.

Two Patterns of Talking about the Future

Working with people coming for an HIV antibody test or those who have been diagnosed as HIV-antibody positive requires medical and paramedical professionals to deal with the individuals' fears of what may happen to them in the future. This is not restricted to formal counselling sessions only, but it is usually most explicit there. In pre-test interviews this means talking about the implications of the possibly positive test result (McCreaner, 1989; Miller and Bor, 1988); in counselling people already diagnosed as HIV antibody positive it entails addressing issues like deterioration in health, disfigurement, pain, loss, and death (George, 1989; Bor and Miller, 1988).

Bor and Miller in particular have argued in favour of addressing these 'dreaded issues' a long time before the person concerned might otherwise confront them. In doing this, the counsellor should first find out what the specific fears are, and then encourage talk about them. By so doing, they argue, counsellors can decrease the possibility of future complications should the issue actually occur. Those prepared well beforehand, for example, are less likely to cut off their relations with their support network (including the counsellors) or to develop psychiatric disorders. Practical issues too — such as decisions about future care and difficulties in preparing wills — can be attended to, provided the difficult situation has been addressed while the patient was in good health. Examining the dreaded issues in advance can help the patient to think positively and to maintain hope.

In recent work which has entailed transcribing and analyzing video and audiotapes from HIV counselling interviews in several different clinics in the UK, it has been possible to identify two different patterns of talking about the future.[1] The difference is very basic: one of the approaches involves the counsellor talking to the client, while in the other pattern the counsellor asks the client questions and the client answers them. These two models can be called the Information Delivery format and the Interview format respectively. Being based on a qualitative analysis, this chapter will focus on the internal dynamics of each of these patterns rather than offering estimates of the frequency of their occurrence.

An excerpt follows which was taken from a session in which the counsellor uses the Information Delivery format in talking about the client's future. It was taken from a pre-test interview in a clinic in the UK, and in it the counsellor presents the social services that the clinic and other organizations can offer should there be a positive result. She also refers to the feelings that the client could have if he were to have that result.

Excerpt 1[2]

Co: And (.2)   [there is
Cl: [.hhh ((coughing))
Co: a *lot of support* (.) in this department for anyone who *does* come up with a positive test result. (.8) .hhhh Pretty obviously (.) it's a great shock.
Cl: [Mmh
Co: We *think* it takes about (.) three months to come to terms with it (.6) .hhh And during that time (.2) there is (.3) a lot of support ( ) this clinic (.) in the health advisors of whom I'm one (.2) .hhh em (.3) in the clinic staff (.) who deal with ( ) the medical – (.2) requirements err when they're required. (.) hhh and we have a *support* group (.3) *outside* (.2) of the clinic...

Here the client's contribution to the exchange is extremely limited: there are only two occasions on which he can be seen to react. Things are quite different in a session where the counsellor concentrates on asking questions and the client on answering them. The following excerpt also comes from a pre-test interview and the topics covered are similar.

Excerpt 2

Co: What for you the worst thing would– (.) be (.5) knowing your
     result, (.) one way or the other,
     (1.6)

Cl: Erm
     (1.2)

Cl: Well I mean obviously (.) (if it wasn't AIDS er–) (1.8)

Co: Um

Cl: that would be *great* (.) or (.6)

Cl: but if it was *positive* I (really) don't know how (.3)

Co: Um
     (.2)

Cl: (sniff, cough) I would be able to deal with this. Er . . .

Co: Um What do you think (2) the problems would be *immediately* on
     hearing it, (.2) just (.6) out of *curiosity*?
     (3.8)

Cl: I don't *know* ( )
     (1.0)

Cl: [how it's gonna-(.8) affect my *life* or

Co: [uhum
     (.3)

Co: Ho-how do you *imagine* that *does* affect people's lives. From what
     you know.
     (4.0)

Cl: I *suppose* it (might) just make you (3.0) just be a little bit more (.4)
     aware of (.8) .hhh *dying* and (1.0) the *way* of dying, you know I
     mean (.6) how you die.
     (.3)

Co: Wh — what it is about how one dies that — (.6) that might be a
     problem, (.7)

Cl: Just becoming dependent on somebody

This interchange begins from the counsellor's general enquiry about the 'worst thing in knowing your result'. The client answers by doubting whether he would be able to cope with a positive result. The counsellor responds by asking what the problems might be were the client to learn they have a positive test result. Via a series of further questions and answers they end up talking about awareness of dying.

While it is possible to identify two dominant ways in which dreaded issues are talked about in counselling sessions, there are occasions when another communication format is used. In the pattern dominated by the Information Delivery model, talk about the future is occasionally followed by the client asking some questions, usually about medical facts or treatments related to HIV. The questions are usually invited when the counsellor offers a 'question time'. Similarly, in sessions where talk about the future is dominated by the Interview model, occasionally at the end of the sequence the counsellor may offer the client information about some relevant medical facts, and /or she or he may offer some comment on the client's way of coping.

Solving Problems of Delicacy

Given the basic differences between these two ways of talking about dreaded issues, attention will now be given to what these two approaches have in common. Aligning as speaker and recipient in the Information Delivery format or as questioner and answerer in the Interview format excludes several other forms of interaction. Most importantly, in sessions favouring either of the two formats, independent patient talk is excluded. It is extremely rare that the clients volunteer any statements without a prior invitation from the counsellor. Moreover, the questions that the clients ask of the counsellor are also quite limited in number.

In an ordinary casual conversation all participants can equally become speakers and recipients, questioners and answerers. Limits on this range of possible roles, and the concentration in Information Delivery and Interview formats, make counselling a particularly institutionalized encounter (Heritage, 1989; Heritage and Greatbatch, 1989). The institutional role of the counsellor entails confining him or herself to delivering information or asking questions, that of the client to receiving information or answering questions.

Shaping the institutional roles of a counsellor and a client in this particular way serves several functions. Clients can rely on counsellors' expertise in having a clear sense of the purpose of the encounter. The counsellor is likely to take care of the topical structure, and plays a key role in opening and closing the session. Being in control of these issues is also of vital importance to the counsellor, who may work under pressure of time and resources.

When it comes to talking about delicate human issues related to the client's future, the focus on Information Delivery or on Interview, and the respective institutional identities associated with each of these strategies, makes it possible for participants to deal with delicate topics with minimal possibility of interactional complications. A counsellor asking questions or one delivering information can relatively easily break through the barriers that surround such topics in everyday conversation. Should there be more room for independent client talk in HIV counselling, then participants would have to engage in much of the conversational manoeuvring which is more characteristic of 'troubles telling' in informal settings.

This is more obviously the case in relation to the Information Delivery format. If the counsellor does most of the talking, and the client is confined to displays of recipiency, the counsellor can, if she or he so decides, introduce delicate topics as part of the flow of the information. Indeed, on many occasions the counsellor's retreat from the Interview format into Information Delivery coincides with the introduction of 'dreaded issues'. By so doing, the counsellor minimizes dependence on the client's contribution to the introduction of the topic. Excerpt 3 provides an example.

Excerpt 3

Co: Erm (.3) do you know (.6) er Betty (.) if any of your sexual partners have been bisexual, (1.0)
Cl: No [no: I don't know
Co: [No
    (1.9)
Co: Right. (1.1) .hhh (1.0) We *have* (1.2) a few people or a nucleus of people that we *know* (.2) are carrying the HIV virus. (.2) .hhh we've found antibodies (.2) in their blood, (.4) now *most* of them are fit and well. (.6) And they look like you and me, and they're about to their normal job.

The Interview format is not as free of the possibilities of interactional difficulties emerging as the Information Delivery is. Nevertheless, as the counsellor confines him/herself to asking questions, and the client to answering them, the counsellor remains in control of the agenda. He or she is much freer to introduce or follow up delicate and sensitive issues than would be a participant in an ordinary conversation.

The general structure of an Interview-based sequence of talk about dreaded issues seems to be very simple. It consists of three parts: (1) the gloss, (2) the unpacking and (3) management. The 'gloss' refers to an open-ended and vague formulation by the client of troublesome issues. In excerpt 2 (p. 251) the gloss that the client produced was, 'if it was *positive* I really don't know how ... I would be able to deal with this.' 'Unpacking' refers to the specification of the content of the gloss: what does it mean to this particular client that, for example, he does not know how he would be able to deal with a positive result? Like the delivery of the gloss, the unpacking is achieved through a series of questions and answers between counsellor and client. The third stage, 'management' refers to questions and answers, and sometimes also the counsellor's talk to the client, through which participants seek to identify remedies for the glossed and unpacked fear(s). In so doing, they can talk about clinical services, patient support networks and so on.

Anssi Perakyla

Even though the Interview format allocates much of the topical control to the counsellor, proceeding through the various stages involved in talking about dreaded issues entails a considerable amount of negotiation between client and counsellor. To achieve a gloss of a fear, to unpack that gloss, and to outline ways in which fearful future possibilities can be managed — all these activities require the active contribution of both the client and the counsellor, and all the professional skills of the counsellor are often needed to facilitate this.

Excerpt 4 offers a glimpse of key features of these dynamics. It is taken from a session involving an HIV antibody positive man (Cl), his wife, (ClW), a counsellor (Co) and a doctor.

Excerpt 4

Co: Can I ask you what are your greatest *concerns* (.) Liz.
Cl: [Liza
Co: [Liza I can't get it [( )
ClW: [((coughing))
Co: Liza about- .hh (.4) at *this moment* in time (.) Can you say aloud.
        (3.0)
ClW: Erm ... the *uncertain*[ty?
Co: [Mmh
        (1.5)
ClW: Obviously (.6) and (3.0) trying to get John to *cope* with it (.2) and
        — (.3) lead as normal a life as possible? (.) I don't see . hhh (1.0) I
        don't really see any feasible realistic alternative.
Co: Mmh
        (.5)
ClW: than (.) (both) to *carry* on (.3) as (.) as nor[mal.
Co: [mmh   [mmh
        (.5)
Baby: gjuu
ClW: And (1.6) what would happen to me?
Co: mmh
ClW: and the *children* (2.1) if he did devel[op
Co: [mmh
ClW: something?
        (.2)
Co: What's your greatest *fear* about that?
        (1.8)
Co: ([ ) (.2) ( )
ClW: [T:here *isn't* anything (.2) *specific* (.) I mean it's just a
        general abstract

254

Co: I mean would you have any *more* worries than you've got now?
       (.4) When he's *antibody positive*?
       (.6)
Co: (Is he) *what* would you *know* about .hh (.2) looking after people
       with AIDS,
ClW: (Well) I *don't*?
Co: (Well) what (.3) do you kno[w ( )
ClW: [I haven't even   [I haven't even
       I haven't even *thought* that far
Co: Um
ClW: Because I feel that (.2) .hhhhh (1.0)
Co: Would you see [(there) ( )
ClW: [( ) ENOUGH
       TO WORRY ABOUT (I'm calm enough to worry abo[ut that
Co: [BUT
       I THINK AS YOU'VE RAI[SED-
?:   [OOH
ClW: something [*should* happen . .
Co: [Liza
Co: As you've raised it (.) I mean, *would* there're any more-(.5) *risks*
       attached (.) for you and the children than there are now
       (.3)
Co: I'm not talking about
ClW: Well—
       (.4)
Co: *future* risks and (.) (.4) *life* ( )
ClW: What you mean risks? You mean (in an-) =
Co: = (well) (.4) yes
ClW: Infection [and that sort of [thing,
Co: [*yes*
ClW: Erm
       (2.6)
ClW: *Not* (.3) that I'm aware of
Co: Yes. Would you confirm that? (.2) Dr. A?

At the beginning of this excerpt there is a general enquiry by the counsellor about the client's wife's 'greatest concerns'. She responds to this by producing a gloss, 'the uncertainty'. Thereafter there is a lengthy section where the counsellor says little, and in response the client's wife raises several issues that unpack, or develop upon, the initial gloss. The counsellor's silence here is very significant. She withholds her response, and an opportunity is provided for the client to engage in discussion of more delicate issues. The existence of these was implied in the initial gloss, 'uncertainty', and both participants seem to orient to the possibility of expanding upon them. As a result, and at the end of the unpacking sequence, the client's wife reveals her concern: 'what would happen to me ... and the children ... if he did develop something.'

So far in this interchange the participants have progressed in broad consensus. But when the counsellor asks another question aimed at further unpacking ('What's your greatest fear about that?'), there is some reluctance to proceed. Instead, the client's wife responds, 'there isn't anything specific ... it's just a general abstract.' There follows a series of questions and answers, all of which are equally unsuccessful in unpacking more of the client's wife's concerns.

We can see analytically in this series of questions and answers the extraordinary power of a question in general and of the professional question in particular. The client's wife does not just refuse to answer, she produces accounts for not being able to answer. She does not know about looking after people with AIDS, she has not thought that far, she has got enough to worry about already. By producing these accounts, she complies to the set of institutional roles where the counsellor is the questioner and the client the answerer. Nevertheless, unpacking the worry goes no further.

Towards the end of the excerpt a fresh start is made when the counsellor offers a formulation of the ongoing talk and thereafter moves into 'management' issues. This move into 'management' was anticipated earlier when the counsellor asked the client's wife about her knowledge of looking after people with AIDS. The formulation of the conversation is one of the devices that counsellors regularly use in facilitating clients' talk. By describing key issues in the preceding talk, a formulation shows that the counsellor has been attending to the difficulties that the client has had in producing answers to previous questions and simultaneously keeps the line of questioning going. Here the formulation is a very simple one: 'As you have raised it.' It conveys that even though issues may be difficult to talk about, they nevertheless are something that the client's wife *herself* raised. The formulation here, as do such formulations in general, serves a double function. It shows that the counsellor is sensitive to the client's point of view; and simultaneously, it maintains the sequence of questions and answers.

The fresh start signalled here is, indeed, a successful one. After some searching for a response, the client's wife ends up by answering the counsellor's question: as far as she knows, she and the children would face no greater risks even were her husband to develop AIDS. The exchange is closed when the counsellor gives the floor to the doctor present who then offers her specialist view about the risks.

In summary, in this fourth excerpt the conversational movement is from a general, open-ended concern with 'uncertainty' to a concern about what would happen to the client's wife and the children if the client did develop 'something'. After sharing this concern, they ended up by estimating the risks attached to them if the 'dreadful' situation occurred. This movement entailed phases of consensus and phases when the counsellor used her professional authority to facilitate more talk.

Concerning both Interview and Information Delivery formats, the conclusion is that professional counselling practice seems to run counter to certain common-sense assumptions. One might expect that good counselling on 'delicate' topics is very informal, like a conversation between good friends. However, the opposite is true: by confining themselves to their institutional roles, both clients and counsellors contribute to the *formal* character of these encounters. This very formality is a central resource in the management of delicacy.

From the point of view of counselling practice, what is important here is that talk about dreaded issues (at least in the interview format) seems to entail a considerable deal of persuasion. It requires not only empathetic understanding, but also the consistent use of professionally authorized questions and other conversational devices like formulations which create an expectation for the client to produce more talk.[3]

Misfortune, Medicine and Language

Michel Foucault once described the development of modern medicine as expansion of the scope of language. The workings of a human body were exposed first to a medical gaze, and thereafter to accompanying speech. As modern medicine has evolved, it has become possible to talk about the body in ways that were not available before. Of course, exposing the body to speech has only been possible in the context of the social institutions and practices of the clinic. Medicine entailed an expansion of the scope of the language: To discover, was 'to push a little farther back the foamy line of language' (Foucault, 1976).

It is tempting to view those aspects of HIV/AIDS counselling that have been described in this chapter from an analogous position. To counsel people seems also to entail pushing the foamy line of language a little further back: not to the workings and organs of the human body, but to the experience of misfortune. Here too, as in the times when medical language expanded into the sphere of the body, the participants act within an institutional context, with their conversational activities trading off and maintaining their institutional roles as professionals and clients.

HIV/AIDS counselling is part of a wide ranging enterprise that began earlier than the present epidemic. As studies by Armstrong (1983), Arney and Bergen (1984) and, most recently, Lindsay Prior (1989) have convincingly shown, in the last few decades the medical discourses of death and dying have shifted their focus from the body to that of experience. The *meaning* of death has become just as important a theme as the *causes* of death in talk about the end of human life.

Accordingly, in clinical practice the dying man or women has been given more opportunity to speak out about his or her experiences to psychologically trained health professionals. Important literary milestones in the evolution of this approach have been the studies by Gorer (1955), Kubler-Ross (1970), Aries (1982) and Elias (1985).

HIV/AIDS counselling is a new arena for this rapidly expanding institutionalized practice (Chester, 1987; Silverman, 1990). Even though the motivation to set up centres for HIV/AIDS counselling has in many cases been linked to efforts to limit the sexual transmission of HIV, these practices have simultaneously created an unforeseen institutionalized sphere for talking about the experiences of illness, death and dying. This is one of the most important, but perhaps less well understood, social consequences — perhaps an unintended one — of the AIDS epidemic.

Acknowledgments

I am grateful to David Silverman (University of London Goldsmith's College) for help and support in analyzing the data. I wish to thank Riva Miller and Eleanor Golman (Royal Free Hospital Haemophilia Centre) and Robert Bor and Heather Salt (Royal Free Hospital District AIDS Unit), whose counselling practice and theoretical work have provided me with a frame of reference for studying the discussions about hypothetical future situations in HIV counselling.

Notes

1 The research project 'Counselling and AIDS' at University of London Goldsmith's College is funded by Health Education Authority and Glaxo Holdings plc and is led by Professor David Silverman. The data that led to these findings are video and audio recordings from over fifty HIV counselling sessions (both pre-test and with people carrying the virus) taped in seven clinics in the UK and two in the USA.

2 All the transcripts presented in this chapter are somewhat simplified from their original form. The simplifications have been restricted to the non-lexical aspects of talk, like intonation and prolongation of sounds. The transcription symbols are presented in Appendix A.

3 Using the professionally authorized questions as a resource as much as in the excerpts above is probably related to the fact that in HIV counselling regular meetings between counsellor and client are not the rule. If the participants spent more time together, the form of the interaction would probably be different.

References

ARIES, P. (1982) *The Hour of Our Death*, New York, Vintage Books.
ARMSTRONG, D. (1983) *The Political Anatomy of the Body*, Cambridge, Cambridge University Press.

ARNEY, W. and BERGEN, B. (1984) *Medicine and the Management of Living*, Chicago, Ill., Chicago University Press.

BOR, R. and MILLER, R. (1988) 'Addressing 'Dreaded Issues': A Description of a Unique Counselling Intervention with Patients with AIDS/HIV', *Counselling Psychology Quarterly* 1,397–405.

CHESTER, R. (1987) *Advice, Support and Counselling for the HIV Positive*, report for the DHSS, University of Hull.

CREANER, A. (1989) 'Pre-test Counselling', in J. GREEN and A McCREANER (Eds), *Counselling with HIV Infection and AIDS*, Oxford, Blackwell Scientific Publications.

ELIAS, N. (1989) *The Loneliness of the Dying*, Oxford, Basil Blackwell.

FOUCAULT, M. (1976) *The Birth of the Clinic*, London, Tavistock.

GEORGE, H. (1989) 'Counselling People with AIDS, Their Lovers, Friends and Relations', in J. Green and A. McCreaner (Eds), *Counselling with HIV-Infection and AIDS*, Oxford, Blackwell Scientific Publications.

GORER, G. (1955) 'The Pornography of Death', *Encounter*, 5, 40–53.

HERITAGE, J. (1989) 'Current Developments in Conversation Analysis', in D. ROGER and P. BULL (Eds), *Conversation: An Interdisciplinary Perspective*, Clevedon, Multilingual Matters.

HERITAGE, J. and GREATBATCH, D. (1989) 'On the Institutional Character of Institutional Talk: The Case of News Interviews', in P.A. FORSTORP (Ed.), *Discourse in Professional and Everyday Culture*, Studies in Communication, SIC 28, University of Linkoping.

JEFFERSON, G. (1980) *Final Report to the SSRC on the Analysis of Conversations in Which 'Troubles' and 'Anxieties' Are Expressed*, No. HR 4805.

JEFFERSON, G. (1985) 'On the Interactional Unpacking of a Gloss', *Language in Society*, 14, 435–466.

JEFFERSON, G. and LEE, J.R.E. (1981) 'The Rejection of Advice: Managing the Problematic Convergence of a 'Troubles Telling', and a 'Service Encounter', *Journal of Pragmatics*, 5, 339–422.

KUBLER-ROSS, E. (1970) *On Death and Dying*, London, Tavistock.

MILLER, R. and BOR, R. (1988) *AIDS: A Guide to Clinical Counselling*, London, Science Press.

PRIOR, L. (1989) *The Social Organisation of Death: Medical Discourse and Social Practices in Belfast*, London, Macmillan.

SILVERMAN, D. (1990) 'The Social Organisation of HIV Counselling', in P. AGGLETON, P. DAVIES and G. HART (Eds), *AIDS: Individual, Cultural and Policy Dimensions*, Lewes, Falmer Press.

Appendix A: The Transcription Symbols

[	Co: quite a [while Cl: [yea	Left brackets indicate the point at which a current speaker's talk is overlapped by another's talk.
(.4)	Yes (.2) Yeah	Numbers in parenthesis indicated elapsed time in silence in tenths of a second.
(.)	to get (.) treatment	A dot in parentheses indicates a tiny gap, probably no more than one-tenth of a second.

——	What's *up*?	Underscoring indicates some form of stress, via pitch and/or amplitude.
WORD	I've got ENOUGH TO WORRY ABOUT	Capitals, except at the beginnings of lines, indicate especially loud sounds relative to the surrounding talk.
.hhhh	I feel that (.2) .hhh	A row of h's prefixed by a dot indicates an inbreath; without a dot, an outbreath. The length of the row of h's indicates the length of the in- or outbreath.
( )	future risks and ( ) and life ( )	Empty parentheses indicate the transcriber's inability to hear what was said.
(word)	Would you see (there) anything positive	Parenthesized words are possible hearings.
(( ))	confirm that ((continues))	Double parentheses contain author's descriptions rather than transcriptions.

Chapter 18

Care: What's in It for Her?

Sheila Henderson

This chapter reports some of the findings of the Institute for the Study of Drug Dependence (ISDD)'s HIV Carer's Project, a short programme of qualitative research funded by the Department of Health and conducted by ISDD and subcontracted researchers between February and June 1989. The project set out to gain a wide perspective on care issues in relation to HIV and AIDS, including the drug dimension. However, since coverage of HIV/AIDS issues gave women a low profile at the time, while a sharp increase in numbers of women becoming infected was predicted, particular emphasis was given to the experiences and needs of women. One hundred and ninety-nine respondents participated either through ten semi-structured interviews or twenty-seven group discussions in seventeen sites (mainly in Britain but also in Ireland and Italy). Included were 'general population' groups, HIV seropositive people, their friends and family, and generic and specialist workers in the voluntary and statutory sectors with drug and/or HIV-related experience. Areas of focus within the research as a whole included the attitudes, needs and/or experiences of HIV seropositive people, of lay and professional carers, of general population and generic professional samples with little or no personal or professional contact with HIV, of 'unanticipated' and of committed HIV/AIDS carers. The differences/similarities between caring for/being someone with life-threatening illness were also explored (Dorn, Henderson and South, forthcoming). The following is an overview of aspects of the research which focused on the prevailing perceptions of women in relation to HIV among general population groups, the experiences and needs of HIV seropositive women and the gender-specific needs of carers.

A brief and predominantly empirical piece of work, the research raised more questions than it answered. The process of conducting the initial research made it clear that a high level of demand for information and discussion existed in the area of women and HIV — a demand which had become more acute, but little nearer to being met, a year later when the research findings were fed back in a number of locations nationally. Hence what follows lends important insight into issues and experiences but also begs a number of questions: Where *are* the in-depth, quantitative and qualitative studies of service development for women in relation to HIV? What *are* the regional, local and gender-specific needs in relation to HIV today, and how can they best be prioritized in policy terms? How can relevant support systems for carers attentive to the dynamics of gender be developed? Why *are* the discussions and analyses on women and HIV which draw upon the wealthy tradition of feminist theory so little in evidence at the time of writing? It is to be hoped that the focus of World AIDS Day in 1990 on women will have galvanized a number of initiatives on these and other counts by the time this book is available.

The Context

It is important that the findings reported here are read with some awareness of public priorities and images in relation to HIV at the time and subsequent shifts. The research took place in a context in which the government anticipated an increase in HIV infection — much of it drug-related — and a corresponding lack of experience and training among HIV/AIDS services in dealing with drug injectors. September 1988 had seen the announcement of a £3 million government allocation to health authorities with the express purpose of preventing the spread of HIV among injecting drug users. The second part of a report by the Advisory Council on the Misuse of Drugs (1989), published during the research period, made recommendations premised on its earlier conclusion that HIV outflanked the injection of illicit drugs as the number one danger to individual and public health. A somewhat different climate prevails in mid-1990, with HIV slipping down the public agenda under the weight of varying claims from Lord Kilbracken[1] to Ann Leslie[2] and Michael Fumento[3] about the 'myth of heterosexual AIDS'. Meanwhile, drugs have made a comeback as number one public health threat via Britain's role in the international 'war on drugs'. Walk down the street, take a bus or tube and it is the horrors of drug taking, not HIV, which will, on an initial siting at least, catch the eye and interest. Moreover, the language of drugs circulating with most currency in the corridors of power has been one of 'demand reduction' rather than 'harm minimization'.

It is also worth bearing in mind the limitation of public images of women in relation to HIV at the time. Those in circulation traded in a currency of women as sexual threat to men, as opposed to informing women of the risks they faced — a discourse with a long historical tradition most graphically illustrated by First World War notions of 'the amateur prostitute'. Pinpointed in the context of fears for the national health aroused by the prevalence of venereal disease among the military, such so-called 'sexual freelancers' (Bland and Mort, 1983; Bland, 1985) were drawn from all social classes, took no sexual precautions and, what is more, gave sex for *free*. The lines of acceptable and deviant female behaviour were redrawn across similar lines in an early TV campaign, for example, which focused upon a woman in low-cut blouse and black stockings in a late night domestic scene. 'It is quite late, can you stay?' she asks her male guest. Here, like the 'amateur prostitute', the sexually active woman spells danger to men. 'Nice girls *don't*' is the familiar moral echo.

Again, however, that seems to be changing with the advent of advertizing like the example from early 1990 shown in Figure 18.1. Here — admittedly in the familiar context of recruiting young women to the task of taking responsibility for the outcomes of penetrative heterosexual sex — women are addressed, in a new departure, as sexually active *without* social sanction. Active and non-reproductive sex, albeit a limited version of the range of sexual options open to women, is represented as normal and socially affirmed. The technique of fear arousal, so familiar in the context of health education campaigns, is tempered by an attempt to reassure and comfort.

The Preconditions of Care: Perceptions of Women in Relation to HIV

A section of the research, which included 'general population' groups, was conducted for us by NOP Research Ltd. Attitudes to HIV were generally negative among these groups. There was still very much a sense of it only happening to someone else, with HIV strongly associated with homosexuality, drug use to a lesser degree and with both homosexuality and drug use seen as outside the experience of so-called ordinary people. There was a strong tendency towards 'just deserts'/'innocent victim' models. HIV still had a predominantly white male image, with race serving as a 'glue' binding together perceptions of social deviance. In the words of one white male respondent: 'Call me racist or otherwise ... there's more homosexuals and drug injectors amongst black people than amongst others.'

General population groups considered the whole concept of the HIV sero-positive woman to be a hypothetical, or at most, futuristic case. When pressed to imagine a close female friend or relative confiding their HIV seropositive status, they accommodated the situation only by assuming the woman to have become infected (in their terms) 'innocently' (i.e. through blood products), while at the same time clearly holding an image of HIV seropositive women, if they existed in reality, as prostitutes or drug users. One woman encapsulated this tension between conflicting images by describing her predicted response as: 'hoping for the best but fearing the worst.' Perhaps not unsurprisingly, however, the predominant language of predicted responses to a friend/relative disclosing their HIV status was one of 'love conquers all' fear and prejudice. How this precarious combination of dedication, fear of ascribed deviance and longing for 'innocence' would shape up in

Figure 18.1 Sex Feels Better When You're Using a Condom

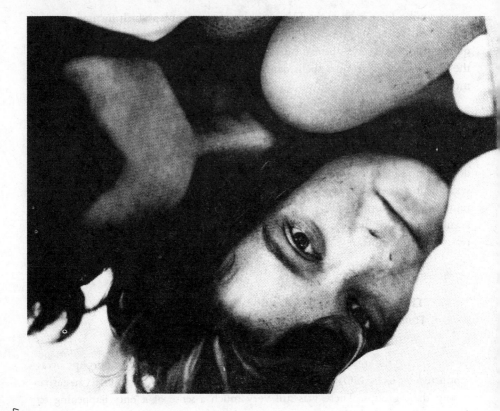

SEX FEELS BETTER
WHEN YOU'RE USING A CONDOM.

You had sex last night.

It was a wonderful experience.

He didn't bother with the condom. He said it would ruin the mood and you were on the pill anyway.

So how do you feel this morning?

Perhaps a little worried?

Well here's something to think about.

In Britain the number of people with AIDS is still on the increase.

And for every person with AIDS, we estimate there are thirty with HIV.

Human Immunodeficiency Virus is the virus which leads to AIDS.

Someone can have it for several years and still look and feel perfectly healthy.

But through unprotected sex, they can pass the virus on to you.

If you choose to have sex (and remember it is your choice) a condom can help protect you.

Let's start again.

You had sex last night.

It was a wonderful experience.

You used a condom. You'd talked about it beforehand and both agreed it was the right thing to do.

Now how do you feel this morning?

What a stupid question.

AIDS. YOU'RE AS SAFE AS YOU WANT TO BE.

FOR MORE INFORMATION OR CONFIDENTIAL ADVICE ABOUT AIDS, FREEPHONE THE 24-HOUR NATIONAL AIDS HELPLINE ON 0800 567 123.

a given real situation is currently left largely to private experience and anecdotal evidence.

The view was generally expressed that women do not constitute a 'special case' in the context of being cared for, except in relation to their reproductive and child-care roles. This stated gender 'equality' was, however, contradicted by other observations. For instance, women predicted that their sex would make better AIDS patients — on the assumption that they are 'harder' and more willing to share with others than their male counterparts (who were, in turn, considered 'soft' with a tendency to 'bottle up'). There was also wide consensus that women were the most likely to take up the caring role within the domestic context, with men providing practical backup in the form of transport and errands.

Much attention was given to the question of knowing the source of transmission: women's concern for the infected woman was in terms of her needing to know in order to deal with her feelings, while men's concern was expressed more in relation to fears for their own status. They also made an interesting distinction between appropriate responses to a woman with whom they had a sexual relationship and one with whom the relationship was non-sexual. In the former context it was assumed (with only one exception) that the woman had become infected outside the relationship. For instance, one man said he would 'have no time' for his wife if she was HIV seropositive, but if it was his daughter, he'd 'give her a big kiss'.

The picture sketched here is composed of the predicted responses of people to a given situation. The limitations of the concept 'general population' should also be recognized, shrouding as it does the existence of specific social constituencies. As such, it can only hint at the underlying attitudes to suggest popular concepts of HIV, women and care which provide the general context in which women have experienced becoming infected with the virus, have (or have not, as the case may be) been cared for or, indeed, have become involved in caring roles in the face of HIV. It does, however, give some foundation to the worst fears of those wishing to change negative public attitudes to HIV that the need for their work, at least in the first half of 1989, was still great.

Women's Experiences of Services

In relation to gender-related problems reported by women living with the virus, it was felt that the major impetus behind public service development for women to date has been a concern over the spread of HIV infection via reproduction. Public concern has focused upon women's reproductive role rather than the overall health of individual women. Reported exceptions to this included voluntary organizations formed in response to the challenge of HIV. Some had sought or were seeking to extend their support services to women at the time of the research, but women reported problems with services which had originally been developed for gay men and still maintained that image — with the consequence of a low service uptake among women.

The strong and underlying perceptions distinguishing between 'nice' and 'bad girls' which were prevalent among general population groups also ran through responses experienced by women with the virus. It was common, for example, for infected women to elicit responses which involved an assumption that they were promiscuous and/or in some way socially deviant, no matter what their lifestyle. Women who injected drugs, had done so in the past or had a drug injecting partner, felt particularly affected by the negative end of care responses. They referred to a triple layer of social stigma confronting them: first, the images of sexual deviance which cling to the whole topic of AIDS; second, the association of deviance and self-infliction with injecting drug use. Finally, the departure from socially prescribed behaviour worthy of the 'good woman', which some connection with the previous two factors still apparently signifies to large sections of society clearly untouched by over two decades of the 'new' women's movement. These dimensions of social stigma were reflected in the experience of women infected through drug use in that they expressed a greater sense of shame (particularly where prostitution had played a part in funding drug use), taking the blame upon themselves.[4]

Women reported the more customary refusal of treatment to HIV sero-positive people by dentists and GPs, but more gender-specific responses revolved around their reproductive role or very particular notions of 'normal' female sexuality. For instance, some so-called post-test counselling sessions were comprised of being advised to 'ask God's forgiveness for being so wicked' (that is, for having five sexual partners in two years) or of being informed of the test result by means of a request to 'promise me you won't get pregnant in the next six months before I see you again.'

Family planning services provided another service area where women were denied proper treatment. For example, one woman was having seriously painful problems related to her coil but was refused treatment upon informing staff of her HIV status. Pregnancy met with pressure from services on the woman to terminate — with little or no support upon which to make an informed decision. Motherhood, in opening women up to contact with a wider range of services, also increased the possibilities for negative responses. Stories of 'space suit' treatment during childbirth, physical isolation and acute 'hazard' treatment after the birth and further conspicuous maltreatment by health care staff in the domestic context (e.g. 'gowning-up' in the street prior to a home visit) were common.[5] Contact with public services through older children was also cause for concern, as the following example demonstrates. This respondent had just moved into a new area and her children had started a new school.

When the children had to start school I had to take them for a medical. The doctor said to me, 'Is there anything in the family?' and I had to say ... she asked the children to go out and asked me all these questions and one of them was what happens to my waste products ... and I thought what does she mean and I said, 'I go to the toilet' and I thought what the hell does she mean. She said, 'What about your periods?' and I said, 'Well I haven't had them for a long while but I flush them away.' She said '... Because we could arrange to collect them' and it came into my head a man walking down the path like ET ... and I thought how ignorant. I said to her afterwards she was totally out of order.

It is difficult to gauge the present extent and exact quality of both specific HIV service provision for women and responses to HIV within the range of generic health and other services of which women are directly or indirectly consumers, since little of the available information has currently been collated and circulated.[6]

Women's Care Needs

A recent paper on proactive media work on HIV referred to the concept of 'customer delight' which has currently superseded the concept of 'customer satisfaction' in the business education world on the ground that 'customer satisfaction' accepts a norm of customer *dis*satisfaction (Kay and Stewart, 1990). This admirable shift in goals could usefully be employed in the context of much health service development and accurately describes the ideals of many potential consumers. The emphasis among respondents in this study was certainly upon building care for women around a positive perspective, but widespread customer *dis*satisfaction and a precarious combination of optimism and pessimism had tempered aspirations somewhat.

High on the agenda was giving women quality services and information in order to give them real choice, as was the development of flexible, consumer-led and accessible services in the community available on one site, thus reducing the number of mainly statutory services which women, particularly from low socio-economic groups have to deal with. However, pessimism accompanied some such suggestions as major blocks to the process were referenced: the conclusion that HIV exacerbates existing problems for women in society — such as their economic, sexual and emotional dependence upon men and their greater dependence upon public services; the present underresourced and precarious state of health and welfare services in general and the predominance of men as consumers *and* providers of services.

On the brighter side, it was felt that, although women lacked a readily identifiable economic base outside the state system upon which to draw in meeting their needs around HIV, they had a long tradition of collective action and support networks. This seemed strangely contradicted by the low incidence of self-help groups for women and the seeming failure of some of the groups to survive. While HIV seropositive, but asymptomatic, some women were able to draw upon their informal networks and 'self-service' (as one respondent put it), but there was widespread reporting of women living in isolation. The coordination of multiple social roles, which results in women 'putting themselves last', together with the high level of social stigma attached to HIV were both suggested as major obstacles to women seeking help and as essential considerations for service development.

Other obstacles to either self-help or good quality services included: (1) the lack of accurate and simple information on how HIV affects women — what to expect in terms of symptomology, the risks to the unborn and existing children, where to get support; (2) lack of support in living positively with the virus — learning to make personal priorities, changing lifestyle to increase personal control, gaining access to holistic health care and having positive and public role models as a resource; (3) lack of assistance with child-care, particularly assistance which did not carry with it the fear of having children removed. Motherhood also spelt worry over the future of children in terms of the mother or child becoming seriously ill or dying. In this particular context it was felt that the need for respite and residential care for mothers with children was acute but provision virtually non-existent. With a view to death, fostering systems which make the transition of the child from one family to another as untraumatic as possible for all concerned were required.

The uptake of HIV issues in family planning clinics, Well Woman clinics and women's health centres was felt to be low but highly necessary, as were women-only services at drug agencies. Women who were, or had previously been, drug injectors and were HIV seropositive reported a lower level of attention from services than male partners, especially in cases where their partner's HIV status was confirmed before their own. Relief upon confirmation of a positive status was expressed in this context.

The subject of safer sex was cause for both optimism and pessimism. More positively, it was felt, HIV could open up the space for women to pursue the sex they have traditionally preferred (i.e. non-penetrative sex). The down side posed questions as to how to support women who clearly had little or no chance of negotiating even the use of a condom. There were, for example, reports of HIV antibody positive women experiencing physical violence in the attempt to negotiate safer sex with male partners, or of women whose internalization of messages of female self-sacrifice rooted in models of love and romance was so fundamentally fixed as to position risking HIV infection as the ultimate form of demonstrating love (see Holland *et al.*, 1990, and Ch. 9, this volume).

Needs of Carers

High on the agenda for all respondents involved in different dimensions of care was the need to change prevailing negative attitudes to HIV. It was predicted that this would be a major source of support to them and remove a considerable amount of stress. Some admitted the need to overcome their own fears and prejudices, to practise what they preached on matters of lifestyle and to overcome a tendency to take over the life of, or idealize, the person cared for. Concern was expressed over both the motivation for some becoming involved in the HIV field — possibly as a way of dealing with their own pain — and over questions of an AIDS hierarchy — where empire building and holier-than-thou attitudes can undermine the quality of services.

The establishment of informal and formal systems of support for people involved in all dimensions of care was seen as essential (for both carer and quality of service), as was learning how to say no and to take a rest. But, whereas some progress had been made with informal networks, formal systems of support, such as non-managerial supervision, still largely awaited translation into reality, appearing as yet another overwhelming DIY task awaiting already overstretched workers. Pessimism was often compounded by the generally uncoordinated, haphazard state of much service development and recruitment which opened the way, it was felt, to lack of commitment. Family members and friends of people with HIV had low expectations of getting outside help, often preferring to 'keep it in the family'. At the same time they admitted that the need for emotional support outside the relationship with the person cared for was great but felt there was little scope for this in terms of service provision or even self-help. Partners and friends, who were themselves HIV seropositive, emphasized the difficulties experienced in the context of informal caring in the hospital setting, where possible future health scenarios for themselves were graphically visually described.

By no means all respondents felt that gender was significant in dimensions of care, other than those directly related to reproduction and/or childcare. However, a frequently recurring theme was the relationship between women's wider social positions and identities and the dynamics of both caring and being cared for.[7] All respondents felt that being involved with women made them aware of the generally low level of support available to women. Inability to give, with any confidence, basic information and advice on topics such as HIV symptomology as it relates to women, the precise risks of sexual practices and pregnancy, and on local support services, were cause for frustration for many. Some workers in HIV-specific organizations also expressed initial, at least, adverse reactions to their first contact with women with the virus. Men and women alike had become involved through a commitment to caring for gay men and were not eager to adjust. Women were particularly affected in that it graphically illustrated that it could actually happen to them.

The gender aspects of caring roles in general, and in relation to HIV in particular, had their loudest voice among paid workers — especially in Edinburgh, where a crisis situation combined with significant numbers of women involved in different dimensions of care has put 'caring for carers' issues high on the agenda. In this context women as copers, managing their multiple roles efficiently, together with women as compassionate carers were the two major themes. Respondents not only recognized them as a major source of identity to large numbers of, if not the majority of, women and certainly themselves, but also as a source of hindrance to getting much needed support in their work. Because of their internalized gender identities as copers and carers, and also because of codes of professionalism in the workplace, they felt they had more difficulty in approaching often male bosses to establish formal support systems. In seeking support outside successful and overtaxed informal systems, the experience of not coping as a woman and a professional had first to be faced. Equally, learning how to say no and admit the need for a break were seen to cut across the feminine grain. 'Granny burnout', usually mentioned in the context of New York, was a depressing phenomenon reported in Scotland with self-evident gender overtones.

Conclusions

The research reported here highlights a number of gender-specific issues and experiences arising in the context of HIV and dimensions of care in early 1989. In roughly sketching the general ideological landscape within which women infected and affected by the virus find themselves (both domestically and within health and social welfare services), it touches upon issues — such as sex and sexuality, domestic roles, access to services — which have long been on the feminist agenda and to which the advent of HIV has lent both a new dimension and a potential for further challenge. Recently, there has been great improvement in some specialist services, as well as a growth in HIV posts with some remit for women, conferences and meetings on the topic and loose networks of women concerned about women and HIV/AIDS issues. However, officially reported numbers of women in this country are growing, and unofficial reports of the poor quality of support and care they receive are still in abundance. The basic issues would appear unchanged (so much evidence remains, however, at the anecdotal level) not only for women with the virus but also for those in 'hidden' caring roles. As for women working in the HIV context with a more public face, a question asked of them nationwide in 1989 speaks volumes: 'What's a nice girl like you doing in a job like this?'

Acknowledgments

Thanks to all who made the research possible: to all the women and men who participated; to the Department of Health AIDS Unit, which provided the funding; to Nigel South and Nicholas Dorn, who initiated and worked on the project; to Karim Murji for his comments; and to all in the Scottish and London Women and HIV/AIDS Networks. I am also grateful to all those who organized and/or conducted group discussions in Britain, Ireland and Italy in early 1989: Joy Awiah, Andrew Bennett, Shane Butler and Marguerite Woods, Malcolm Colledge and Sandy Maddison, Amadeo Cottino, Isobel Freeman/Moira Paton and Avril Taylor, Sarah Jones and Robert Power, Jane McLoughlin, Valerie Morrison, National Opinion Poll Market Research Limited, Kamlesh Patel. Most of this work is more fully reported in Dorn, Henderson and South (forthcoming).

Notes

1 In November 1989 *The Sun* with its usual vigour picked up on the latest wave of attempts to sway the official line on HIV and AIDS away from the notion that it affects us all and sweep it to the margins. The headline on 18 November 1989 was typical of the rekindled media coverage: 'AIDS — The Hoax of the Century'. These headlines were sparked off by words, attributed to Lord Kilbracken (a member of the All Party Parliamentary Group on AIDS and whose previous eccentric campaigns without the HIV ingredient had gone unnoticed), to the effect that 'straight sex cannot give you AIDS.' The precise substance of his words was later debated but was in the end immaterial since they were utilized to insinuate that previous campaigns against the spread of 'heterosexual AIDS' had been nothing other than a phoney war.

2 In *The Daily Mail*, 18 November 1989, Ann Leslie bewailed the waste of public money spent on informing heterosexuals they were at risk for AIDS, suggesting that a 'Lightning Doesn't Discriminate' campaign would have been more cost-effective.

3 Coverage of his book, *The Myth of Heterosexual AIDS* (1990, Basic Books), particularly in *The Sunday Times*, has kept public messages on the subject of 'heterosexual AIDS' very mixed, despite the eventual screening of a Health Education Authority TV campaign postponed in November 1989 and some revived AIDS coverage in popular magazines (e.g. *Take a Break*, 5 May 1990; *Hello!* 28 April 1990; *Cosmopolitan*, 19 May 1990; *Company*, May 1990).

4 For an eloquent account of the dynamics of socially affirmed and socially sanctioned forms of dependency as they relate to women drug users in the context of HIV, see Roulston (1988).

5 Although there has been great improvement in some major hospitals at the time of writing, Positively Women, the support organization for HIV positive women, was still reporting fresh cases of such treatment in local hospitals in London in May 1990.

6 *Rights and Humanity* (1989) A Survey of British Women's Organizations with AIDS Programmes in Britain and Overseas, prepared for the Global Programme on AIDS, WHO, Geneva, was the only completed survey of service provision for women in relation to HIV in this country known to the author at the time of writing beyond the *National AIDS Manual* and local leaflets. Those in process include *Women, Drugs and Alcohol: A National Survey of Service Provision*, conducted by DAWN (Drugs, Alcohol, Women, Now) and funded by the Department of Health (this includes an HIV section),

and a survey of service provision in the south-east, conducted by the Women and HIV/AIDS Network Information Project.

7 Although raised in the context of the everyday and general discussion, analyses which draw upon feminist debates over the gender dynamics of caring and wider social relations have still to be widely pursued in the public arena. (For an exception to this, see Wilson, 1989).

References

ADVISORY COUNCIL ON THE MISUSE OF DRUGS (1988) *AIDS and Drug Misuse Part One*, London, HMSO.

ADVISORY COUNCIL ON THE MISUSE OF DRUGS (1989) *AIDS and Drug Misuse Part Two*, London, HMSO.

BLAND, L. (1985) 'Guardians of the Race or Vampires on the Nation's Health? Female Sexuality and Its Regulation in Early C20 Britain', in Whitelegg *et al.* (Eds), *The Changing Experience of Women*, Oxford, Blackwell.

BLAND, L. and MORT, F. (1983) *Look Out for the Good Time Girl*, Formation of Nation and People, London, Routledge and Kegan Paul.

BOR, R. (1989) 'AIDS and the Family', paper presented to the Fifth International Conference on AIDS, Montreal, Canada.

CORBY, N. (1989) 'Needs of Family Caregivers of Persons with AIDS', paper presented to the Fifth International Conference on AIDS, Montreal, Canada.

DORN, N. HENDERSON, S. and SOUTH N. (Eds) (forthcoming) *AIDS: Women, Drugs and Social Care*, Lewes, Falmer Press.

HOLLAND J., RAMAZANOGLU, C. and SCOTT, S. (1990) 'Managing Risk and Experiencing Danger: Tensions between Government AIDS Education Policy and Young Women's Sexuality', *Gender and Education*, 2, 2, 125–146.

KAY, J. and STEWART, S. (1990) 'Don't Just Sit There — Do Something: Proactive Media Work around HIV and AIDS', paper presented at the First International Conference on the Reduction of Drug-related Harm, April.

McCANN, K. (1990) 'Informal Care of People with HIV Infection', paper presented at the Fourth Social Aspects of AIDS Conference, South Bank Polytechnic.

RESEARCH INSTITUTE FOR CONSUMER AFFAIRS AND DISABILITIES UNIT (1990) *Caring for Someone with AIDS*, London, Consumers Association.

ROBINSON, D., MAYNARD, A. and SMITH, G. (1990) 'Investigating HIV/AIDS and Social Care', *International Journal on Drug Policy*, 1, 6, 14–15.

ROULSTON, J. (1988) 'Social Implications of HIV Infection for Women', in *Needs, Issues, Awareness*, report of the First Women and Aids Conference, Edinburgh.

ROULSTON, J. (1990a) 'Implications of Safer Drug Use and Safer Sex Strategies for Women Drug Users', paper presented at the First International Conference on Drug-Related Harm, Liverpool.

ROULSTON, J. (1990b) 'Scotland: A Snapshot of the Future?' paper presented at Women, AIDS and the Future, a National AIDS Trust Conference, London.

ROULSTON, J. (1990c) 'Women in Perspective', paper presented at the NOVOAH Conference, Birmingham.

SEGAL, L. (1989) 'Lessons from the Past: Feminism, Sexual Politics and the Challenge of AIDS', in A. CARTER and S. WATNEY (Eds), *Taking Liberties: AIDS and Cultural Politics*, London, Serpent's Tail.

SMALL, N. (1990) 'Autobiography and AIDS', paper presented to the British Sociological Annual Conference, University of Surrey.

WILSON, J. (1989) 'Women as Carers', paper presented at the Second National Women and AIDS Conference, Edinburgh.

Notes on Contributors

Peter Aggleton is Senior Lecturer in Policy and Management in Education at Goldsmiths' College, University of London. He is a director of a number of major projects concerned with HIV/AIDS health promotion. His recent publications include *Nursing Models and the Nursing Process* (with Helen Chalmers, Macmillan, 1986), *Deviance* (Tavistock, 1987), *Social Aspects of AIDS* (ed. with Hilary Homans, Falmer, 1988), *AIDS: Social Representations and Social Practices* (ed. with Graham Hart and Peter Davies, Falmer, 1989), *AIDS: Individual, Cultural and Policy Dimensions* (ed. with Graham Hart and Peter Davies, Falmer, 1990) and *Health* (Routledge, 1990).

Mary Boulton is Lecturer in Medical Sociology at St Mary's Hospital Medical School, London. Her research interests include the health beliefs and health behaviour of gay men in response to AIDS, and the sexual identity and sexual behaviour of bisexual men. She is the author of *On Being a Mother* (Tavistock, 1983) and *Meetings between Experts: An Approach to Sharing Ideas in Medical Consultations* (with D. Tuckett, C. Olsen and A. Williams, Tavistock, 1985).

Stephen Clift is Senior Lecturer in Educational Studies at Christ Church College, Canterbury. He is Co-director (with D. Stears) of the HIV/AIDS Education and Young People Project.

Mitchell Cohen is a Research Fellow at the Institut Nationale de la Santé et de la Recherche Médicale (INSERM) in Paris. He is presently developing and testing models of safer sex behaviour change, using data on knowledge, attitudes and behaviour from an international UK/US/French study of HIV/AIDS. As a consultant for the World Health Organization, he is working with nationals from several African countries to develop a condom component as part of their national AIDS prevention programmes.

Peter Davies is Senior Lecturer in Social Sciences at South Bank Polytechnic. He is the Co-director of Project SIGMA (Sociosexual Investigations into Gay Men and AIDS) and author of *Key Texts in Multidimensional Scaling* (Heinemann, 1982), *Images of Social Stratification* (Sage, 1985), and the editor (with Peter Aggleton and Graham Hart) of *AIDS: Social Representations, Social Practices* (Falmer, 1989), and *AIDS: Individual, Cultural and Policy Dimensions* (Falmer, 1990).

Jill Dawson is a Research Officer at the University of Oxford, on a study of the behaviour of gay men in response to AIDS.

Kate Dolan is a Research Fellow at the Centre for Research on Drugs and Health Behaviour, Charing Cross and Westminster Medical School, London. She is currently the project manager of the Cohort Study of Clients Attending Syringe-Exchange Schemes and Comparison Groups of Drug Injectors.

Martin Donoghoe is a Research Fellow at the Centre for Research on Drugs and Health Behaviour, Charing Cross and Westminster Medical School, London. He is currently the project manager of the National Syringe Exchange Monitoring Study, in England, and has been involved in similar work since 1987.

Clare Farquhar is a Senior Lecturer in the School for Independent Studies at the Polytechnic of East London. While working at Thomas Coram Research Unit (Institute of Education, London University) she carried out research on 8-10-year-olds' knowledge, attitudes and beliefs about HIV/AIDS. She has co-authored (with P. Sanders) a book for 10/11-year-olds about AIDS and materials designed to help teachers address HIV/AIDS-related issues in the primary school.

Ray Fitzpatrick is University Lecturer in Medical Sociology and a Fellow of Nuffield College, Oxford. His research interests include the health beliefs and health behaviour of gay men in response to Aids, and the sexual identity and sexual behaviour of bisexual men. His publications include *The Experience of Illness* (with J. Hinton, S. Newman, G. Scambler and J. Thompson, Tavistock, 1984).

Graham Hart is Lecturer in Medical Sociology at University College and Middlesex School of Medicine, London. His research interests include sexual and injecting risk behaviours for HIV infection, and he has recently published papers on these subjects in the *British Medical Journal*, *AIDS* and *AIDS Care*. He is editor (with Peter Aggleton and Peter Davies) of *AIDS: Social Representations, Social Practices* (Falmer, 1989), and *AIDS: Individual, Cultural and Policy Dimensions* (Falmer, 1990).

Richard Hartnoll is Senior Research Fellow with the Drug Indicators Project, Department of Politics and Sociology, Birkbeck College, and is currently Visiting Scientist with the Institut Municipal d'Investigatió Mèdica, Barcelona. His research interests include epidemiology of drug misuse, international comparisons of drug policy and studies of hard to reach populations.

Sheila Henderson is currently working in a research and development role at ISDD on HIV/AIDS-related projects. A long-standing interest in gender issues has been pursued largely in the context of health and social policy-related research. She has also lectured on gender perspectives in history, sociology and cultural studies.

Janet Holland is a Research Lecturer in the Department of Policy Studies, Institute of Education, London. Her general research interests are in the area of gender, youth and class. Her current research is into young women's sexuality with the Women, Risk and AIDS Project, and the evaluation of street drug agencies.

Andrew Hunt is a Senior Researcher for Project SIGMA at South Bank Polytechnic.

Hilary Kinnell is Manager of the 'SAFE' Project, an HIV outreach project working with prostitutes and injecting drug users in Birmingham. Funded by the West Midlands Health Authority, this project has been engaged in action research directed towards sexual and injecting risk behaviour since 1987.

Rachel Lart is a graduate in social policy and has worked in the National Health Service as a nurse. She worked with the Monitoring Research Group at Goldsmiths' College, London focusing on aspects of service delivery in syringe exchange schemes and issues of policy. She currently teaches courses in health policy and the sociology of health, and is completing a doctoral thesis on British drugs policy and HIV.

John Mclean is a Research Officer at St Mary's Hospital Medical School, London, on a study of behaviour of gay men in response to AIDS.

Amina Memon is Lecturer in Psychology in the Department of Psychology at Southampton University. Her research interests include health psychology, legal psychology and ethnicity.

Anssi Peräkylä is Glaxo Research Fellow at Goldsmiths' College, London. His research interests include the interaction between health professionals and seriously ill patients. He has recently published a book on the care of the dying in Finnish, and articles in *Sociology of Health and Illness* and *AIDS Care*.

Caroline Ramazanoglu is a Senior Lecturer in the Sociology Department, Goldsmiths' College, University of London. Her research interests are in the area of gender, race and power and methodology, and she is a member of the Women, Risk and AIDS Project team. She is author of *Feminism and the Contradictions of Oppression* (Routledge, 1989).

Tim Rhodes is Research Fellow with the Drugs Indicators Project at the Department of Politics and Sociology, Birkbeck College, University of London. He is currently involved in a Department of Health funded study examining models of HIV outreach health education in the United Kingdom and United States, and in outreach evaluation work in central London.

Tim Robinson is currently researching a series of programmes called *Sextalk* to be broadcast on Channel 4. Before completing one and a half years of ethnographic research on homosexual male prostitutes, he wrote extensively as a freelance journalist for such magazines as *City Limits* and *New Statesman and Society*, on topics ranging from theatre, dance and film to social issues.

Zoe Schramm-Evans is a Research Associate at University College and Middlesex School of Medicine, London. She has worked for the Terrence Higgins Trust and the National AIDS Helpline. Her research interests include the lifestyles and health behaviour of bisexual men, and she is currently concluding PhD research to be entitled *AIDS: The Failure of Ideology*. She co-authored and edited *AIDS Help* (Thames Television, 1987).

Sue Scott is a Lecturer in the Sociology Department, University of Manchester, and Director of CRISAH, Centre for Research into Social Aspects of Health. A member of the Women, Risk and AIDS Project team, her other major research interests are in feminist methodology, the application of sociology to evaluation, and the sociology of mind, body and emotions.

Sue Sharpe is a freelance writer and researcher, currently working with the Women, Risk and AIDS Project team. Her main research interests are the lives and experiences of young women, and her books include *Just Like a Girl* (Penguin, 1976), *Falling for Love* (Virago, 1987) and *Voices from Home* (Virago, 1990).

Gerry Stimson is Director of the Centre for Research on Drugs and Health Behaviour at Charing Cross and Westminster Medical School, London. He has conducted numerous studies of drug problems, and investigations into the effectiveness of British drug policies. Recent work includes the evaluation of the UK government sponsored syringe exchange programme. He has published widely in international journals, and is joint editor of *AIDS and Drug Misuse: The Challenge for Policy and Practice in the 1990s* (Routledge, forthcoming).

David Stears is Senior Lecturer in Educational Studies at Christ Church College, Canterbury. He is the Co-Director (with S. Clift) of the HIV/AIDS Education and Young People's Project.

Rachel Thomson is a Research Assistant in the Sociology Department, University of Manchester. She is currently doing research into young women's sexuality on the Women, Risk and AIDS Project and completing an MA in applied social research.

Simon Watney has been a long-term member of the Health Education Group of the Terrence Higgins Trust. He is the author of *Policing Desire: Pornography, AIDS and the Media* (Methuen, 1987; University of Minnesota, 1989). He has also co-edited with Erica Carter *Taking Liberties: AIDS and Cultural Politics* (Serpent's Tail, 1989).

Peter Weatherburn is a Senior Researcher for Project SIGMA at South Bank Polytechnic. His former research includes an AVERT funded study of the effects of alcohol and other drugs on HIV risk behaviour.

Tamsin Wilton is a research, training and development officer in the Department of Education at Bristol Polytechnic. She is a joint author (with Peter Aggleton, Chrissie Horsley and Ian Warwick) of *AIDS: Working with Young People* (AVERT, 1990). Her research interests also include lesbian feminism, equal opportunities and feminist art practice. She is currently helping to set up a proposed MA in women's studies at Bristol Polytechnic.

Index